CORAM'S CHILDREN

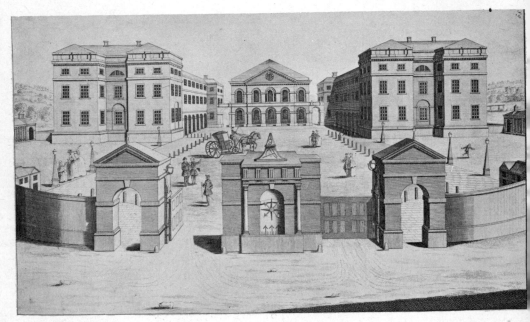

A View of the Foundling Hospital, engraved by B. Cole

CORAM'S CHILDREN
THE LONDON FOUNDLING
HOSPITAL
IN THE EIGHTEENTH CENTURY

RUTH K. McCLURE

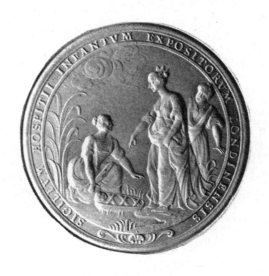

YALE UNIVERSITY PRESS
NEW HAVEN & LONDON
1981

Set in Monophoto Plantin by Thomson Press (India) Ltd., New Delhi.
Printed in Great Britain by Ebenezer Baylis and Son Ltd.,
The Trinity Press, Worcester and London.

Published in Great Britain, Europe, Africa, and
Asia (except Japan) by Yale University Press,
Ltd., London. Distributed in Australia and
New Zealand by Book & Film Services, Artarmon,
N.S.W., Australia; and in Japan by Harper & Row,
Publishers, Tokyo Office.

Library of Congress Cataloging in Publication Data

McClure, Ruth K   1916-
    Coram's children.

    Bibliography: pp. 298–310
    Includes index.
    1.   London.   Foundling Hospital-History-18th
century.   I.   Title.
HV 844.G72165   362.7′32′0942142   80-21375
ISBN 0-300-02465-7.

*To my Husband
and
in Memory of my Grandparents,
Mott and Anna Brower*

PREFACE

HORACE WALPOLE PUT it best when he coined a punning Latin motto for Captain Thomas Coram in 1782, more than thirty years after Coram's death: '*Coram, quem quaeritis adsum.*' As Walpole suggested, Coram was indeed the man that eighteenth-century English philanthropy needed, for not only did he establish England's first foundling hospital, but in doing so he also created a new form of charitable institution, the eleemosynary corporation.

In the early eighteenth century no country conducted its charitable enterprises under such a form. Catholic nations regarded organized charity as a function of the Church; Protestant countries treated it as a function of government. England was no exception. After Henry VIII took his country into the Protestant fold, the burden of carrying on most charitable activities fell upon the local parish officials, who financed them by land taxes, although later the charity schools operated under the aegis of the Church of England. There was also a long tradition of individual benevolence: wealthy Englishmen used testamentary trusts to endow almshouses, schools for poor children, and hospitals for the care of the sick. But by the eighteenth century England's growing population and expanding cities required a new form of philanthropy to meet multiplying and changing needs. The genius of Thomas Coram was that he gave to this increasingly commercial and industrial world the most appropriate charitable structure possible, an adaptation of the joint stock company already in use by British entrepreneurs, whereby individuals acting together in a voluntary corporate body not only could undertake philanthropic projects of greater magnitude than any of them could support alone but also could form a legal entity capable of receiving legacies. Once the utility of the eleemosynary membership corporation had been demonstrated by the successful operation of the Foundling Hospital in London, it became the prototype for thousands of successors in England and the United States because such corporations proved to be ideal channels for the benevolence of a growing middle class.

Today these corporations come into existence virtually overnight, but for Captain Coram, with no models to guide him and with many difficulties to overcome, the task of obtaining a Royal Charter for a foundling hospital stretched out over seventeen years. To understand what obstacles stood in his way and how, by a daring innovation, he surmounted them, we must also understand the man himself as well as the society in which he lived. The life and character of Thomas Coram cannot be divorced from the origins of the institution he founded.

Beyond the intriguing questions of why a semi-retired sea captain should want to establish a home for abandoned infants, and why it took him seventeen years to do so, the story of the Foundling Hospital itself is well worth telling. For it is a story that touches upon many aspects of eighteenth-century social history: morals and manners, music and medicine, economics and education, clothing and cuisine, politics and poverty, art and architecture, the apprenticing of children and the role of women. Hogarth made the Hospital London's first art gallery. Handel gave annual performances of his oratorio, *Messiah*, in its chapel. Mid-century saw it a centre of scandal and controversy during the four years that it functioned as a quasi-public body receiving Parliamentary support. And the development of its estate late in the century added two new squares and many new streets to the expansion of London. In short, the Foundling Hospital reflected in microcosm the world of eighteenth-century England. Yet it was more than a reflection. Over the years the institution took on a personality of its own, compounded of tradition well mixed with innovation, for its Governors, although very much men of their time, showed a remarkable willingness to experiment with new methods. And some of the methods they introduced can be considered forerunners of today's social casework with children.

In telling the Hospital's story, I have included some information about similar institutions on the Continent, so that Captain Coram's 'Darling Project' may also be seen from a comparative point of view. Above all, however, the perspective from which I have tried to write this book is that expressed by G. M. Trevelyan when he urged all who read history and all who write it to remember that 'the dead were and are not. Their place knows them no more and is ours today. Yet they were once as real as we, and we shall tomorrow be shadows like them'. The Captain and the children and all the others who people this book were once as real as we.

The writer of any scholarly work must necessarily be debtor to many—those who ease archival research, those who generously share their knowledge by answering thorny questions in their fields of expertise, those who provide constructive criticism and advice during the stages of writing, and those who sustain the writer's efforts with financial support, comforting assurances, and encouragement along the way. Therefore, to all the librarians and archivists, who have never failed me, I acknowledge my first debt. They include the staffs of the Rare Books Division of the Boston Public Library, the Massachusetts State Library, the Office of Massachusetts Archives, the Massachusetts Historical Society, the Offices of the Court Clerk and Register of Bristol County, Massachusetts, the American Antiquarian Society, the Department of Archives and History of the State of Georgia, the Henry E. Huntington Library, the Lewis Walpole Library, the Newberry Library, the Butler Library of Columbia University, the Library of the University of Georgia, the Houghton Library at Harvard University, the Kenneth Spencer Research Library at the University of Kansas, the Vassar College Library, the Yale University Libraries, the New York Public Library, the Kingston Area Library, and the Hyde Park Free Library, and in London, the Royal Commission on Historical Manuscripts, the Institute for Historical Research, the Lambeth Palace Library, the British Library, the University of London Library, and the Library of the Wellcome Research Institution.

In addition to those persons whom I have thanked in the notes for supplying specific information, I must also acknowledge my indebtedness to Miss M. E. Holmes, Dorset County Archivist; Mr John D. Cushing, Librarian, Massachusetts Historical Society; Dr Robert G. McPherson, Head of the Department of History, University of Georgia; Mr John Earl of the Greater London Council Department of Architecture and Civic Design; and Dr Arthur W. Hazenbush, of Kingston, New York. And I am much indebted to Miss Marchien Prinsen for her excellent translation from the Dutch of a long eighteenth-century manuscript. I am also most appreciative for the assistance of Miss A. L. Reeve, Senior Assistant Archivist of the Greater London Record Office, and the members of her staff, in guiding me through the Foundling Hospital's archives on deposit in that office.

I am especially grateful to Mr J. G. B. Swinley, former Secretary and Director of the Thomas Coram Foundation for Children, and to all the members of his staff, not only for their complete cooperation, which made possible and pleasant the basic research for this book, but also for the personal kindness and friendship he and they extended to me during my stay in London. I also wish to thank his successor, Mr C. P. Masters, and the Thomas Coram Foundation for Children for graciously granting me permission to quote from the Foundling Hospital archives.

I am grateful, too, to Professors John H. Middendorf and Trygve Tholfsen, Dr Warren Hunting Smith, Dr Edwine M. Martz, and Dr John C. Riely, and the late Dr James L. Clifford for good advice and much encouragement. No words of appreciation are adequate to express my gratitude to Professors Robert K. Webb and Sheila Biddle, whose detailed criticisms have been invaluable and whose friendship has been a special joy. Nor can my debt to Professor Donald J. Olsen ever be repaid: he introduced me to eighteenth-century England and has watched over my research with sympathy and advice for a dozen years.

To the American Association of University Women I express my gratitude for the fellowship awarded me for 1973–4 that made my research in London possible.

And finally, I happily own my debt to my husband, Walter McClure, Jr, for his never-failing patience, help, and constant encouragement.

New Haven, September 1979.   R. K. M.

TABLE OF CONTENTS

LIST OF ILLUSTRATIONS

Except as noted below, the originals of these illustrations are in the possession of the Thomas Coram Foundation for Children, which has graciously given permission to reproduce them. Grateful acknowledgment is also made to the Greater London Record Office for permission to reproduce Section C1(a) of Rocque's 1746 Map of London and Section C of Horwood's 1799 Map of London. The original of B. Cole's View of the Foundling Hospital is in the possession of the author.

PART I

Coram

Sisyphus, with toil and sweat,
And muscles strain'd, striving to get
Up a steep hill a ponderous stone,
Which near the top recoils, and rolls
   impetuous down.

John Dyer, 'An Epistle to
a Famous Painter', 1726.

The Treatment of Foundlings
at Home and Abroad

A LEGEND OF THE London Foundling Hospital relates that the children, accustomed to seeing daily Hogarth's great portrait of its founder, believed that when they prayed 'Our Father, who art in Heaven', they were addressing Captain Thomas Coram.[1] If the legend is not true, it should be, for it cost seventeen years of the old sea captain's life to bring the Foundling Hospital into existence.

Coram began, said Dr Brocklesby, 'in respect to this Design as he did in all others, with making it the Topic of his Conversation, that he might learn the Sentiments of other Men; and from thence form some Notion, whether what he had in view was practicable'.[2] In the course of such conversations, he probably learned, if he did not already know it, that England lagged far behind Continental nations in the institutional care of foundlings. Addison had pointed this out in the *Guardian* nine years before Coram became interested in the plight of these children:

> Since I am upon this Subject, I shall mention a Piece of Charity which has not been yet exerted among us, and which deserves our Attention the more, because it is practised by most of the Nations about us. I mean a Provision for Foundlings, or for those Children who for want of such a Provision are exposed to the Barbarity of cruel and unnatural Parents . . . .
>
> I shall therefore show how this Evil is prevented in other Countries, as I have learnt from those who have been conversant in the several great Cities of Europe.
>
> There are at Paris, Madrid, Lisbon, Rome, and many other large Towns, great Hospitals built like our Colleges.[3]

In France, official concern for the foundling began in 1586 with the Ordinance of Moulins, which required the *seigneur*, or, in towns, the *seigneur haut justicier*, to support any foundling within his jurisdic-

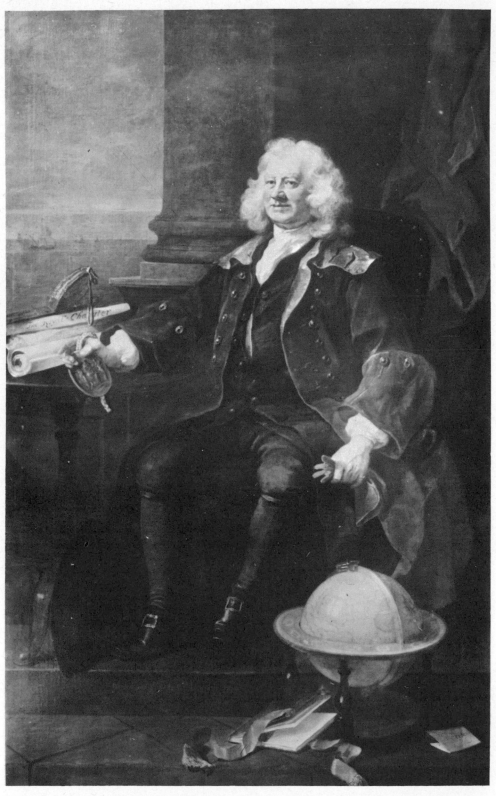

1. Portrait of Captain Thomas Coram by Hogarth, 1740

tion. Since the *seigneurs* paid such charges reluctantly, if at all, the effect of the ordinance was non-existent in some areas; erratic, or modified to conform to local custom, in others.[4] L'Ordre Hospitalier du St Esprit de Montpellier, however, maintained asylums for illegitimate infants, the earliest having been established at Marseilles in 1188. By 1372 this Order was operating more than a hundred such institutions throughout France.[5]

But in Paris little was done for foundlings. In 1445 Charles VII, in *lettres patentes* granted to l'Hôpital du St Esprit en Grève, declared that that institution, founded in 1362, should continue to care for legitimate orphans only. As for foundlings,

> . . . ja soit ce que de tout ancienneté cen ait accoutumé pour les dits enfans ainsi trouvés et inconnus, quêter en l'Eglise de Paris, en certain lit étant à l'entrée de la dite Eglise, par certaines personnes, qui des aumônes et charités qu'ils en reçoivent, ils les ont accoutumé gouverner et nourrir, en criant publiquement aux passants, par devant le lieu où iceux enfans sont, ces mots: *faites bien à ces pauvres enfans trouvés.*[6]

Thus, the care of abandoned children was relegated to La Couche, a little house located near the Cathedral of Notre Dame and loosely supervised by the Cathedral's dean and chapter. And for almost a hundred years it received no support except the alms of the charitable. Probably because these alms were proving insufficient, the Parlement of Paris in 1552 ordered the *seigneurs hauts justiciers* of that city to support the institution, but under the pressures of the religious wars at the end of the century, virtually all support and supervision ceased.[7]

By the 1630s La Couche had become a scene of neglect, cruelty and exploitation. St Vincent de Paul, describing the manner in which the infants were cared for, told Les Dames de la Charité:

> . . . que ces pauvres petites créatures étaient mal assistées: une nourrice pour 4 ou 5 enfants! Que l'on les vendait à des gueux huit sols la pièce, qui leur rompaient bras et jambes pour exciter le monde à pitié et leur donner l'aumône, et les laissaient de mourir de faim . . . qu'on leur donnait des pilules de laudanum pour les faire dormir, qui est un poison . . . qu'il ne s'en trouve pas un seul en vie depuis 50 ans . . . et enfin, qui était le comble de tous maux, c'est que plusieurs mouraient sans être baptisés.[8]

Having discovered these frightful conditions, St Vincent, like Thomas Coram a hundred years later, set out to remedy the evil. He succeeded in doing so by, first of all, inducing the Daughters of

Charity to rent a house in 1638 and take in a dozen of these children. Two years later, in order to expand the project, he turned to the women, many of the highest social position, whom he had been organizing since 1617 into local societies called Les Dames de la Charité. But the contributions of these women, who devoted both their time and their money to good works, could not meet the need. Application was then made to the King for assistance. Louis XIII responded with a grant of 4000 *livres* a year, and in 1644 Louis XIV gave the charity an additional annual income of 8000 *livres*. The Queen donated the château of Bicêtre for the charity's use, but it was soon seen to be unsuitable for the project. And additional funds were granted by the Parlement in 1667 to what was still a private charity.

Finally, in 1670 the King issued an edict officially establishing the charity as L'Hôpital des Enfans-Trouvés and uniting it to the Hôpital Général of Paris. He continued its prior revenues and augmented them by a monthly lottery and by a share in the revenues received by the Hôpital Général from a duty on wine imported into the city. Private and church charities had failed to meet the need, so that, in the end, the state was obliged to shoulder the total support of the institutions caring for foundlings, not only in Paris but also in the provincial cities where such institutions were similarly merged with the local Hôpitaux Généraux. In Paris the number of foundlings cared for—virtually all of them illegitimate—mounted steadily from 312 in 1670 to 1441 in 1720. But small villages and towns in France still lacked local provision for such children.[9]

In Lisbon the Brothers of the Misericordia had cared for foundlings ever since Sebastian I entrusted responsibility for such children to them in the sixteenth century. According to Jonas Hanway, about three thousand infants were received annually into the institution known as the House of the Wheel, a name derived from the device by which the infants were admitted to the hospital.[10]

The Conservatorio della Ruota in Rome also took its name from the turning-box by which the infants were admitted. This institution, large enough to care for six hundred children, was founded early in the thirteenth century by Innocent III, who, according to tradition, was shocked to learn of the many drowned newborn infants that fishermen in the Tiber were finding in their nets. Florence, Milan, and other Italian cities also had institutions to care for foundlings, most of them supported and operated by the Church. The exception was Venice where the Doge and forty members of the nobility managed the Pio Spedale della Pietà for illegitimate children.[11]

And in Amsterdam the Burgomasters committed the management of the Almoners' Orphanage to eight gentlemen regents and six lady regents. This institution, founded in 1666, accepted children of all ages and religious backgrounds, including orphans, half-orphans, deserted children, and foundlings. Its support came from the charges made for boarding children whose absent fathers could afford to pay for them, from charitable gifts and legacies, and from a wide variety of local fees, licenses, permits and taxes, known as *precarios*.[12]

The common feature of all these institutions was that they owed their origin and continuance either to the Church or to the State, or, as in France, to a combination of the two. None had arisen through nongovernmental secular associations; none derived support exclusively from private secular charity. In short, the Continental institutions could, and in time did, provide models for the day-to-day operation of a foundling hospital in London, but they could offer no pattern to a layman who proposed to establish such an institution outside the aegis of Church or State.

The history of earlier attempts to provide for foundlings in England gave no greater guidance and little encouragement. There had, of course, been some attempts to take care of orphaned children of legitimate birth, such as the Royal Asylum of St Anne, founded in 1702 for children whose parents had seen better days.[13] Interest had also been shown in the plight of those vagrant orphans known as the 'Black Guard', the ragged children who stole and begged in the streets of London by day and slept where they could at night. Sometime after 1662, the President and Governors of the Poor for the City of London fitted up a house for them in Bishopsgate Street Without. By 1704, 368 of these children were being fed, clothed and educated, but by 1739 'the Citizens withdrawing their Contributions, this great and truly good Work, is very much decreas'd, . . . And for want of a proper Fund for its Support, 'tis like to be intirely lost, to the great Dishonour of the City, whose Streets were never more pester'd with such deplorable Objects than at present'.[14]

Another effort to provide for poor orphans had been made in 1686 when the Justices of Middlesex set up a nursery or 'Infantory' for such children in a large house at Clerkenwell that cost the parishes involved in the project at least £5000 to build.* Apparently operating

---

* The parishes involved in the enterprise were: St Giles-in-the-Fields, St Andrew Holborn, St James Westminster, St Margaret Westminster, St Martin-in-the-Fields, St Paul Covent Garden, St Clement Danes, St Mary le Savoy, Roles Liberty, St James Clerkenwell, St Giles Cripplegate, St Ann Westminster, Tower Hamlets, plus others outside the Bills of Mortality.

costs were underwritten in part by private donations, in part by parish funds, and in part by the charges made for boarding children of seafaring men and others whose work took them away from home. But, Jonas Hanway tells us, the enterprise was short-lived because 'it is very apparent, that altho' the Justices of Middlesex and Westminster had much zeal, they were not vested with sufficient authority to accomplish the work they undertook', so that 'in this case it is evident that too much was attempted at once'. The Clerkenwell experiment lasted only sixteen years.[15]

But none of these institutions had concerned themselves with foundlings. The only genuine attempt to do anything for the abandoned infant in London had ended some fifty years earlier and had flourished for only a short time. For the care of such children had been one of the original purposes of the famous grammar school, Christ's Hospital, which opened its doors on 23 November 1552 to 380 children, including 100 infants. Its building was the gift of Edward VI; its support came in part from private benefactions and in part from the City. Proof that it functioned as a foundling hospital in its early years comes from the London City Archives: on 13 September 1554, officials agreed that 'the yonge tenter infant' found in the church porch of Saint Pancras should be delivered to 'Xristes hospytall within Newgate and theire nerysshed op at the Cyties chargies'. Another entry in December of the same year records a like disposition of a 'poore yonge mayden chylde'.[16]

Soon the parishioners of Christ Church were objecting to the Hospital's activities because a child left at the gates of the Hospital or in its cloisters was technically in the Parish of Christ Church and chargeable to it. Pressure, therefore, was exerted on the Hospital's governors to reconsider their policies, and gradually they took in fewer and fewer foundlings. In 1572 the Hospital received only twenty-three children between the ages of two weeks and twelve months; by 1653 the number had dwindled to three, although by then the Hospital was caring for close to a thousand children.

Still, the situation created by people trying to leave infants in the Hospital's cloisters remained a source of friction between Hospital and parish all through the seventeenth century, and the beadles were constantly admonished to be watchful 'to prevent the laying downe of children'. In 1696 the whole question was argued out before the Court of Aldermen, but, in the end, nothing was done except to give the churchwardens of the parish leave to post at the Hospital's gates a notice stating 'These are to certify that no Child or Children who are dropped in Christ's Hospital can receive any benefit from thence'. But, in fact, the Hospital had done nothing to relieve the needs of

8

abandoned children since 1676 when new rules prohibited the admission of such infants.[17] Parochial parsimony had defeated the cause of the foundling.

The absence of an institution to care for foundlings had not gone unnoticed. In June 1687 Mrs Elizabeth Cellier addressed to King James II a proposal to establish a Royal Hospital to care for foundlings and also to train midwives. The institution was to be supported by the annual license fees that would be paid by the members of a corporation of practicing midwives, by the fees paid to twelve subsidiary lying-in hospitals for poor women, by fees received from doctors and surgeons for the privilege of attending monthly lectures on midwifery, by one-fifth of all voluntary charity bestowed in the parishes within the Bills of Mortality, and by gifts, legacies, and poor-box contributions. Nothing came of Mrs Cellier's scheme.[18]

According to Hanway, during the reign of Queen Anne several merchants proposed the opening of a subscription and solicitation of a charter for a hospital to receive 'such infants, as the misfortunes, or inhumanity of their parents, should leave destitute of support'. Before the plan reached fruition, however, the merchants were dissuaded from their scheme by public opinion, 'ill grounded prejudices that such an undertaking might seem to encourage persons in vice, by making too easy provision for their illegitimate children'.[19]

Elihu Yale, a wealthy merchant, one-time governor of the East India Company's settlement at Madras and the generous benefactor of Yale College, had also pondered, after his return to England from India in 1711, 'on Founding such an Hospital for Cast-off Children, and in order to that End, proceeded far towards an Agreement . . . for the Duke of Beaufort's great House at Chelsey; But he dying without a Will, the Design dropt with him'.[20] At about the same time Robert Nelson, philanthropist and energetic promoter of the charity school movement, was urging, to no avail, the establishment of a 'House of Charity to receive poor exposed Infants; whereby many Murders and Abortions might be prevented'.[21] The history, then, of public concern for foundlings in England gave little ground for believing that longstanding prejudice, penny pinching and apathy would be easily eradicated.

The most difficult obstacle to overcome, as Coram soon found out, was prejudice because, for the most part, the attitude of the average Englishman toward foundlings was not recognized as a prejudice. Everyone took for granted the equation: foundling equals bastard; and except at the very highest or very lowest levels of society, everyone also took for granted the corollary: bastard equals disgrace.

That was the accepted order of things in God's universe and all decent English society; few questioned it.

The attitude of the aristocracy constituted the major exception to the general loathing of the illegitimate child. Bastard birth was, in fact, remarkably common among them, and it in no way interfered with marriage chances nor, usually, with preferment to high office. Nor were the parents of such children disgraced by their birth. To cite only a few examples: Henrietta Needham, illegitimate daughter of the Duke of Monmouth (himself one of the many illegitimate children of Charles II), married the second Duke of Bolton. The first Duke's wife was also illegitimate. The fifth Earl of Berkeley did not trouble himself to marry his Countess until after she had borne him seven children. Henrietta Godolphin, Duchess of Marlborough, gave birth to Congreve's daughter in 1723, yet the Duchess and Congreve were both buried in Westminster Abbey. Sir Robert Walpole had two illegitimate daughters by two mistresses before he was created Earl of Orford.[22] The explanation for the tolerance with which the aristocracy viewed illegitimate births probably lies in their unquestioning acceptance of what Lawrence Stone has called the aristocratic ethic[23]—one traditionally indifferent to sins of the flesh—based on the arrogant self-confidence possible to those whose great wealth protected them from any economic threat, including that posed by bastards, and whose position at the top of the social pyramid was unchallenged.

But most respectable people at any social level below the aristocracy would see nothing strange in Mrs Deborah's reaction when Mr Allworthy discovered the infant Tom Jones in his bed. She cried:

> . . . for my own part, it goes against me to touch these misbegotten wretches, whom I don't look upon as my fellow creatures. Faugh! how it stinks! It doth not smell like a Christian. If I might be so bold to give my advice, I would have it put in a basket, and sent out and laid at the churchwarden's door. It is a good night, only a little rainy and windy; and if it was well wrapt up, and put in a warm basket, it is two to one but it lives till it is found in the morning. But if it should not, we have discharged our duty in taking proper care of it; and it is, perhaps, better for such creatures to die in a state of innocence, than to grow up and imitate their mothers; for nothing better can be expected of them.[24]

Among such folk of the middling sort, the shame of bastard birth pursued the innocent victim for life. Even modest wealth and merit could not wipe away the obloquy of illegitimacy:

For frequent Experience shews, that personal Merit and Wealth are hardly sufficient to obtain that general good Reception for illegitimate Persons which other Persons have of course; and as to illegitimate People of the lower Classes, they always labour under Disadvantages on that Account, nor is there any Scruple made of branding them with Bastardy; but the Masters and Mistresses of well-regulated Families are very scrupulous of employing such People, for though they may behave well, yet Experience is against them; and if this be the Case of illegitimate People who know their Parents and Relations, what must be the Case of Foundling-Children, the most wretched of all Illegitimates?[25]

This observation of Joseph Massie is confirmed by the experience of the writer of a letter to the *Universal Spectator* on 30 August 1735:

I endeavour to live innocently, and never, to my Knowledge, refus'd being serviceable where an Opportunity offer'd; not even to men who without Reason have shewn me Ill-will; I have had a liberal Education, and did not lose the Time of my Youth; I owe no Man a Groat; I live within the Compass of my small Fortune, and this enables me to relieve some real Objects of Charity, . . . But all this will not skreen me from Contempt; I was illegitimately born, and suffer for the Crimes of others, which I was neither Partner in, nor in Being to prevent; I am worse treated by the Relations of my Parents than by any others; my Mother's esteeming me a Badge of her Infamy, and my Father's as a Robber who has unjustly deprived them of a small Estate he settled upon me.[26]

The letter writer suggests, by implication, two reasons why most people despised the bastard child: he was the living and undeniable proof that his parents were sinners and lawbreakers; they had transgressed God's laws in any event and those of England if they could not provide for the child. And he was a threat to the natural order of inheritance. It was quite true that *filius nullius* possessed no legal right of inheritance under English law, but men sometimes, whether moved by threat of blackmail, feelings of guilt, or affection for the child or its mother, settled a decent competence on their illegitimate children, thereby disappointing the legal heirs by reducing the size of the estate they had counted on.

Not only did such a child appear as a disturbance of the established family pattern in what was still essentially a patriarchal society—one inclined to regard female chastity as the guarantor of family purity—but it also appeared, at a more subtle level, as a break in the natural order of things. To a society deeply impressed by the

Newtonian idea of order as a governing principle of the universe, any threat to traditional ways was felt as a danger to the very structure of society itself.[27] And no society views complacently defiance of authority and failure to conform to its established patterns of behaviour.

It is also probable that among certain groups, which had been strongly influenced by Puritan mores, sexual jealousy helped to shape the prejudice against illegitimate children. To such persons the notion that an erring couple might indulge in the fleshly pleasures of which they scarcely dared to dream and then escape paying the piper was too painful to endure. Someone should be made to pay for sin—if not the parents, then the child.

For the illogical consequence of all these reasons for prejudice was that the average Englishman directed his aversion not only against the parents but also against the child who had committed no sin, broken no law, and knew nothing of breaks in family patterns or disturbances of social order. Why, then, should he be treated as a wrongdoer? According to Professor Gordon W. Allport, who made an exhaustive study of prejudice, 'in every society on earth the child is regarded as a member of his parents' groups . . . . if the parent because of his group-membership is an object of prejudice, the child too is automatically victimized'.[28] In short, if society is prejudiced against unwed parents, the child of the illicit union will also be tarred with the brush of prejudgment. Having thus coated the bastard child with its parents' faults and sins, society could feel free to vent its jealousies and fears on him along with them except that—gnawing thought—he was, if a foundling, a totally unprotected and helpless infant. Could one actually be indifferent to such a child's needs? One could, says Dr Allport, if one evades one's feelings of guilt for doing so by projecting one's own motives or traits on the victims so that they become wholly to blame for their own predicament, thereby justifying one's treatment of them.[29] This may not be logical but, according to psychologists, it is a common phenomenon of human behaviour, one which, lacking evidence to the contrary, we might accept as at least a partial explanation for the cold hostility that greeted the foundling.

To make matters worse for bastards and foundlings, prejudice walked hand-in-hand with penny pinching because someone always has to bear the expense of bringing up a child. Since 1576, if not before, that expense had fallen upon the parish in respect to any bastard child born within its boundaries and not provided for by its parents.[30] If the parents were known, the parish officials could sometimes, by one means or another, compel them to support the child, but in the case of foundlings, there was no hope of extracting money for their care from any source save the poor rates, and no one wanted to see those rates increased.

Overseers of the Poor in the eighteenth century served their one-year, unpaid terms of office reluctantly. Well-to-do men avoided this legal responsibility by paying fines; farmers and small tradesmen, on whom the burden chiefly fell, tried to shuffle through the year with only two objectives: to take as little time away from their own businesses as possible, and to keep the rates down. None of these men had any training, of course, for such positions, and many of them were illiterate. They took, therefore, the easiest and cheapest way possible to deal with all problems, including foundlings, whom they turned over to the parish poorhouse, the parish nurse, or, after 1722, to the parish workhouse. By none of them would the child be well cared for.

Parish poorhouses, which usually provided nothing but shelter, had existed for several centuries. Some had been legacies to their parishes from charitable persons; others were buildings that had formerly belonged to the Church; a few were built after 1601 by parish officers, who financed them out of the poor rate. All were filthy, disorderly habitations for mixed groups of able-bodied paupers, unmarried mothers, neglected children, vagrants, beggars, idiots, lunatics, the blind, the aged and the ill, where pandemonium and vice ruled jointly. In such surroundings, the foundling could expect only the care some feeble crone might choose to give it for the short period that it usually survived.[31]

The workhouses authorized by Parliament in 1722,[32] or which some parishes built earlier, were little better. Older children might survive the overcrowding, foul air, vermin and rampant disease that prevailed in most of such establishments, but the mortality rate of infants stood at nearly a hundred percent. As Hanway says, 'In the open Court at Guildhall, it was declared by the master of a work-house of a very considerable parish that not a single child was reared in his parish in fourteen years because the parish had no proper place to keep them in'.[33]

Parish nurses were just as lethal as parish workhouses. Some of them were even called 'killing-nurses' for 'no child ever came out of their hands alive'.[34] A Parliamentary committee, appointed in 1715 to investigate the poor rates in London, examined the records of the parish of St Martin-in-the-Fields, said to be one of the better managed parishes, and learned that more than three-quarters of the infants cared for by the parish's nurses died every year. The Committee reported to the House:

That a great many poor Infants, and exposed Bastard Children, are inhumanly suffered to die by the Barbarity of Nurses, especially Parish Nurses, who are a sort of People void of Commiseration, or Religion; hired by the Churchwardens to take off a Burthen from the Parish at the cheapest and easiest Rates they can; and these know the Manner of doing it effectually, as by the Burial Books may evidently appear.[35]

Hanway cites the example of the parish of St Clement's where, of twenty-three infants committed to the care of Mary Poole, a parish nurse, eighteen died within a year. He also reports the comment of a parish officer who, when asked to allow a poor young woman 2s 6d a week to nurse her own child, on the ground that this was the usual rate paid a parish nurse, refused, saying: 'Yes, that is very true, but then after a month or six weeks we hear no more of the child, whereas your young woman will probably preserve hers'. The parish nurses, who continued to bury infants week after week with no criticism and no lessening of the number of children given to them, took the hint, said Hanway, that it was 'very fit and convenient that a child should die'.[36] Few, in short, favoured any expenditure of time or money on an object that society at worst loathed and at best ignored.

For we should not discount public apathy as an additional reason for the failure to provide properly for foundlings after Christ's Hospital closed its gates to them. From that day on, a woman who was forced by the power of prejudice to conceal the existence of an illegitimate child had no alternative, save infanticide, to abandonment of the child in a public place with the desperate hope that some compassionate person would rescue it.[37] Everyone knew this if they thought about it, but most did not trouble themselves over other people's problems. Even the good-hearted find it hard to overcome inertia and exert themselves to relieve the difficulties of a faceless group remote from their own lives: it is always easier to pass by on the other side.

Prejudice, apathy and inertia are probably universal human phenomena, but on the Continent they were offset by the active interest of Church and State: the former wanted souls, the latter soldiers. In Catholic countries there existed, of course, the desire to combat Protestantism by increasing Church membership, but, in addition, religious doctrines provided two strong motives for organizing the care of foundlings: the importance of preserving infants' souls through baptism, and the value of good deeds to the doer as a means toward earning his own salvation. Calvinist influence on religious thought largely undermined both motives in England.

From the point of view of the Continental state, foundlings as potential soldiers and colonists seemed a good investment. Louis XIV, in his Edict of 1670, made the point precisely in stating why he and his father had made grants to support such children. They had done so 'considering how advantagious their preservation really was, since some of them might become soldiers, and be usefull in Our Armies or Troups, some to be Tradesmen, or Inhabitants in Our Colonys, which we are settling for the advantage of the Trade of Our Kingdome'.[38] While the British shared the mercantilist view implicit in the King's statement, they had little interest in maintaining a large standing army.

Moreover, France and Holland had both found ways to finance the cost of supporting foundlings by less direct and painful means than raising parish poor rates. State lotteries, taxes on wines paid at the wholesale level, license fees and the bounty of the King's purse, although still coming out of the people's pockets, tended to conceal the objects for which they would be used, thereby avoiding the opposition that arose in English parishes where the link between poor rates and the number of bastards to be cared for was only too clear.

Nothing in English attitudes or experience, therefore, offered Coram much encouragement when he began in 1722 the task that was to consume a large part of his energies for the next seventeen years.

2

Thomas Coram:
The Years of Preparation,
1694–1735

THOMAS CORAM WAS fifty-four when he became interested in the plight of foundlings,* but his life had prepared him well for the disappointments that were for many years to attend his efforts on their behalf. He had met with rejection and failure more than once since his first encounter with prejudice a quarter of a century earlier. In 1694 he had gone out from England at the head of a company of shipwrights to establish a shipyard in Boston, acting as agent for a group of London merchants who were favourably impressed by his abilities.[1] In Massachusetts he ran head on into religious bigotry, for the men of that colony, led by their Puritan pastors, for the most part regarded members of the Church of England with a mixture of superstition and fear.[2] Moreover, the new charter for Massachusetts, brought to Boston only two years earlier, in augmenting the authority of the Crown at the expense of popular participation in government, had afforded the Anglican residents opportunities for power and appointive posts long denied them—a state of affairs certain to increase the anti-Anglicanism of the majority of the population.[3]

Although young Thomas Coram was a good Anglican, at first he encountered no unpleasantness. He began to find friends, not only among Boston Anglicans but also among the more tolerant Congregationalists, so that the next three years, during which he and his workmen built ships in Boston, passed quietly. But mindful that his mission in Massachusetts was to promote shipbuilding, he began

* Coram was born in 1668 in the Dorset coast village of Lyme Regis. The parish registers indicate that his parents were probably John Coram and his wife, Spes (Hope), who died on 13 September 1677. This chapter does not purport to be a full scale biography of Captain Coram. Apart from his efforts to establish a foundling hospital, the incidents related have been selected to illuminate his motivation and character and to indicate his circle of acquaintances.

to look about for ways to expand his activities. Upon learning that large oak planks, fir timber, and iron could be had much more conveniently at Taunton, located on a navigable river about forty miles south of Boston, he moved some of his men there in 1697, set up a shipyard, and started to build Taunton's first ship. Between 1697 and 1700 he built four more.[4]

But by this time Coram was feeling the pressure of anti-Anglican prejudice. For the people of Taunton, he discovered, were as bigoted as those of Boston and even more xenophobic. His torment in Taunton began in 1699 with a series of failures on the part of local men to live up to agreements he had made with them. The broken contracts led to multiple lawsuits, countersuits, and appeals to higher courts from the decisions of hostile judges and juries. And in the midst of all this litigation Coram was also sued for slander because he had let his hasty tongue run away while in court and, in the presence of a jury, had accused one of his presecutors of lying under oath.[5]

Outside the courtroom Coram was constantly harassed by his opponents and their friends, who prevented his men from cutting and hauling lumber into his shipyard and interfered with their work in various ways. Finally, upon the pretext of executing a judgment, a deputy sheriff, as one of Coram's shipwrights later related, 'came to Mr. Corams yard againe & a great crew of Taunton men with him both Horss & Foot & then he Read his execution againe & turned me & other of Mr. Corams work folks out of Mr. Corams house & made such Havock of his things & at such an Inhuman manner'.[6] Two of Coram's ships worth at least £1000 each were seized, together with his shipyard, dwelling, furniture, and orchard. In the end he regained his property only by an appeal to the General Assembly of Massachusetts.[7]

This did not stop the men of Taunton, who started their lawsuits all over again.[8] Once more one of Coram's ships was attached,[9] and this time local feeling ran even higher against Coram: someone fired a shot at him as he rode past a thicket. A week later the deputy sheriff attempted to murder him in a lonely spot in revenge for a judgment Coram had procured against him, but no judge would issue a warrant for the attacker's arrest.[10]

In the fall of 1702 Coram gave up his struggle against Taunton* and returned to Boston where he continued unsuccessfully to seek redress for the injustices he had suffered.[11] Early in 1704, defeated by

---

* By this time, however, shipbuilding was firmly established as a Taunton industry, and unusually large ships continued to be built there for many years.

Taunton's small-town cliquishness, its fear and jealousy of an ambitious and successful newcomer, and the colony's anti-Anglican prejudice, he sailed for England. His ten years in Massachusetts had given him, however, a great fund of knowledge about American colonial affairs, a strong sense of what it means to be an underdog, and a wife.

For on 27 June 1700, Thomas Coram had married Eunice Wayte, the oldest child of a good Congregationalist family of Boston. A gentle person, content to remain in the background and devote herself to her husband's interests, Eunice Coram nevertheless adhered firmly to her Puritan faith and, with no objection from her husband, went to meeting regularly during the forty years of their life together.[12] It was apparently a happy marriage, but it produced no children.

Coram's first humanitarian project, undertaken after his return to England, proved to be just as disappointing as his experiences in Taunton. At the end of the War of the Spanish Succession he became concerned about the welfare of discharged soldiers and officers: would there be work enough for all of them? It seemed unlikely. The answer to the problem, he thought, lay in relocating the men in America on a tract of land that is today situated for the most part in the State of Maine but which the Province of Massachusetts then claimed to own.[13] The Board of Trade considered Coram's scheme highly advantageous both to the soldiers and to Great Britain,[14] but Coram's efforts to set the plan in motion met with repeated delays. First there was the virtual paralysis of the ministry resulting from the constant struggles between Oxford and Bolingbroke.[15] Then came the death of Queen Anne and the consequent reorganization of the government. Scarcely had this been achieved when the Jacobite rising in Scotland made unthinkable any notion of sending out of the country trained soldiers who might be needed to put down insurrection at home.

Then, too, there were the recurring claims and counter-claims—which Coram characterized as 'Cobweb Pretensions'—to ownership of the land proposed for the soldiers' settlement.[16] The agent for Massachusetts, Jeremiah Dummer, also opposed Coram's plan, partly to protect the interests of Massachusetts residents and partly because Coram had offended him by tactless remarks about New England men.[17] Dummer's opposition to the plan melted away, however, when he conceived of a scheme whereby he might exploit the proposed settlement to his own financial advantage and that of his associates. To this end he induced Coram to withdraw a petition at a critical moment, apparently by misrepresenting the nature of his own plan. When Coram learned the truth, Dummer reported to the General Court of Massachusetts, 'he ran about in a mad rage declaring . . . the whole design was only a trick in me to save that fine country for the villainous people of New England'.[18] But even as he wrote in September 1720, the South Sea Bubble was bursting, and with it hundreds of lesser schemes that had bubbled forth from the spring of human ingenuity and greed were deflated. Dummer's scheme shared their fate, and Coram's unselfish plan also failed to survive. Thus, all of the time and thought that Coram had devoted from 1713 to 1720 to his work for the benefit of discharged soldiers came to nothing.

But he had learned—and not easily—patience, persistence, and the art of petitioning. Perhaps he had always been, as Jeremiah Dummer said of him, 'a man of that obstinate, persevering temper, as never to desist from his first enterprise, whatever obstacles lie in his way',[19] but these fruitless years strengthened the trait. There were some gains, however, for Coram's efforts had made him known to a vast number of influential men both in commerce and in government. And his reputation for honesty and disinterestedness had also grown and now guaranteed that at least men would listen to him if not necessarily agree with him. Two years later Sisyphus started the long uphill climb again. He was well prepared.

Coram had given up seafaring some years earlier and had settled down in that part of London which was 'the common Residence of Seafaring People'—probably Rotherhithe. His business took him into the City early; often he returned late. And in winter, daylight comes late to London and leaves early. 'Both of these Circumstances afforded him frequent Occasions of seeing young Children exposed, sometimes alive, sometimes dead, and sometimes dying', at the side of the roads and streets over which he walked. Shocked at the spectacle, he made up his mind in the spring of 1722 to do something about it.[20]

He realized at once that he could not afford to endow an institution for foundlings as an Elihu Yale might have done, and he learned very quickly that neither the English government nor the Anglican Church was interested in sponsoring such a project. The joint stock company, then so much in the public mind, seemed the only solution to the problem of means. If the King would grant a charter to a non-profit corporation, whose members agreed to support it by their subscriptions, a legal entity would be created that could undertake the care of foundlings and also the solicitation of further donations and legacies for that purpose.

To obtain such a charter, Coram would certainly have to demonstrate substantial support for his project and would require powerful advocates to present his plan to the King. But, as he later wrote to his friend, Dr Benjamin Colman, pastor of the Brattle Street Congregational Church in Boston,

> . . . I found it was Impossible to be done, for I could no more prevaile on any Arch Bishop or Bishop or Nobleman Britain or Foreigner or any other Great Man, I tryed them all, to speake to the Late King or his present Majesty on this affair than I could have prevailed with any of them, if I had tryed it, to have putt doun their Breeches and present their Backsides to the King and Queen in a full Drawing room such was the unchristian Shyness of all about the Court.[21]

Unquestionably, his timing was bad. A proposal for a chartered corporation to care for foundlings coming on the heels of the South Sea Bubble affair, which had included among its lesser bubbles the 'Company for erecting houses and hospitals for maintaining and educating bastard children',[22] was bound to evoke suspicion. In fact, joint ventures of all kinds received such a bad name from the Bubble episode that it appears to have affected for some years the erection of any form of associational charity. Not one of the charitable institutions still operating in London in 1810 had been founded between 1720, when the Bubble burst, and 1739, when the Foundling Hospital came into existence, although prior to 1720 associational charity in non-corporate form had flourished in the heyday of the charity school movement.[23] Moreover, it is likely that the Bubble fiasco increased conservatism and suspicion of innovation at the same time that it decreased the ability of many who had suffered financial ruin to commit themselves to the support of any charity.

Nor was it a propitious time for presenting such a project at Court. Some of the men whom Coram approached probably refused to act as intermediaries with the King because they themselves disliked the idea, but others may have thought it futile and a possible source of personal embarrassment. Although George I's court and the monarch himself were not celebrated for chaste behaviour, nevertheless the King had refused at the beginning of his reign to appoint Charles Churchill Groom of the Bedchamber to the Prince of Wales, despite the pleas of the Dukes of Marlborough and Argyll, solely upon the ground of Churchill's illegitimacy.[24] This episode might well deter any approach to him on behalf of lesser bastards. And it was by no means easy to gain access to George I's presence in any event. After 1720 he became more and more reclusive, and in the summers of 1723 and 1725 he was away from England for months visiting Hanover.[25]

George I died on 11 June 1727; the coronation of George II took place in October, but, of course, no one could be expected to approach the new King immediately with so dubious a proposal. By the end of 1727, however, Coram had enlisted the help of Dr Thomas Bray with whom he had become acquainted while residing in Bray's parish, St Botolph Without Aldgate.[26] After receiving an account from a friend in Paris of the provision made for foundlings in that city, Bray wrote a pamphlet incorporating this information and advocating the establishment of a 'like Charitable Foundation' in London.[27] How much the tract affected public opinion cannot be measured, but support from the widely respected divine, who had already founded the Society for Promoting Christian Knowledge as well as the Society for Propagation of the Gospel in Foreign Parts, must have carried weight in some quarters. Be that as it may, the tract decisively affected the course of Coram's endeavours because it suggested to him a new method of approach. Toward the end of his tract, Bray pointed to the example of charitable Parisian women and recommended that

> . . . as to the Management of this whole Design, I humbly presume, it cannot be recommended to any so proper as those of the other Sex, both Persons of Quality, and other Women of an inferior Rank, as those whose Bowels are most tender towards Children, and who best understand how to order what is fitting for them. And to induce Persons even of the highest Rank, to condescend to the taking these, the meanest of their Fellow Creatures under their Care and Management, I cannot offer to their Consideration any Thing more Moving than to propose to their Imitation what is done by the Dames and Sisters of Charity in Paris, in the Hospital of the very same Kind with this proposed to be erected . . . even Princesses and Dutchesses, and other Ladies of the Prime Nobility of Paris, to the Number of Two Hundred and above, have associated themselves, and entered into a Confraternity to manage this Affair.[28]

Bray probably intended no more than that the day-to-day operation of the hospital, after it had been established, should be handed over to a committee of Lady Managers, but Coram was a 'Man, whose Head was fertile in Expedients', and 'bethought himself at last of applying to the Ladies'.[29] He knew well the technique of petitioning, and by an imaginative extension of Bray's suggestion, he conceived the unheard-of idea that ladies of the nobility should—if they would—become petitioners to the King for a charter establishing a foundling hospital. He secured his first signature on 9

March 1729, when the Duchess of Somerset signed his petition at Petworth.[30] In the course of the next six years, seven more duchesses, eight countesses, and five baronesses followed her example.

Because the Ladies' Petition proved to be the key to Coram's success, the women who signed it merit some attention. Chart 1 in Appendix I lists them in the order in which they signed. Chart 2 in the same Appendix indicates the web of relationships that existed among them. Thirteen of these women were related to each other either by blood or by marriage, a fact that goes far to explain how Coram obtained introductions to many of them. The earlier signers, obviously, interested themselves sufficiently in his project to recommend him to their relatives, and they continued the chain. True, the aristocracy was not a large group, so that many of them would be more or less related in any event. But among these lady petitioners the relationships were close. As an examination of Chart 2 will show, among blood relationships none were beyond the degree of first cousin once removed; in-law connections followed a similar pattern.

Who introduced Coram to the first signer, the Duchess of Somerset, or to the second, the Duchess of Bolton, who was not related to the Duchess of Somerset, is not known. Henry Newman, Secretary of the S.P.C.K., whose acquaintance Coram would have made through their mutual association with Dr Bray, if not earlier in Boston, may have provided the introduction to the Duchess of Somerset, since he had been in the service of the Duke from 1703 to 1708. Or Dr Richard Mead, physician to both George I and George II, may have provided letters of introduction recommending a project that he favoured.[31]

There are also eight of the lady petitioners who do not fit into the chains of relationship at all, although there are some remote family links not shown in Chart 2. Coram probably obtained introductions to some of these women from his friends. Almost certainly, his introduction to Lady Torrington came from Henry Newman, who had long collaborated with her in caring for the children of the improvident Marquis DuQuesne.[32] Similarly, his introduction to Lady Onslow probably came from her husband's cousin, Arthur Onslow, Speaker of the House, with whom Coram had been acquainted for many years. Friendships among the women themselves, however, provide the most likely explanation in other instances: it would account for the Dowager Baroness Torrington and Lady Byron signing the petition on the same day and for the Countess of Huntingdon and the Duchess of Leeds signing only three days apart. But this is speculation, not certainty.

The charts, then, cannot tell us exactly how Coram secured the support of all of these women for his project. But Chart 2 does explain how a man of modest origins was able to gain a hearing from at least a dozen of these titled ladies: the 'cousinhood' of the aristocracy in eighteenth-century England could be employed as effectively among women as among men in order to further a cause that seized their interest.

An analysis of Chart 1 shows that thirteen of the petitioners were not over thirty-five years of age—six were in their twenties. Three were in their forties, and only one of those for whom information is available could be called elderly: Lady Trevor, who was sixty-four. Brocklesby tells us that Coram did not find it difficult to persuade these women to sign his petition: 'They did not listen much to his Arguments; for the Sweetness of their own Tempers supplied a Tenderness that rendered Arguments unnecessary'.[33] Perhaps it would be truer to say that a youthful openness to new ideas and the novelty of what they were doing combined happily with the security of their own positions and the aristocratic tolerance for bastards to encourage whatever humanitarianism they possessed. For it should be noted that most of these women were members of the aristocracy by birth as well as by marriage: fifteen of the twenty-one were daughters of dukes, marquesses, earls, or barons.[34]

In the course of the first five months of 1730 Coram obtained twelve signatures to his petition. But by the summer he found himself increasingly diverted from the foundling hospital project by the pressures of a new commitment. His friend Dr Bray had died in February. While on his deathbed, Bray had executed a deed of trust creating the Associates of Dr Bray and had named Coram to be one of them. This group was charged with carrying on several of Bray's projects, the most important of which was to apply for some part of a legacy left by Joseph King for unspecified charitable uses and to employ such funds in establishing a new colony for debtors and other poor persons south of the Savannah River in America.[35] The Associates never succeeded in obtaining any part of the Joseph King legacy, but their efforts to secure a grant of land in Georgia and a charter for the establishment of a colony there eventually overcame all obstacles. Yet when the charter was signed by the King on 12 April 1732, the newly created Trustees for the Colony of Georgia, of whom Coram was one,* found themselves without means for carrying out the charter's purposes.[36]

* The Trustees for the Colony of Georgia was identical in membership with the Associates of Dr Bray.

23

Help finally came from an unexpected source: a number of prominent and wealthy merchants saw the commercial possibilities of the new colony and contributed generously to get it under way. By the end of October 1732 their subscriptions totaled £2000, and the Trustees thought themselves able to send out the first settlers.[37] Coram went to Gravesend to watch them sail for Georgia on 17 November.[38]

Perhaps because his own plans to colonize upper Maine had come to nothing, Coram from the first enthusiastically supported the Georgia project. Nothing could discourage his activity in soliciting funds for the new colony, and few could match his record of attendance at Trustees' meetings. His activity continued throughout 1732 and 1733.[39] He took so keen an interest in the welfare of a group of emigrating Salzburgers that he spent Chrismas 1733 at Dover in order to see to the comfort of these forty-five German settlers, led by the Reverend John Martin Bolzius and Baron Philip von Reck, when 'contrary winds' delayed their sailing for four weeks. Coram welcomed them to England with a dinner and visited them every day. He wrote to Henry Newman, 'I carry the Children a few apples, and sometimes give them a few plumbs, a pound of malaga Raisins which costs 3d. fills them with above 5 pounds worth of Love for me. They shew it by a Dawn of Joy in their faces as soon as they see me coming'.[40] Little wonder that the Salzburgers remembered for years his 'fatherly care & love'.[41]

Earlier in 1733 while visiting Rotterdam, Coram had spread the word of the opportunities that Georgia afforded to those driven from Europe by religious persecution,[42] but he was already beginning to have misgivings about the system of land tenure that the Trustees had imposed upon the new colony. The question involved was whether daughters should inherit lands granted to the male settlers, each of whom received a fifty-acre tract in a form of tenure not unlike a military fief. Each recipient of land was required to perform military service in time of war and guard duty in time of peace. He could neither mortgage nor sell his land, and it could be inherited only by a male heir who would similarly be capable of military service.

Coram sympathized fully with the colonists who complained of this system. In the spring of 1734 he read to the other Trustees a written declaration expressing his views and predicting that the outcome of the Trustees' policy would be 'that the Inhabitants would desert from that Province like leaves from a Tree in Autumn'.[43] But his arguments did not move the other Trustees. In his annoyance, he then committed the unpardonable sin: he talked about the affair publicly. As a consequence, he was subjected to a tongue lashing from

Thomas Towers, a close friend of Oglethorpe, who favoured retention of the system of tail male. Describing the scene, the Earl of
Egmont wrote in his journal on 29 May, 'Mr. Towers . . . fell severely
on Capt. Coram for being the occasion of the dissatisfaction which
was risen against the exclusion of female heirs. He told him . . . that
we Should hear his opinion at all times with pleasure, but he ought to
know himself bound by the decisions of the board'.[44]

After this public reprimand, Coram attended only five meetings
during the rest of 1734 and early 1735. On 5 February 1735 he made
one more effort on behalf of the settlers: he moved at the Trustees'
meeting to set a day on which to consider whether or not it was
expedient to exclude female heirs from inheriting lands in Georgia.
No one seconded his motion. He stayed away from the Trustees'
meetings for nearly four months, and thereafter his participation in
the affairs of Georgia virtually ceased: he did not attend another
meeting until 1738.[45]

However hurt by the treatment of the Georgia Trustees, Coram
was not a man to be incapacitated by feelings of rejection. True, he
did not forgive readily those who injured him nor forget the injury,
but his natural bent to look toward the future coupled with his knack
for involving himself in new schemes guaranteed that he would have
little time left for brooding or self-pity. He never mourned for what
might have been while the world held so much that still might be.

Within a few weeks after his humiliating rejection by all of the
Georgia Trustees, he began once more to pursue his dream of a new
province in the northern part of America. He had resigned himself to
the impossibility of obtaining consent to colonize upper Maine.
Accordingly, on 3 April 1735 he addressed a memorial to the King
proposing the establishment of a colony in Nova Scotia. To it he
attached a petition signed by 102 persons who described themselves
as 'Labouring handy Craftsmen whose respective Trades and Callings
are over Stock'd by great Numbers of Artizans and work-men who
resort from all parts of the Kingdome to this Metropolis Whereby
your Petitioners are unable to procure work sufficient to maintain
themselves and Families'.[46] But once more Coram's colonizing
efforts failed. After requests by the Board of Trade for further
information, proposals and counter-proposals, and the delays occasioned by the death of the Queen, which for a time held all public
business in abeyance, the threat of war with Spain put an end to
Coram's hopes.[47] No further thought was given to establishing a
colony in Nova Scotia until after the War of the Austrian Succession
in 1748.

Nova Scotia, Georgia, and plans for a foundling hospital, however,

were not Coram's sole preoccupations in the 1730s. Among other
projects, he also interested himself on behalf of two Mohegans from
Connecticut, whom John Mason and his son, Samuel, had brought to
London to plead with the King for redress of wrongs perpetrated
upon their tribe whereby they had been defrauded of their lands.
Coram appealed to Sir Charles Wager, and through Sir Charles's
intervention, not only was their complaint referred for examination
to a commission of the Governors and Councils of New York and
Rhode Island, but in addition, the younger Mason—his father having
died while in London—was given £300 out of the Exchequer to pay
his expenses and those of the Indians.[48] The Reverend Samuel
Smith, who had succeeded Dr Bray at St Botolph Without Aldgate,
summed up this period of Coram's life when he wrote to Dr Colman
in 1735: 'Mr. Coram is animated with so generous and extensive a
Zeal, that he has a share in forwarding the Progress of almost every
good Undertaking, that is set on Foot by publick spirited Persons
amongst us'.[49]

3

The Royal Charter
for a Foundling Hospital Obtained,
1735–39

IN SPITE OF ALL THESE activities, Coram continued his efforts to secure a royal charter for a foundling hospital in London. After a hiatus from May 1730 to April 1734, during which the only signature that he obtained to the Ladies' Petition was that of the Countess of Harold, he prepared a second petition to be signed by noblemen and gentlemen and began soliciting signatures. In the course of the next year, he induced thirty-one men to sign. He also added the signatures of four more ladies to the first petition.[1]

Fortunately one of the early subscribers to the second petition was Dr Richard Mead, and undoubtedly the interest of this prominent physician in the project procured the signatures of six other men associated one way or another with the medical profession. Twelve of the signers were dukes or earls, eight of them being closely related to the lady petitioners. The remaining twelve included several merchants, a Master in Chancery, a powdermaker, a captain, and several men of whom nothing is known.

Later in 1735, Coram also began gathering signatures of Justices of the Peace residing in or near London and of other 'Persons of Distinction' on a third petition. In all, he persuaded fifty-three men to sign, among them the Earl of Derby, whose signature he travelled to Lancashire to obtain. But, as he later wrote to the Countess of Huntingdon, he 'could never have obtained the Charter had not the Great Ladies Subscribed the Book . . . . But the Great Ladies Subscribing the Declaration in the said Book Induced Several Noble Lords & Gentlemen to Subscribe another Book after the Example of the Great Ladies'.[2]

To these three petitions Coram added his own. The prestige of the signers of the first two petitions was, of course, sufficient to ensure that all would reach the King, and they came before him in Council on 21 July 1737. He ordered that they be referred to a committee of the Privy Council, which, eight days later, directed that Coram's petition be transmitted to the Attorney General and Solicitor General for their opinions on the clauses of a charter that Coram was to lay before them.[3] This by no means concluded Coram's responsibility: he had also to provide the names of the first governors to whom the charter would be granted.

He presented his list of 375 men to the Privy Council on 13 February 1739, and it was confirmed by the King in Council on 22 March without change. He divided the names on his list into three categories: those who had consented to act as governors or had subscribed one of the petitions; those who, he says, 'I have been well Inform'd approve of the Design'; and those who 'are well known to be Persons highly proper to Promote this Desirable Work'.[4] An analysis of Coram's roster of proposed governors shows that he had obtained the signatures or consents to act of 172 of the 375 men named. This included the consent of the Duke of Bedford to be the first president, the consent of six others to be vice-presidents, and Lewis Way's consent to fill the office of treasurer. Calling upon so great a number of men was, in itself, a formidable task, especially for a man now over seventy who travelled about London on foot, even though, as he told Dr Colman in the autumn of 1738, he could walk ten or twelve miles a day.[5]

Beyond revealing Coram's enormous expenditure of energy, the list of proposed officers and governors tells us, by inference at least, his criteria for selecting them. Appendix II sets forth the data from which such inferences may be drawn.[6] It indicates, first of all, that nearly 25 percent of the men named were members of the nobility. Most of them, however, are included in Group III, that is, Coram had not secured their consent to be named and probably had never met them. Nevertheless, he regarded them as suitable persons to promote the charity, obviously because their social position and wealth could be helpful to it.

Wealth also seems to have been of prime importance in selecting the other governors. Thirty-one of them were extremely wealthy men, of whom fifteen are in Group III. Almost certainly they were chosen because Coram hoped for their generosity to the new institution. Doubtless this also explains in part the preponderance of merchants selected by Coram to be governors. His own business affairs, of course, would have made him personally known to many merchants, as Group I testifies. But in addition to the thirty-seven merchants in Group I, there are eight in Group II and twenty-one in Group III, making in all sixty-six, by far the largest numbers in any occupational category. And Coram's knowledge of the role played by the merchant community in the establishment of the colony of Georgia had certainly made him aware of the wealth and power that such men possessed. Indeed, he took care to secure the consent of the great merchant, Sir Joseph Eyles, who had exerted much influence on behalf of the Georgia project, to act as a governor.

For Coram's second measure of a man's suitability to be a governor was, it would seem, his potential for exercising influence. If the need for political action should ever arise, the nobles he named could apply a good deal of pressure. Of more immediate importance, however, was the fact that these men, by virtue of their position, constituted society's natural leaders. They could sway public opinion by example and, if they chose to do so, could make a charity fashionable. In somewhat different circles, powerful merchants and country gentlemen could exert similar influence. Men who held important posts at court or in various departments of the government also possessed the capacity for political and social influence; significantly, this group stands third in the occupational categories represented in Coram's list. Finally, we must note that seventy-two of the men named—more than half that number being in Group III—were members of the House of Commons at the time Coram submitted his list to the Privy Council and could, in varying degrees, be politically useful.

Almost certainly Coram chose some men because of their close ties of kinship with one or more of the lady petitioners. Probably the ladies themselves had something to do with the inclusion of thirteen such men named in Group I and seven listed in Group II. The others may well have been named as compliments to the women to whom they were related.

Age was not, evidently, a controlling consideration: the nominees ranged in age from twenty-one to eighty. But, in fact, few were in their twenties, and they tended to be either members of the nobility or wealthy young country gentlemen. The eighty-year-old was the Archbishop of York. For the most part, however, the men in all groups were in their mid-forties, the age by which they would normally have acquired wealth and influence.

This emphasis on Coram's criteria of wealth and influence may seem excessive, for today the organizers of any new charitable enterprise automatically seek as members of its governing board those persons whose social position will guarantee the project's respectability and attract as supporters people who enjoy at least the illusion of being in the company of society's leaders. And such leaders are, most often, wealthy men and women. We take for granted, for example, that the treasurer of almost any governing board will be a banker. And we make these assumptions because our notion of the proper persons to sit on the board of a charitable institution was fixed long ago. But Thomas Coram had no model to work from in making up his list. No one had previously been called upon to compile a list of governors for an incorporated secular associational charity. The problem had to be thought through for the first time. It is, therefore, of some importance to analyse how Coram dealt with it, for what he did in 1739 established many of the precedents for the composition of governing boards of charities that we today take as a matter of course.

Coram did not, we should observe, simply propose a list of his own personal friends and the early supporters of his project, although, looked at from a short-range point of view, this might have seemed the easy and obvious solution to his problem. Instead, his choice of so many men whom he did not know at all and, indeed, of whose support for his project he had no positive assurance, clearly indicates that he was employing criteria in making his selections other than emotional ties and indebtedness for previous help. When we consider, then, whom he selected, especially in Group III, it becomes apparent that his sound sense of what was needed to assure the Hospital's future success led him to commit his project to men who, he believed, possessed the means to support it, the influence to promote it, and the power to protect it. He realized that the force of prejudice was far from dead and that his new institution would require the patronage of the powerful. He told Dr Colman, 'I have found Many weak persons, more Ladies than Gentlemen, say such a foundation will be a promotion of Wickedness'.[7]

This realization, perhaps, accounts for one significant omission: Coram named as governors no members of the clergy except the Archbishops of Canterbury and York and the Bishop of London, and they were included only by virtue of the words 'The Rt. Honble. The Lords and others of His Majesties Most Honble. Privy Council for the Time being' following the list of nobles. This omission could not have come about by pure chance: Coram always acted with a purpose. What makes the omission even stranger is that Coram and his wife had been residing in the rectory of All Hallows London Wall since 1736 by invitation of the Reverend Samuel Smith.[8] Since the Smiths and the Corams were close friends, one would expect Coram to have nominated Smith to be a governor just as he nominated a few of his other close friends.

It would be odd indeed if Coram did not discuss the matter with Smith before completing his list, and if he did, Smith must have declined the honour. There are several possible explanations for such a refusal. Perhaps Smith was too busy. Yet he was not too busy later to baptize the foundlings after they were admitted into the Hospital.

Perhaps—and this seems more likely—Smith feared that narrow-minded people would construe his appointment to an official position on the governing body of a foundling hospital as approval by the Church of unwed motherhood or as a winking at fornication. Since it behoved the ministry to preserve the Church from any possible imputation of scandal and keep it safe from even the appearance of evil, Smith might well have concluded that becoming a governor of a foundling hospital would be inconsistent with his duty to the Church. If this was his reason, Smith would probably have suggested to Coram that he refrain from asking other clergymen to serve as governors in order to spare them the embarrassment of refusing.

Certainly, there is no evidence to support a conclusion that Coram deliberately set about to create a totally secular institution with no members of the clergy involved, even minimally, in its government. Nor is there any evidence to the contrary. But taking into account Coram's stout Anglican sentiments and his friendships with both Anglican and Dissenting clergymen, it seems probable that the clergy were omitted by their own choice rather than by Coram's.

Whatever the reasons for omissions and inclusions, compiling the list of nominees required a vast expenditure of time, not only in calling on possible supporters, but also in keeping records of those who signed petitions or agreed to be named governors, and lists of those recommended by others or who ought, for one reason or another, to be included. Then, the lists had all to be put in alphabetical order and copied out by hand. The wonder is that Coram found time for anything else. Yet, almost simultaneously, he was obliged to seek funds to pay the costs of having the charter prepared. What these expenses were Coram detailed to the Countess of Huntingdon in explaining why the charter lay 'fee-bound':

> The Expence for Stamps & Fees are so Excessive high That besides the Attorny & solicitor Generals Fees Several Times wch they had for Examining the Proposals & Making Reports & preparing a Draught of the Charter &c. I also paid Seventy one pounds for the said Bill or Charter for the King to Signe, & it will Cost much more for that which the Chancelor must fix the Great Seal unto, The Stamps for each of the Skins of Vellom will be Six pounds, it has already Cost above 150£ for Fees & Rewards, wch are unavoidable, to the Several Officers & offices and it requirs near as much More.[9]

He had hoped for the Queen's help to meet these expenses, but, as it turned out, he never had an opportunity to ask for it.* His own long illness in the autumn of 1737, following shortly after the Privy Council's approval of the foundling hospital project, confined him to his home for several months; by the time he was able to go out again, the Queen had died.[10] Thinking that the Queen's daughter might be as inclined to charitable deeds as her mother, Coram decided to approach Princess Amelia with a petition setting forth the events leading up to the present need and asking for her help. He chose Holy Innocents' Day to take his petition to St James's Palace. Having been told that the proper procedure was first to address his request to the Lady in Waiting, he presented the petition to Lady Isabella Finch. But, he noted later, she 'gave me very rough words and bid me be gone with my Petition, which I did without opertunity of presenting it'.[11] He drafted an identical petition addressed to the Princess of Wales, but there is no indication that he had any greater success in presenting it.[12]

Coram then began to write letters to the lady petitioners and to the men who had signed the other two petitions, asking for contributions toward the costs of preparing the charter. He soon found that writing so many letters was too great a task and arranged for the printing of 500 form letters. Some of the ladies responded; the Lord Mayor, one of the Aldermen of London, and the Duke of Bedford contributed five guineas each; and Lord Vere Beauclerk promised contributions of £50 from Lady Betty Germaine and £20 from his wife. In spite of all Coram's efforts, however, the costs exceeded the contributions.** In the end, he paid the difference out of his own pocket.[13] The Charter establishing the Hospital for the Maintenance and Education of Exposed and Deserted Young Children was, at last, signed by the King on 14 August 1739, and the Great Seal was affixed to it on 17 October.[14]

The first meeting of the new corporation—now, although no one realized it, the world's first secular associational philanthropic corporation—was held on Tuesday, 20 November 1739, at Somerset House in the Strand. Standing before an audience of 170 Governors that included six dukes and eleven earls, Thomas Coram presented the institution's charter to the young Duke of Bedford, its first president, with a 'handsome speech' that Governor Belcher's son, Jonathan, had written for him.[15]

More than seventeen years had passed since Coram began his project. During those years he had encountered overt opposition and

* The Queen died on 20 November 1737.
**In all he collected only £217 toward payment of the costs.

covert indifference, the distractions of other worthwhile causes, bureaucratic delays, personal illness, and the discouragement that attends repeated disappointments. He had become heavier, he found it increasingly harder to write, and his hair had turned white; he had grown old along the way and no longer expected to see the full accomplishment of his plans.[16] But he was satisfied with the outcome and told Dr Colman, 'I am the better pleased with myself that every Step I have taken in this affair has been exactly what I would do if I had life enough before me and was to begin it again so that I cannot find room to repent my doing this or that about it'.[17]

Inevitably the question arises: why could Coram accomplish in the 1730s what he could not achieve in the 1720s? The answer lies in the combination of circumstances rather than in any single reason. In the first place, if the corporate form of the enterprise had aroused suspicion in the 1720s, this feeling may well have subsided by 1734–36 when Coram obtained most of the signatures to his second and third petitions. By then the South Sea Bubble affair lay fifteen years in the past, and after the passions it aroused had had time to cool, reflective men probably learned to distinguish a truly charitable project, regardless of its technical form, from the corporate schemes that they still distrusted.

A second factor that may have influenced public acceptance of the need for a foundling hospital is the probability that the 1730s saw an upsurge in infanticide, resulting from the marked increase of illegitimacy during these years. This would have given greater prominence to the problem. According to the recent study of bastardy in England made by Peter Laslett and Karla Oosterveen, the ratio of illegitimate births, which had remained fairly constant from the late seventeenth century up to 1720, began to rise in the years 1721–30, and in the 1730s continued sharply upward to a level that had not been reached in a hundred years. Logically, one would expect a sharp rise in illegitimate births to produce a similar rise in infanticide, but concrete evidence of such a correlation is lacking. Furthermore, Laslett and Oosterveen's study does not include London, and whether the trend in the countryside held true in the capital we do not know. They themselves remark that such evidence as they had gathered seemed to imply a lower incidence of illegit-imacy in cities than in the country.[18] But most aristocratic families and wealthy Londoners owned country seats and might have been influenced in their views by knowledge of what was happening in the parishes where their country houses were located if a rising illegit-imacy rate there was producing an unusually large number of cases of infanticide or having a marked effect on the parish poor rates.

We must also keep in mind that some of the difficulties in approaching George I did not exist at the court of George II. That the King himself approved a foundling hospital is shown by the fact that in 1749 he contributed £2000 to it and in 1758 became its patron.[19] He was, perhaps, no more available than his father, for he, too, visited Hanover frequently. But the Queen always had his ear, and her counsel carried great weight. Apparently she had been interested in such a project before her death, for in 1739 a pamphlet was published in London entitled *An Account of the Foundation and Government of the Hospital for Foundlings in Paris Drawn up at the Command of her late Majesty Queen Caroline*. Its preface stated that 'this Account was drawn up at the Command of her late Majesty Queen Caroline; and would then have been publish'd, if there had been a sufficient Prospect that the Design, which was then much thought of, would have succeded. In Her the Hospital for Foundlings has lost a Protectrix and Benefactrix'. Certainly she had ample opportunity to be influenced in favour of the project by four of her Ladies of the Bedchamber who were signers of the first petition.* Perhaps, then, she had already paved the way for the King's well-disposed attention to the petitions when, at last, they reached him in the Privy Council.

The Ladies' Petition was, of course, the crucial factor. There can be no doubt that it influenced the signers of the other two petitions and that the combined prestige of all the petitioners virtually assured the grant of the charter, just as, later, the continued patronage of important people made the Foundling Hospital London's most fashionable charity. Once Coram had discovered how he could channel the influence of society's leaders in favour of his project, he had laid hold on a tremendously potent force: the power of the example that can move others to emulation, reinforced, moreover, by a tradition of benevolence. For conspicuous giving to charities approved by society, such as almshouses, grammar schools and funds for the poor, had long been not only a means of furthering the aspirations to higher social status of those whose positions were not yet securely established, but also a way of confirming an established position by acting out the role expected of the fashionable and well-to-do.

Whether motives other than a desire to follow the ladies' example

* These Ladies were the Countesses of Albemarle, Burlington, and Hertford, and the Duchess of Richmond. The Countess of Burlington stood proxy for the Queen at the christening of Princess Augusta in 1737, and the Countess of Hertford had sufficient influence with the Queen to save the life of the poet Savage when he was found guilty of murder.

or concern over problems caused by increasing numbers of illegitimate births prompted the signers of the second and third
petitions to pledge their support cannot be said with any certainty.
Coram's one-man campaign produced no literature prior to 1739
other than Dr Bray's pamphlet. Without knowing how wide a
circulation this pamphlet enjoyed, we cannot assess its influence. It is
apparent, however, that Dr Bray, like many other eighteenth-
century pamphleteers, believed that an appeal to secular and
materialistic reasons was as needful as one directed to religious and
humanitarian motives, for his appeal was twofold. First, he urged the
Christian duty of saving the lives of innocent children, but in the
second place, he pointed out that the children so preserved and
properly trained up would not only tend to lower parish rates but also
'will be every one of them rendered useful and fit for Services, and
Apprenticeships to the meanest Trades, instead of being innured to
Beggary, Pilfering and Stealing'.[20]

Finally, of course, there was Coram's own patient perseverance
and capacity for innovative action. No man, of course, can transform
social institutions singlehandedly. The social and economic conditions that breed the ills the reformer seeks to remedy must first
change, must catch up, so to speak, with his too early vision. But
those conditions over which he has no control will change in any
event. In Coram's time, George I would die and George II would
succeed him; the years would pass and people would reassess the
experiences of 1720 with greater discrimination; for whatever reasons
the numbers of illegitimate births throughout England would mount
rapidly in the 1730s. Coram had nothing to do with these events, all of
which may have been prerequisite to his success. Yet without him the
fire would have been laid with no match to light it, and England might
have waited another fifty years for a foundling hospital.

To concede the importance of the individual is not, however, to
explain him, to say why Coram should be more interested than
another man in the fate of foundlings, or whence he derived his
energy, persistence and resourcefulness. Perhaps, having no children
himself, he felt toward all childen a vicarious fatherhood—consider
his way with the Salzburgers' children. Certainly, over the years
a remarkably large number of the most active Governors of the
Foundling Hospital were childless men, a verification of Bacon's
observation that 'the noblest works and foundations have proceeded
from childless men. . . . So the care of posterity is most in them, that
have no posterity'.[21] Furthermore, having lost his mother at an early
age, Coram may well have felt some sense of kinship to those deprived
of the care of both parents from birth. And, having been himself the

victim of prejudice in Taunton, he thereafter empathized with the underdog in every situation—witness his concern for unemployed soldiers, women disinherited of property rights, and exploited Indians.

These aspects of his life may account for Coram's interest in foundlings. Probably his physical energy was a matter of genetic inheritance and early conditioning to hard work. His persistence and ingenuity were, doubtless, Dorset cultural traits like his other yeoman characteristics. But there is no explanation for the charm that gained him the support of the lady petitioners.

4

The Foundling Hospital Begins, 1739–1741

THE GOVERNORS OF THE NEW institution—at least some of them—lost no time in setting to work. A General Committee of fifty members, charged with transacting all of the Hospital's business except matters involving major policy decisions, had been elected at the first meeting on 20 November 1739. Nine days later this Committee met for the first time in Mr Manaton's Great Room at the Crown and Anchor in the Strand.

The first concern of the thirty-one men present was to find out how other countries managed similar hospitals; the second was to collect any moneys that might be payable to the Hospital from the estates of persons whose wills had provided for legacies contingent upon such an institution coming into existence; their third concern was to find a house in which to begin caring for the abandoned infants of London. It seemed that this last problem might be readily resolved: the Duke of Montagu, one of the earliest signers of Coram's second petition, had already offered to lease Montagu House (the present site of the British Museum) to the new corporation for twenty-one years at £400 a year, with the first seven years to be rent free.

During the next three months the secretary wrote to the British Ambassadors and Ministers in Paris, Florence, Venice, Turin, and Holland, asking them to gather data about foreign foundling hospitals; by 23 February 1740 reports had been received from Amsterdam and Paris. The treasurer advertised for legacies payable to the Hospital in the *Daily Advertiser* and other newspapers and even investigated rumours of such legacies. He also received, as one of the first benefactions to the Hospital, £21 from the Free Masons Lodge that met at the Prince of Orange's Head in Jermyn Street. A committee of Governors inspected Montagu House, and John Milner, one of their number, sought legal advice as to whether the Duke of Montagu, who possessed the life use of the property rather than absolute ownership of it, had a right to lease it. The General Committee also decided to obtain an estimate of the cost of the alterations required to convert Montagu House to their purposes and, for comparison, an estimate of the cost of buying land and building a hospital.

Captain Coram had anticipated this development. In the summer of 1739, while the Hospital's charter still lay fee-bound, he had written to Dr Colman that he was sure of having thirty-four acres of land 'in the fields before Queens Square in Ormond Street for a Scite for our Hospital'. He had also anticipated the need for a corporate seal and had one ready for the Committee's approval at its first meeting. The design, he told Dr Colman in the same letter, 'I chose out of the affair Mentioned in the 2d of Exodus of Pharoah's Daughter and her Maids finding Moses in the ark of Bulrushes which I thought would be very appropo for an hospital for Foundlings Moses being the first Foundling we read of. The Motto round the Seal is vizt. Sigillum Hospitii Infantum Expositorum Londinensis'.[1] The Committee approved his choice, and the General Court officially adopted it. Coram had also anticipated the Governors in seeing the need for information about foundling hospitals abroad. In 1732, long before he had any assurance of success, he had asked his friend Henry Newman to write to Sir Erasmus Philipps, who was then traveling in Italy, requesting him to find out everything possible about the institution for foundlings at Rome that Addison had mentioned in the *Guardian*.[2]

While the surveyor,* Mr Sanderson, was engaged in inspecting Montagu House and preparing plans and estimates for a new building,[3] the Governors asked Coram to ascertain what price the Earl of Salisbury would demand for his land adjoining Queen Square. He reported on 25 January 1740 that he, the treasurer, and another Governor had visited the Earl's agent, who told them that he believed the Earl would not sell the land at all unless a foundling hospital were to be built on it, in which case he would charge the going rate for land near London. On the same day, Mr Sanderson

* American readers should note that the functions of British and American surveyors are not identical. The term in the United States is usually applied to men qualified to determine boundaries of lands or the lines of roads by mathematical measurements. In Britain, however, surveyors are men qualified to inspect real property and to ascertain its condition and value, to superintend large properties, to give estimates of costs of repairs and replacements, to estimate costs of building, and to supervise construction. In short, they combine the skills of a land agent, appraiser, engineer, and practical architect.

reported that it would cost £2005.10.8 to repair Montagu House and £666 to convert it into a hospital; a new building of comparable size would cost £10,000 plus the expense of paving, fences, and drains. Unable to reconcile so large an estimate with its inadequate funds, the Committee resolved not to build for the present.

Two weeks later the Committee learned that Montagu House did not offer an alternative to building. The Attorney General, the Solicitor General and an independent solicitor all agreed that the Duke of Montagu, as a life tenant, could not legally permit the major alterations required for the Hospital's purposes because such alterations would change the building from its original use. This, it was pointed out, a Court of Equity might construe as waste and prohibit by injunction.[4]

During these months it had become apparent that the corporation would require more powers than its charter contained. The Governors, therefore, decided to solicit an Act of Parliament to remedy the deficiencies and to resolve any ambiguities. Among other things, the proposed Act granted the Governors the right to purchase lands not exceeding in rental value £4000 per annum, and it directed that any lands so acquired should be taxed at 1739 rates regardless of any hospital buildings subsequently erected. To prevent the controversies with parish officials that Christ's Hospital had experienced in its early years, the Act also provided that no child or employee of the Hospital should acquire a settlement in the parish where the Hospital was located. On the other hand, no parish could claim any fee for christening or burying a child, nor might any parish officer exercise authority within the Hospital or prevent persons from bringing children to it on penalty of a forty-shilling fine. The Act further empowered the Governors to apprentice the children, to receive the profits from work performed by them, and to punish them for idleness, disobedience, or misbehaviour. Another provision eliminated any requirement for an oath or other test prerequisite to serving as a Governor or officer of the corporation. This, of course, was a shrewd bid for the support of philanthropic Dissenters and wealthy Jews, several of whom later became Governors—for example, Sampson Gideon and Francis Salvador. But it also underlined the independence of the institution from Church and State.

Not everyone agreed that the clause which prohibited the children from gaining a settlement by virtue of their residence in the Hospital was a good one. Some argued that such a law would deprive the children of any settlement at all since, ignorant of their parentage, they could not turn to their parents' place of settlement for relief if needed; the Hospital, therefore, owed them the duty of providing a settlement. Others objected that the result of the Act would be to compel any parish where the children in later life might become destitute to relieve them, since their lack of a settlement would prevent their removal to any other parish; this would place an unfair burden on the parish obliged to furnish relief. In spite of such objections the Act was finally passed, and the King gave his assent to it on 29 April 1740. The Lord Chancellor and the officials and clerks of both Houses charitably remitted all customary fees in connection with its passage.[5]

Meanwhile, the Governors had received offers of several houses for the Hospital's use, and funds were accumulating. By 1 May the treasurer was able to invest £3000 in New South Sea annuities, thereby establishing a pattern of keeping any surplus funds invested in income-producing securities. By 22 May the Committee thought itself ready to formulate a plan of operation. To this end, a special committee of six Governors was appointed to study the information received from Paris, Amsterdam, and Lisbon and then to prepare such a plan.

During the summer, members of the General Committee inspected houses—newspaper advertisements brought in at least twenty offers at rentals ranging from £6 to £80 a year—but found them either too small or too dilapidated. Coram, the treasurer, and one of the Governors, William Fawkener, were asked to discuss again with the Earl of Salisbury's agent the possibility of purchasing the two fields near Queen Square. With typical impatience, Coram, finding the treasurer and Fawkener both out of town, called on Mr Lamb, the Earl's agent, alone. Five days later he reported back that Lamb had said that the Earl was disposed to sell the land to the Hospital and suggested that the Governors choose an 'honest Man well skilled in Land Affairs'; the Earl would choose another, and the two should agree upon the price to be paid for the land. Coram's eager report met with cool reproof: 'Resolved that it be referred to Mr. Fawkener and the Treasurer to wait on Mr. Lamb about the said Land, and to join Mr. Coram in a Report concerning the same being proper for the use of this Charity'.[6] A week later, on 2 July, Coram presented a report from himself, Fawkener, and the treasurer identical with his previous report. But no action was taken until 17 October except to open a subscription book for contributions to be used specifically for the purchase of land and construction of a hospital.[7]

On 17 October 1740, the first anniversary of the Hospital's charter, the Committee revolved to buy the Earl of Salisbury's two pasture

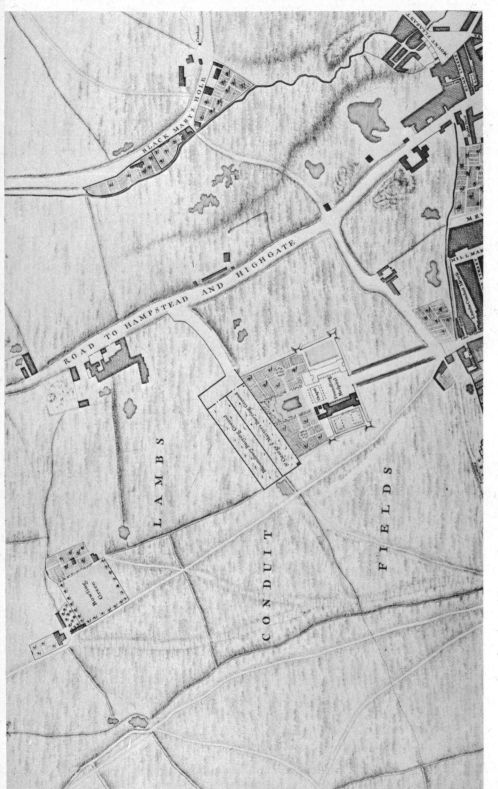

2. Section of Rocque's 1746 Map of London showing Location of the Foundling Hospital

fields containing thirty-four acres, located on the north side of Ormond Street between Lamb's Conduit and Southampton Row, and to build a hospital. On the same day they appointed a committee of three to find a house that could serve as a temporary hospital until a permanent building was erected on the Hospital's own land.

After so many delays, affairs now began to move more rapidly. By 31 October Mr Milner had learned of a suitable house in Hatton Garden; by 13 December the Committee had completed negotiations for leasing it at a rental of £48 a year for six years. Coram and three other Governors were asked to inspect the premises and to arrange at once for any work necessary to ready it for the Hospital's use.

Negotiations with the Earl of Salisbury's agent were also progressing. It now appeared, however, that the Earl owned four fields instead of two adjacent to Ormond Street and that he was unwilling to sell only the two best fields. Forced to accept this change, the Governors, after considering the reports of the Earl's appraiser and their own, decided to offer £6500 for the entire property. The Earl countered with a demand for £7000 but simultaneously promised to contribute £500 to the building fund. On 31 December the General Court authorized the purchase on the Earl's terms.[8]

During the summer the special committee had presented its plan for the operation of the Hospital. Five hundred copies of it were ordered to be printed and delivered to all the Governors for their consideration before the next quarterly Court.[9] Meanwhile, in June, anticipating the need for wet nurses for most of the children, the Committee ordered one thousand questionnaires to be printed and sent to the Governors and 'such other persons most likely to obtain . . . answers'. The purpose of the questionnaires was to locate healthy nurses in the country and to ascertain what fees they would expect for the care of a child in their own homes during its first four years. The questionnaires also asked what wages both wet and dry nurses would want for residing in the Hospital, and how supervision over the country nurses might be best effected.[10]

The plan of operations was adopted at the quarterly General Court on 1 October 1740. The committee that prepared it had used the reports on the foundling hospitals in Paris, Amsterdam and Lisbon as their guides but found that 'these Institutions, being accomodated to the Laws and Governments of their respective Countries, were unfit or impracticable to be wholly executed in this Kingdom'.[11] Not only did law and custom affect their decisions but also the fact that, with a current income of barely £600 a year, they were planning for a much smaller institution than those abroad. So small a sum would require, they said, 'the greatest Frugality to maintain even Sixty Children' without diminution of capital. They hoped, of course, to be able to expand their work later, but except for a few years at mid-century when it received support from Parliament, the Foundling Hospital in London never reached the size of its Continental counterparts. In 1740, for example, the Paris institution was caring for 3150 children, while the orphanage in Amsterdam had a population of 1183.[12]

The necessary limitation of numbers led to restrictions on admissions not found abroad. The plan adopted by the General Court specified that the infants received must be under two months old and free of venereal disease, scrofula, leprosy, or other infectious diseases. In order to carry out this directive, the mother or some other person would be required to bring the child to the Hospital and to wait while the chief nurse and the apothecary examined it. If it did not meet the requirements as to age and freedom from disease, it would be returned to the person who brought it, but no questions would be asked respecting its identity or circumstances.

Heartless though this system might seem to a mother whose child was rejected solely because it was a few months older than the specified age, nevertheless it represented a sensible decision by governors working within a straitened financial framework. Since they could not provide for all, it was logical to use the available means to care for the youngest. And it was realistic to refuse children with diseases regarded as infectious: not only would they probably die before much could be done for them, but also, it was feared, they might start an epidemic among the other children.

In Paris, Lisbon, and Amsterdam, on the other hand, there was no restriction either of age or of physical condition. Indeed, their systems of reception made restriction impossible. In Paris and Amsterdam, mothers were not required to bring their children to the hospitals. Instead, they usually abandoned them in a public place; officials and others, who were alert to watch for such children, would then report the matter. In Paris an abandoned infant was taken first to one of the *commissaires du châtelet* or to an *officier de justice*, who made an official report, a *procès-verbal*, before the child was admitted to the hospital. A child found to be diseased was then transferred to a special hospital for infectious diseases. In Amsterdam whoever found an abandoned child reported the fact to the head provost (*schout*) of the orphanage. A nurse then went to get the child, accompanied by the *schout*, who tried to collect information about the infant by inquiries in the neighbourhood or by questioning the child if he or she was old enough to answer. The matter was also reported immediately to the *Burgermeesteren*. In Lisbon, however, children were brought to the

House of the Wheel by their mothers or by other persons and placed in the revolving device that whisked the child through the institution's walls without anyone seeing or questioning the person who brought it.[13] Only the Dutch made any effort to learn a child's identity. Probably this was because the orphanage was a municipally operated institution, and the good *Burgermeesteren* had no intention of being imposed upon. For the basic fact of what body operated an institution directly affected its policies and methods.

The effect of dissimilar administrative structures can be seen most clearly, perhaps, in the extent to which women participated in the management of these institutions. The House of the Wheel in Lisbon, where thirteen Brothers of the Misericordia saw to every detail, allowed no administrative role at all to women and employed them only as nurses and maids. On the other hand, both Amsterdam and Paris accorded women some managerial responsibility.

In Paris the First President of the Parlement and the Attorney General, as Chief Governors, assisted by four Directors chosen by the Board of the Hôpital Général out of its own number, constituted the policy-making authority. But, reflecting the combination of Church and State sponsorship of Les Enfants Trouvés, day-to-day operation was left, for the most part, in the hands of the Order of the Daughters of Charity and the Association of Ladies of Charity. The *religieuses* visited every two years the children placed in the country for nursing, supervised the hospital's wet nurses, and saw to it that older children were employed in knitting. The Sister Superior paid the wages of the country nurses and the lower servants in the institution, purchased food, materials for clothing, and other necessaries, and also acted as receiver of alms. The Ladies of Charity met annually to audit the Sister Superior's inventory of cloth and linens and to give orders for the purchase of such items for the following year. One of the Ladies verified the tradesmen's bills for these purchases every quarter, and the Ladies, acting as a board, fixed the amount of the monthly wages of the country nurses.

In Amsterdam the *weeshuijs* was managed by eight male and six female Regents, who met separately and performed different functions. The Lady Regents met as a board every Thursday. They supervised and paid the nurses with whom infants were boarded outside the hospital; they looked after the children's clothing, minor provisions, and fine linens; and they regulated the hospital's workshops in which the girls were taught sewing, knitting, and lace-making. In addition to a large number of women working in minor capacities, the orphanage also employed a woman as house-mother to superintend the whole institution and to report directly to the two Boards of Regents.[14]

Obviously, the history of the institutions on the Continent and local tradition account for the role, or non-role, played by women in their government. The care of foundlings in Lisbon had been committed to a monastic order in the sixteenth century, and these Brothers would certainly have found it unseemly to share their administrative responsibilities with women. On the other hand, it will be remembered, when St Vincent de Paul sought to establish a home for the abandoned infants of Paris, he turned first to an order of nuns for nurture of the children and then to Les Dames de la Charité for financial assistance. In 1670, when the King merged St Vincent's foundling hospital into the Hôpital Général of Paris, the existing pattern of operation was preserved by specific enactment.[15] In the Netherlands a long tradition of strong-minded women, accustomed not only to taking an active part in business and public affairs but also to governing charitable institutions, virtually guaranteed that they would participate in administering any orphanage or foundling hospital.[16]

In contrast to Amsterdam and Paris, the plan for operating the Foundling Hospital in London delegated the duties of the Parisian Sister Superior to a male steward, and although it provided for the employment of female nurses and servants, it expressed no intent to turn over to women any managerial duties beyond empowering the chief nurse to supervise the work of the other women employees. Day-to-day overall supervision, it was contemplated, would rest in the hands of a Daily Visiting Committee of Governors serving on a rotating schedule. On 20 June 1740, the committee to prepare bylaws for the corporation had proposed

That twelve or more Ladies or other Gentlewomen of Good and Benevolent dispositions, Circumstances and Characters be Annually requested by the General Court to Inspect the Behaviour of the Matron, Nurses and other Female Servants of this Corporation; And that they be also desired to acquaint the Grand Committee from time to time with their Observations thereon; and to propose such Rules and Regulations as they shall think proper to be observed by the said Servants.[17]

But nothing came of this suggestion, and the final plan of operation allowed for no group comparable to the Lady Regents of Amsterdam or the Ladies of Charity of Paris. It merely expressed the hope that

. . . we may receive the Assistance of the Fair Sex, who, although excluded by Custom from the Management of publick Business, are by their natural Tenderness and Compassion peculiarly enabled to advise in the Care and Management of Children; and they may, without Trouble to themselves, see the Oeconomy of the Hospital, and communicate their Observations to any Governor, or to your Committee, by a Memorandum put into the Charity Box, or in such Manner as they shall think fit.[18]

By this statement the Governors clearly indicated that their exclusion of women from responsible participation in the government of London's foundling hospital was also the product of history: there was no tradition in England of female government of charitable or other public institutions. The Governors may also have thought their new project sufficiently controversial without risking any additional criticism that disregard of the customary ways of doing things might provoke. Moreover, in a country that had been overwhelmingly Protestant for two hundred years, there existed no readily available reservoir of women comparable to non-contemplative orders of Catholic nuns vowed to lives of charitable service and trained to shoulder administrative duties. For it seems likely that English women, unaccustomed to the burdens of governing a public charity, might have refused nomination to official positions had they been asked. True, over the years many women contributed generously to the Foundling Hospital, visited it, served as godmothers to its children and as inspectresses of its country nurses, and offered suggestions to improve the conduct of its affairs, but none of them ever sought to participate officially in its administration. On the contrary, when Lady Vere and Lady Betty Germain, both of whom had taken great interest in the Hospital, were asked, one after the other, in 1752 to assume the title of Patroness or Chief Nurse, they declined. Lady Betty gave poor health as her reason; Lady Vere asserted that her duties to her family prevented her from making any commitment that would require regular attendance.[19]

In other matters, however, the English plan closely followed Continental practice. The hospitals abroad, for example, boarded nearly all of their infants with nurses—usually wet nurses—outside the institution. The Paris hospital placed its children with country-women in Picardy and Normandy so that the Sisters from the hospital might visit them easily, although respectable local citizens also supervised the women. The children remained with their nurses until they were five years old, when they were brought back to the hospital in Paris. The Brothers of the Misericordia placed Lisbon's foundlings, too, with outside nurses, but these women lived in the city itself. This made easier the task of the six Brothers who supervised the nurses' care of the infants until the children reached the age of seven. The Amsterdam orphanage also boarded out its infants until they were four, under the supervision of the Lady Regents.

The Governors of London's Foundling Hospital decided to follow the Parisian plan and place the infants as soon as possible after their reception with country nurses, who would care for them for three years and then return them to London. Although the plan did not specify who should supervise the country nurses, in practice the local clergy and gentry most often performed this task.[20]

All of the institutions made some provision for the education and vocational training of their children. Lisbon's method was the most dependent upon public participation since the House of the Wheel possessed no facilities for housing or educating the children after completion of the nursing period. Instead, the Brothers disposed of the children by inducing charitable persons or the children's nurses to bring them up, or if need be, they paid suitable persons to take the children, educate them, and 'put them in a way of Life'. Those who adopted the children out of charity reaped certain benefits: the husband and sons of the family gained exemption from military service. In Paris, on the other hand, the children were housed in a large building in the Faubourg St Antoine and were instructed in reading, writing, and the Catholic faith; boys were taught to knit; girls learned to spin and sew. At about fifteen or sixteen the boys were apprenticed without fees to tradesmen in the city, and the girls were placed in domestic service. Similarly, in Amsterdam the children lived in the orphanage and learned reading, writing, and the catechism of the Reformed Church. Between the ages of thirteen and fifteen the boys were apprenticed to a trade, often one related to ship-building; later some of them would go to the East Indies. The girls learned sewing, knitting, and lace-making in the hospital's own workshops, so that upon leaving the orphanage, they could earn a living either in domestic service or in needlework.

The English plan proposed, upon the children's return from the country to London, to teach them reading but not writing and, at proper ages, to apprentice the boys to husbandry or to the sea service, and to indenture the girls as domestics.[21] For the Governors, as they said on many occasions, intended that the children

> ... learn to undergo with Contentment the most Servile and laborious Offices; for notwithstanding the innocence of the

Children, yet as they are exposed and abandoned by their Parents, they ought to submit to the lowest stations, and should not be educated in such a manner as may put them upon a level with the Children of Parents who have the Humanity and Virtue to preserve them, and the Industry to Support them.[22]

They did not propose, in short, that the foundlings be given sufficient education to enable them to compete on an equal footing with the children of London's smaller merchants and substantial artisans for situations likely to lead to future advancement. To some extent this attitude reflected the Governors' acute sensitivity to public opinion. Even more, their policy reflected the old conviction that children of sin did not deserve at society's hands the same opportunities afforded to legitimate children. Prejudice dies hard.

What, if anything, the Brothers of the Misericordia did about preserving the identity of the children placed in the wheel does not appear in the report of regulations. But the institutions in Amsterdam and Paris took elaborate measures to ensure that a child's identity was not lost. Both kept records of when and where the child was found and of any distinctive marks on the child's body. If a note was left with the child, it was carefully copied into the official registers. In Paris a copy of this identifying data was placed in a small leather pouch attached to a little bead necklace, which was placed around the child's neck when it was turned over to its country nurse. London adopted a similar procedure, except that the identification attached to the child was a small leaden tag bearing a number that referred to a sealed packet containing the identifying records. Both French and English nurses were forbidden to remove these identifications.[23] The stated purpose of such precautions was that parents who later applied to reclaim a son or daughter might be sure that the child given them was, in fact, their own. But it may be, too, that the persons in charge of these institutions felt an unspoken need to preserve whatever tangible shreds of identity these children possessed as an affirmation of their—and, by implication, all men's—individuality.

With a plan of operation adopted and the house in Hatton Garden being readied for occupancy, the Committee began to advertise for staff. By the end of January 1741, they had engaged a messenger, watchman, porter, cook, laundress, housemaid, and four dry-nurses. Soon afterwards a steward and chief nurse were added. The Committee also ordered bundles of clothing for the first sixty children. During February they ordered table and bed linen, blankets, and other supplies; prepared lists of Governors to serve in turn on the Daily Visitation Committee; and arranged with a clergyman at Hemsworth, in Yorkshire, to provide a dozen wet-nurses in his neighbourhood willing to care for children at the rate of 8s a month for each child. On 28 February, the Governors resolved to receive the first children 'upon Lady Day next'.

Preparations continued through March: Dr Nesbitt provided medicines with instructions for their use; Rev. Samuel Smith offered to baptize gratis all children taken in during the first three months; William Hogarth, who had given to the Hospital in May 1740 the full-length portrait of Captain Coram, now painted a shield, which was put up over the Hospital's door; Sir Joseph Hankey presented a Church Bible, and Captain Coram gave a large Common Prayer Book—one that he had received in 1736 from the Speaker of the House, Arthur Onslow. The Committee settled upon a daily diet for the employees, ordered two barrels of beer for them, arranged for a cowkeeper to supply milk, bought coal, engaged wet nurses, and advertised in the daily press the time and date of the opening of the institution.

Meanwhile, the anxious vestrymen of the Parish of St Andrew Holborn were viewing the situation with great uneasiness, fearing that children rejected by the Hospital would be dropped in their parish. After several conferences, the Governors and vestrymen agreed that the latter would direct the Overseers of the Poor, two watchmen, and two constables to be on duty in the area of Hatton Garden on the night the children were to be received; the Governors would order the Hospital's porter or watchman to give a signal to these officials whenever a child was refused, so that they might watch the person carrying it away to prevent its abandonment in the parish.[24]

At last, on the evening of 25 March 1741, the Foundling Hospital opened its doors to receive children for the first time. Gathered at Hatton Garden for the important occasion were the Duke of Richmond, Lewis Way, Theodore Jacobsen, Taylor White, William Hogarth, Samuel Skinner, Peter Godfrey, Dr Robert Nesbitt, Captain Robert Hudson, and Captain Coram. What happened that night is best told in the words of the Daily Committee's minutes:

> The Committee met at 7 o'clock in the Evening. They found a great number of People crowding about the door, many with Children and others for Curiosity. The Committee were informed that several Persons had offer'd Children but had been refused admittance. The Order of the Gen'l Committee being that the House sho'd not be open'd till Eight o'Clock at Night. And this Committee were resolved to give no Preference to any Person whatsoever .... At Eight o'Clock the Lights in the Entry were Extinguished, the outward Door was opened by the Porter, who

was forced to attend at that Door all night to keep out the Crowd. imediately the Bell rung and a Woman brought in a Child. The Messenger let her into the Room on the Right hand, and carried the Child into the Stewards Room where the proper Officers together with Dr. Nesbitt and some other Govrs. were constantly attending to inspect the Child according to the Directions of the Plan. The Child being inspected was received Number'd and the Billet of its Discription enter'd by three different Persons for greater Certainty. The Woman who brought the Child was then dismissed without being seen by any of the Govrs. or asked any Questions whatsoever. Imediately another Child was brought and so continually till 30 Children were admitted 18 of whom were Boys and 12 Girls being the Number the House is capable of containing. Two children were refused, one being too old, and the other appearing to have the Itch.

About Twelve o'Clock, the House being full the Porter was Order'd to give Notice of it to the Crowd who were without, who thereupon being a little troublesom One of the Govrs. went out, and told them that as many Children were already taken in as Cou'd be made Room for in the House and that Notice shou'd be given by a Publick Advertisement as soon as any more Could possibly be admitted. And the Govrs observing seven or eight women with Children at the Door and more amongst the Crowd desired them that they wou'd not Drop any of their Children in the Streets where they most probably must Perish but to take care of them till they could have an opportunity of putting them into the Hospital which was hoped would be very soon and that every Body would imediately leave the Hospital without making any Disturbance which was imediately complyed with with great Decency, so that in two minutes there was not any Person to be seen in the Street except the Watch. On this Occasion the Expressions of Grief of the Women whose Children could not be admitted were Scarcely more observable than those of some of the Women who parted with their Children, so that a more moving Scene can't well be imagined.

All the Children who were received (except three) were dressed very clean from whence and other Circumstances they appeared not to have been under the care of the Parish officers, nevertheless many of them appeared as if Stupifyed with some Opiate, and some of them almost Starved, one as in the agonies of Death thro' want of Food, too weak to Suck, or to receive Nourishment, and notwithstanding the greatest care appeared as dying when the Govrs. left the Hospital which was not till they had given proper Orders and

50

seen all necessary Care taken of the Children.[25]

The next day, the record continues, 'many Charitable Persons of Fassion visited the Hospital, and whatever Share Curiosity might have in inducing any of them to Come, none went away without shewing most Sensible Marks of Compassion for the helpless Objects of this Charity and few (if any) without contributing something for their Relief'.[26]

Two of the children died before the first baptismal service, which was held after Evening Prayer on 29 March. 'There was at the Ceremony a fine Appearance of Persons of Quality and Distinction; His Grace the Duke of Bedford, our President, their Graces the Duke and Dutchess of Richmond, the Countess of Pembroke and Several others honouring the Children with their Names and being their Sponsors'. The first two children baptized were named Thomas Coram and Eunice Coram.[27] The dead infants were buried in the churchyard of St Andrew Holborn; two nurses were engaged at once to care for the sick children; the healthy ones were dispatched to nurses in Yorkshire, Staines, and Egham; and the chief nurse and two others were found almost at once to be unfit for their duties and were discharged—one for 'disobedience and sawciness'.

Although no one dropped a child in the Parish of St Andrew Holborn on 25 March, an abandoned infant was found and carried to the parish workhouse on 1 April; the young woman who had deserted it was apprehended and sent to Bridewell. Obviously, the parish would need additional watchmen and this, the churchwarden and Overseers of the Poor were quick to remind the Governors, meant additional expense. The Governors agreed to contribute £12 a year toward the extra wages.

On 17 April thirty more children were received in the evening, and, the occasion having been well advertised, once more a great number of people gathered in the street in front of the Hospital's doors, so many, in fact, that the Governors feared some of the infants might be hurt. Already the Governors were encountering the problem that was to haunt them for the rest of the century: a demand for help beyond their power to supply. The evident need for expansion, however, led them almost at once to hire the adjoining house. With more space available and substantial benefactions—some of them anonymous—steadily coming in, the Governors concluded that they could take in additional children: thirty were received on 8 May and twenty-three on 5 June.[28]

Over the summer the Hospital settled down into a steady routine. But in the fall the Governors found themselves confronted with a potential scandal.

5

Thomas Coram:
The Last Years, 1741–1751

IN OCTOBER 1741, the Governors received a letter signed G. W.,
which charged that many irregularities existed in the Hospital and
slandered the characters of two Governors, Martin Folkes and
Theodore Jacobsen. A committee was appointed immediately to
investigate the charges. Within two weeks this committee filed its
report, and a special meeting was called to consider it on
9 November. Apparently the charges had originated in information
given to Dr Nesbitt and Captain Coram by several of the nurses, who
accused the chief nurse, Sarah Wood, of dishonesty, immodest
behaviour and drunkenness, and insinuated that she had suffered a
miscarriage while in the Hospital's employ. Their accusations also
implicated the two Governors, Folkes and Jacobsen. But, said the
report, Captain Coram had been the person principally involved in
spreading these scandalous imputations.

Upon receiving this information, the Governors did what
publicity-conscious members of eleemosynary institutions always do
on such occasions: they passed a series of resolutions declaring the
charges against the two Governors 'unjust, false, groundless, and
malicious'; praising the diligence and zeal of the two men; placing
responsibility for the affair on Coram and Nesbitt; and ordering all
records of the matter to be sealed up. Six weeks later they discharged
Sarah Wood. The charges against her were 'groundless and malicious', the Governors stated, but it was necessary to dismiss her
because under her care the affairs of the Hospital had been 'very
improperly managed'. They also directed that a notice be posted up
advising the Hospital's staff that in the future any complaints must be
made to the General or House Committee and not to any single
Governor.[1]

Unfortunately, so far as Coram was concerned, the matter did not
end with the Committee's resolutions. The Governors reproved

Dr Nesbitt for not taking proper measures to discountenance the unsavoury allegations as soon as he heard them from the nurses, but they could not forgive Coram for 'promoting and spreading the said Aspersions on the said two Governors'. Although he continued conscientiously to attend every meeting, from that time on the Governors virtually ostracized him. The purchase of the Earl of Salisbury's fifty-six acres of land was completed on 16 February 1742, and a committee was appointed the following week to consider plans for the new hospital building; Coram was not included. Another committee was appointed to review the leases of the tenants who occupied portions of the newly acquired lands; Coram was not named to it. A third committee was selected by ballot to choose the site for the new building; Coram was not elected. Moreover, his efforts to by-pass this committee by inducing the General Court to fix the site in accordance with the written opinion of several residents of the neighbourhood met with failure: the March quarterly meeting voted unanimously to leave the selection of the site to the General Committee. Finally, at the annual meeting on 12 May 1742, although Coram was present, the Governors failed to re-elect him to the General Committee, thereby excluding him from any further voice in the day-to-day management of the hospital he had founded.[2] Of all the disappointments in a life that had known many, this must have been the hardest for Coram to bear, for he had given to the Foundling Hospital more time, more thought and more concern than to any other project.

The rights and wrongs of the affair of the chief nurse cannot now be known: the sealed file has been missing for over a hundred years. But the formal words of the minutes clearly indicate that Coram had brought about his own rejection in the same way that he had antagonized the Georgia Trustees: he had talked publicly about something that the governing body of the organization considered a private matter, and in so doing, he had laid the enterprise itself open to public criticism that might jeopardize its income from bene-factions. Coram was not a malicious man or one who enjoyed repeating salacious gossip for its own sake. And he had worked too hard and loved his Hospital too much to endanger its future de-liberately, but he had never learned to think before he spoke or to put discretion ahead of candour when he believed in the truth of what he said. And men who do not hesitate to speak without guile and without reckoning all the consequences and possible personal costs seldom get along well with those who do.

Perhaps, too, some irritation had been building up on both sides. Coram had long thought that the Governors were moving too slowly. In September 1740, he had written to Dr Colman that 'Benefactions are at a Stand because we have not began to Build yet which I think we should have done before now'.[3]

For their part, the Governors may have felt uneasy working in harness with a man whose single-minded interest in the Hospital and eagerness to accomplish everything at once far exceeded their own more leisurely approach—the approach of men who were involved in numerous other activities and who were accustomed in the conduct of their own affairs to weigh every move thoughtfully and at length. Most of the Governors were still too young to understand the impatience of an old man who wants to see the fulfillment of his dream before he can dream no more. Perhaps some of them wished that he would stay home occasionally and do less for the Hospital, so that their own lower levels of interest and activity might not evoke a sense of guilt. For he was always there. No other Governor could match his attendance record. From the first meeting on 20 November 1739 to 12 May 1742, he missed only two meetings of the General Committee (in the summer of 1741). During the first three months after the Hospital opened, he served as a member of the Daily Committee eighteen times in addition to attending fifteen meetings of the General Court and General Committee, several of which had to be adjourned for lack of a quorum. Even his wife's death in mid-July 1740 and his own illness in the same month[4] did not prevent him from attending a Committee meeting on 16 July. During this whole period, in fact, he had thought of little else, his only other public activity being to attend five or six meetings of the Georgia Trustees.

Undoubtedly his wife's death gave Coram still more reason to devote all his time to the Foundling Hospital. Not only would her death remind him how few years he, too, could count on, but also it would incline a man of Coram's temperament to seek escape from his grief in increased activity. How deeply he felt his loss is revealed in a letter to Dr Colman:

> It having pleased the Almighty God to remove my dearly beloved Wife from hence by death in the Middle of July Worn out by long Sickness, I was Marryed to her a little above 40 years during which time she never once gave me Cause to be angry or vexed at her, she was always a Sincere Christian of an humble meek and Quiet Spirit and Wisely Study'd my Peace and Comfort and was to her Life's End a vertuous kind and Prudent Wife without fault. She Chearfully bore an affectionate part in all my Toyls and affections. By her Death I am bereaved of one of the best of Wives.[5]

One other reason suggests itself to account for the harshness with which the Governors dealt with Captain Coram: he was still, *au fond*, an outsider. He did not share with his fellow Governors that

54

common base of formal education, social graces, and bonds of kinship and friendship that distinguished their level of society from lower orders. He might call himself Thomas Coram, Gentleman; he might deserve admiration as the founder of the Hospital, but he could never cross the invisible line that separated 'one of us' from lesser men.

From May 1742 to the end of his life, Coram had little official contact with the Foundling Hospital. Occasionally he still received contributions for it, which he turned over to some member of the Committee, but he had been asked to hand over the subscription books that he used to solicit donations for the Hospital's benefit and had surrendered them to Dr Mead.[6] He was present at the annual meeting on 11 May 1743 but was not elected to the General Committee and never again went to a General Court meeting. In 1747, however, he began to attend the baptismal ceremonies for the foundlings and continued to do so to the end of his life, missing only five such occasions between October 1747 and March 1751. During these years he stood godfather to twenty children.[7] It is also told of him that in these later years he was often seen sitting in the Hospital's arcade, dressed in his well-worn red coat, 'distributing with tears in his Eyes Gingerbread to the Children, himself being at the time supported by Subscription'.[8]

For the fact was that in his last years Coram's financial resources became completely exhausted. The reason, according to Dr Brocklesby, was that after his wife's death he spent so much time upon public affairs that he neglected his own. But his friends saw to it that he was not obliged to spend his last days in poverty. Headed by the Jewish financier, Sampson Gideon, they raised a subscription in 1749 large enough to provide him with an annuity of 161 guineas a year. Most of the subscribers—chiefly merchants—pledged a guinea, but the Prince of Wales contributed twenty guineas a year 'and paid it with as much punctuality as any of the rest'.[9]

Neither declining fortunes nor advancing age, however, could dampen Coram's irresistible urge toward good works. Just as he had done when the Georgia Trustees rejected him, he put the rebuff of the Foundling Hospital's Governors behind him and started over again: he would establish a second foundling hospital, this time in Westminster. Sometime between 1742 and 1745, he drafted a petition addressed to the Princess of Wales and set about gathering signatures from members of ten Westminster parishes.* Before he

* The Westminster parishes represented were St Margaret, St Martin-in-the-Field, St Paul Covent Garden, St Clement Danes, St Ann, St James, St Mary le Strand, St John Evangelist, St George Hanover Square, and the Precinct of the Savoy.

finished, he had obtained 120 signatures, twelve from each parish. It was, no doubt, easier to secure signers now than it had been in the 1730s: the initial breakthrough had been made, and men could see a foundling hospital already operating successfully. As the petition pointed out, they could also see that it was not big enough to care for half of the children brought to it. Nevertheless, obtaining 120 signatures from men, none of whom were signers of his earlier petitions, represented a great expenditure of time and effort on Coram's part.

Unlike the signers of the earlier petitions, none of these men were members of the nobility, and the absence of information about them in the usual sources leads to the conclusion that they were mostly undistinguished men of the middling sort. Such an assumption also follows logically from the statement at the head of the petition that it is made by the 'Church Wardens, Overseers of the Poor and other Principal Inhabitants of the Ten Parishes in the City & Liberties of Westminster'.[10]

There is no record indicating whether or not Coram ever presented this petition to the Princess. On 9 February 1750, George Bubb Dodington recorded in his journal that he had seen that evening at Carlton House 'Dr. Lee who brought old Coram with propositions for a vagabond hospital', and that 'they were to go up to the Princess'.[11] Was this the petition for a second foundling hospital being presented some five years after it was drawn up, or was it a petition that Coram had asked Mr Austin, Master of the Charity School in Bartholomew Close, to prepare for presentation to the Princess of Wales in 1749 and which probably related to another project* he had afoot at that time?[12] We do not know, but it is certain that nothing came of his efforts to found a hospital for abandoned infants in Westminster.

In these last years of his life Coram did, however, enjoy the satisfaction of seeing the fulfillment of his long cherished dream of a colony in Nova Scotia as well as the vindication of his stand for a fairer system of land tenure in Georgia, although he himself took no direct part in bringing about either event. In May 1749 a fleet of eighty-four transports loaded with three thousand colonists—many of them soldiers discharged at the end of the War of the Austrian

---

* *Read's Weekly Journal*, 13 April 1751, states that at the time of his death Coram was interested in a project for the employment of vagrants, idle persons, and the distressed poor, and that a building was shortly to be erected for their reception. The *Penny London Post* and *London Advertiser* carried the same item.

Succession—set sail for Nova Scotia. This time the settlement project had been fathered by Lord Halifax, whose plan for the colony displayed many similarities to Coram's earlier schemes. The government had acted with extraordinary speed, and the result was the establishment of the town of Halifax in Nova Scotia.[13]

At the other extremity of the Atlantic coastal colonies, Georgia, too, was receiving attention in the years following the War of the Austrian Succession. The system of land tenure to which Coram had so violently objected was finally abandoned in 1750, although the change had begun in 1739. Under considerable pressure from dissatisfied colonists in Georgia and adverse public opinion in England, the Trustees passed a series of resolutions on 25 July 1739 that permitted, among other things, a daughter to inherit her father's lands if he left no male descendant. The new system applied, however, only to those who owned over eighty acres. Coram, who attended several Trustees' meetings in 1739, was pleased with the improvement, and the Earl of Egmont recorded in his diary that 'I gave my consent thereto; and did it the more readily because Captain Coram was present and approved it, who had much prejudiced us in the town's opinion because we did it not before'. But the resolutions by no means granted full ownership, and the struggle continued until 1750 when the Trustees finally adopted a resolution granting the colonists absolute ownership of their lands with no restrictions on inheritance.[14] Time had proved Coram's ideas sound.

By the spring of 1750 Coram had moved from the All Hallows rectory to lodgings in Spur Street (now Panton Street) off Leicester Square. There he died on Friday 29 March 1751, and 'passed from doing to enjoying Good'.[15] In his lifetime Coram had expressed a desire to be buried in the vault under the Foundling Hospital Chapel, which had been in use, although not formally opened, since 1749. Upon learning of his death, the Governors agreed at once that his wishes should be carried out and quickly made their plans for holding the funeral service in the chapel.

On Wednesday, 3 April, the Governors, clad in deep mourning, gathered at five o'clock in the Court Room of the Hospital to await the arrival of the hearse. Inside the chapel a great number of fashionable ladies and gentlemen, all dressed in mourning, were filling up the galleries. About six o'clock the hearse carrying Thomas Coram's body in a plain elm coffin, followed by a single mourning coach, arrived at the Hospital's gate, where a crowd had assembled in the expectation of seeing a magnificent and imposing funeral cortege. They were greatly disappointed, the *London Advertiser* reported the next day, for only the meanest of funerals did not include at least two or three mourning coaches and other trappings, but Coram left no funds to pay for pomp. He ended life with as little as he began it.

At the gate the hearse was met by the Governors, the children, and the choirs. The funeral procession formed in the courtyard with the porter of the Hospital at its head, followed by the girls and then the boys, walking two-by-two. After the children came the choirs of St Paul's Cathedral and Westminster, clad in their surplices. Behind the choirs and immediately in front of the coffin walked the secretary carrying the Hospital's charter on a crimson velvet cushion. Eight Governors (including two vice-presidents) supported the pall over the coffin,* and following it the treasurer, as chief mourner, walked alone. At the end came Coram's relatives and many more Governors of the Hospital.

As soon as the procession entered the chapel, which had been draped with mourning, the chattering congregation grew very still, and the choirs began to sing the solemn service for the burial of the dead. Dr Boyce, who had composed it, accompanied them at the organ. Near the end of the service the choirs sang his funeral anthem with its Pauline words of promise and of comfort. The clergyman read the last Collect, ending 'Come, ye blessed children of my Father, receive the kingdom prepared for you from the beginning of the world . . .', and the body of Thomas Coram was carried down into the vault and laid under the altar.[16] Sisyphus at last could rest. But as Camus put it, 'il faut imaginer Sisyphe hereux', for 'la lutte elle-même vers les sommets suffit à remplir un coeur d'homme'.[17]

---

* The Governors who carried the pall were Peter Burrell, Joseph Fawthrop, John Milner, Sir Joseph Hankey, Sampson Gideon, Paul Joddrell, Samuel Clarke, and Stephen Beckingham.

PART II

The Children

Whoever is under my power is under my protection.

Lady Mary Wortley Montagu,
Letters and Works, 1753.

6

Hogarth, Handel, and Hospital Routine, 1742–1756

CAPTAIN CORAM GAVE HIS next-to-last vote, as a Governor of the Foundling Hospital, at the annual meeting on 12 May 1742 against a contract with Thomas Scott for making 400,000 'well-burnt' bricks at 12s a thousand for the Hospital's use in the construction of its new building;* the bricks were to be made in the north-east part of the Hospital's recently acquired property.[1] This would be near the intersection of Gray's Inn Road and Heathcote Street (which did not then exist), where today iron markers driven flush with the pavements still indicate the former corner of the Foundling Hospital's property.

From that corner the line of the Hospital's estate ran southward along Gray's Inn Road (at that time often referred to as the Road to Hampstead and Highgate) to a point near its present intersection with Guilford Street, which had not yet been built in 1742. Then, turning westward, the boundary continued along an irregular line more or less parallel with Great Ormond Street but far enough north of it to border on the north side of Queen Square, left open to afford its residents 'the beautiful prospect of the hills, ever verdant, ever smiling, of Hampstead and Highgate'.[2] The Duke of Bedford's estate, which extended along Southampton Row and today's Woburn Place (then a field), constituted the west boundary. And on the north side the line approximated the course of what is now Tavistock Place and then veered southward to the burying grounds of St George Bloomsbury and St George the Martyr, now metamorphosed into St George's Gardens.[3]

These fifty-six acres formed a part of the area generally known as

* All of the other forty-two members present voted in favour of the agreement. Why Coram voted against it we do not know, but since he had just been denied re-election to the General Committee, perhaps his hurt pride lashed out in the negative vote.

Lamb's Conduit Fields because many years earlier a man named Lamb had built a water conduit there. In the fifteenth century, the Prior and Convent of the Charterhouse had owned the property, but after the dissolution of the monasteries, it became Crown land and then passed through several hands before its acquisition by the sixth Earl of Salisbury.[4]

In 1742 it was a lonely spot. The nearest populated area, Queen Square and Great Ormond Street, then lay on the northern frontier of London. Here, in large houses, lived a cluster of well-to-do, fashionable families seeking escape from London's smoky air. The back doors of the Ormond Street houses opened directly into the Hospital's fields, and thus its neighbours included, among others, Dr Richard Mead and the Lord Chancellor, who had rented Powis House in 1739 from Lord Powis. This elegant residence, the largest in Ormond Street, occupied the site of what is today Powis Place.[5] To the rear its gardens adjoined Powis Well, a chalybeate spring equipped with a pump house, pleasure walks, and a Long Room for music and dancing. Although it never enjoyed widespread popularity, Powis Well had been patronized since the 1720s by a considerable number of Londoners eager to drink its waters, alleged to be 'of a sweetning, diuretic, and gently purging Quality, and . . . recommended by many eminent Physicians and Surgeons for the Cure of Breakings out on the Skin, sore Legs, Inflammations of the Eyes, and a great Number of other Scorbutic, Scrophulous and Leporous Disorders'.[6]

Powis Well stood on the lands sold to the Hospital, which acquired with its fifty-six-acre purchase not only the mineral spring but also the tenant, Mr Bell, who was busily exploiting the spring's commercial possibilities—so much so, in fact, that when his son requested a renewal of the lease in 1745 at £9 a year, the Governors insisted that he promise to prevent the playing at skittles and all disorderly behaviour by his patrons.[7] Bell was not the only tenant on the lands purchased by the Hospital. Among others were the Coach and Horses Alehouse and a cowkeeper, who provided the Hospital with a convenient source for its milk supply but later provided it with an inconvenient source of embarrassment when he made a laystall* immediately behind the wall of the houses in Great Ormond Street.[8]

Unfortunately the Hospital did not acquire with its purchase adequate access to its property. The portion of Gray's Inn Road that adjoined its east boundary was not yet paved; the nearest paved carriage-way leading into London was Red Lion Street. In order to connect the Hospital's property with this street, the Governors were

* A laystall was a place for laying dung.

obliged to negotiate for a right of way with the Trustees of the Rugby School, the owners of the intervening land. This became Lamb's Conduit Street and the Hospital's main entrance. Not until later in the century did the Hospital open a way into Gray's Inn Road.

There were, of course, a few footpaths: one ran across the north-west corner of the property leading to the two burying grounds, and another wandered northward to the St Pancras bowling green, which was located just south of the present St Pancras Station, but that was all. For the rest, open fields, more thickly populated with cows than with people, stretched northward from the city in quiet isolation that gave the area a not unwarranted reputation as a dangerous place. There had been, after all, a number of murders and robberies among the brickyards at the north end of Gray's Inn Road.[9]

On the other hand, the estate's remoteness offered the advantages of clean air, the means for keeping the children cut off from the physical and moral contagions of London, and space for expansion. The crowded conditions at Hatton Garden made space seem the most important benefit, and the Governors were eager to take advantage of it. They envisioned a hospital large enough to house four hundred children plus officers and servants but realized that they could pay for a building only half as large. Nevertheless, with an eye to the future, they sought a design for a hospital that could be built in stages, as funds became available, until it reached the desired capacity.

One of the Governors, Theodore Jacobsen, a Steelyard merchant and architect, and three other gentlemen presented plans, which the Committee then submitted to builders for their opinions. One proved to be too small, another too expensive, and a third too difficult to maintain. In the end, the Governors adopted Mr Jacobsen's plan, which provided for a plain brick building with two wings and a chapel built around a courtyard open toward Red Lion Street. Each wing would accommodate 192 children, two in a bed, and would measure 54 feet by 187 feet; the chapel would be 48 feet square, and the courtyard would be 146 feet square; the cost was estimated at approximately £6500. Most important of all, the design lent itself to construction in stages. The Governors, therefore, decided on 30 June 1742 to proceed at once to build the west wing and advertised for bids on digging the foundation and laying up the bricks. James Horne, later elected a Governor, volunteered to act as surveyor for the project without charge.[10]

The bids came in; contracts were let; Mr Scott was authorized to manufacture a million bricks, using clay from the foundation excavation; plans were made for running 'a great Sewer' to join the drain in Red Lion Street—a distance of 712 feet; and on Thursday,

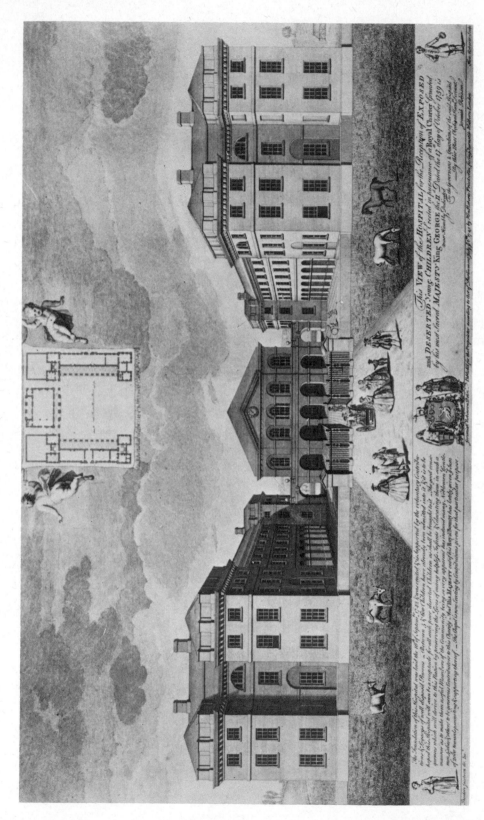

3. Plan and Perspective View of the Foundling Hospital, 1749

16 September 1742, John Milner, one of the vice-presidents, laid the cornerstone at the south-east corner of what would become the west wing. A year later the building was ready for its Westmorland slate roofs and lead gutters. As soon as the gutters were installed, the Governors thought it necessary to hire a watchman, for theft of lead was a common occurrence.

By February 1744 the exterior was complete, and the carpenters and joiners arrived to start the interior work. By May the Governors considered it advisable to insure the building against fire with the Hand & Hand Fire Office, which issued four policies, each for £1000, at a total premium of £25 2s 6d. In June the glaziers began to set the 'best crown glass' in the window frames, and the 'plaisterers' commenced their work. Meanwhile, other workmen were putting down Purbeck stone paving in the kitchen, the two necessary houses, and the arcade on the east side of the building, while still others installed the Portland stone chimney-pieces and hung two-inch-thick deal doors in oak frames. The overall effect, both inside and out, was one of simplicity and utility, except for the Court Room on the ground floor. In contrast to the plainness of the rest of the building, this room displayed great elegance, with an elaborate ceiling, plaster embellishments on the walls, and handsome woodwork.*

In the spring of 1745 work on the building was progressing so well that the Governors could start to think about bedsteads, mattresses, 'coverlids' and other furnishings. They also arranged to pipe water from a nearby spring into the building. At last all was ready. On 25 September 1745, three years after the laying of the cornerstone, the Governors held their last meeting at Hatton Garden. On 1 October 'the Children and family removed from the house at Hatton Garden to the New Hospital in Lambs Conduit Fields'.[11]

The children had hardly moved into the new building when two projects that were to prove of major importance in promoting the Hospital's popularity got under way. One was the beginning of the Hospital's famous art collection; the other was the erection of its chapel. The subscription roll for the latter enterprise was opened on 9 April 1746 with an advertisement published once a week for a month in the *Daily Advertiser*, the *London Courant*, and the *General Evening Post*.[12] Meanwhile, the Governors directed Theodore Jacobsen to prepare building plans, from which Mr Horne estimated

---

* When the Foundling Hospital was torn down, this room was carefully preserved and faithfully reconstructed in 1937 in the new building at 40 Brunswick Square that today houses the Thomas Coram Foundation for Children.

that the cost of a chapel would be £4195 17s 4d. Pledges and gifts mounted up rapidly, however, and within a year the Committee considered it safe to begin construction. Jacobsen laid the corner-stone on 1 May 1747, and the Governors turned the occasion into a festive celebration and money-raising affair with a public breakfast at the Hospital for the 'great concourse of Nobility and Ladies of Distinction' who attened. At the breakfast the children presented baskets of flowers to the ladies and afterward, under the Governors' supervision, took up a collection. The affair was a great success: although the expenses came to nearly £4 more than the receipts from selling 675 tickets at 2s 6d each, the collection brought in £596 13s for the building fund, and the breakfast became an annual event.[13]

Almost simultaneously William Hogarth, who had been a Governor from the beginning, conceived the idea of adorning the bare walls of the Court Room and other public rooms of the Hospital with works of art by English painters and sculptors eager to prove to the fashionable world that their skills equalled those of the foreign artists so much favoured by critics and connoisseurs. His motive, undoubtedly, sprang from a combination of benevolence and self-interest. His engravings depicting the degradation of London's poor, his interest in St Bartholomew's and Bethlem Hospitals, his asso-ciation with the Parliamentary Committee on prison reform in 1729, and his willingness to serve as an inspector for the Foundling Hospital's children at nurse near Chiswick—all testify to his humani-tarian concerns. On the other hand, since no academy where artists could display their works then existed in London, he would have been more than human had he not hoped that a permanent exhibition of works of art at the new Foundling Hospital, joined with the opportunity of seeing the children, might prove an irresistible attraction to the upper levels of society—Londoners, after all, were mad for the new and the curious—and from their visits not only benefactions to the charity but also commissions for the participating painters and sculptors might result.

Hogarth brought into the scheme the sculptor, John Michael Rysbrack, who had become a Governor on 27 March 1745, and Rysbrack's aristocratic connections, as well as his influence with other artists, assured the success of the plan. Sometime in 1746 Hogarth and Rysbrack interested a number of London painters in the proposal, and each began to work on his own project. No announce-ment was made, however, until the General Court held on 31 December, when the treasurer told the assembled Governors that fifteen 'Gentlemen Artists had severally presented and agreed to present Performances in their different Professions for Ornamenting the Hospital'.[14] Whereupon they were all* elected Governors and, together with Hogarth, Rysbrack, Theodore Jacobsen, and the miniaturist George Frederick Zincke, who had become a Governor in 1740, were appointed a committee to meet annually on 5 November 'to consider of what further Ornaments may be added to this Hospital without any expence to the Charity'.[15]

By February some of the paintings were finished and hung, but they were not unveiled to the public until 1 April 1747. On that day, according to the engraver George Vertue:

> Wensday the first of April. 1747. at the foundling Hospital was an Entertainment. or publick dinner. of the Governors and other Gentlemen that had inclination—about 170 persons great benefactions given then towards the hospital—at the same time was seen the four paintings newly put up, done Gratis by four eminent painters—by Hayman. Hogarth Hymore. & Wills—& by most people generally approved & commended. as works in history painting in a higher degree of merit than has heretofore been done by English Painters—some other portraits are done & doing by Ramsay Hudson. & landskips &c.[16]

The four paintings to which Vertue referred hung in the Court Room, and all centred around the theme of the rescue of young children. Highmore's painting was *Hagar and Ishmael*; Hayman's, *The Finding of the Infant Moses in the Bullrushes*; and Wills's, *Little Children Brought to Christ*. Hogarth decided to use the theme of Captain Coram's design for the corporation's seal: *Moses Brought to Pharaoh's Daughter*.

Rysbrack's contribution was a marble bas-relief of *Charity* to go over the Court Room fireplace. The portraits 'done & doing' by Ramsay and Hudson, which Vertue mentioned, were Hudson's portraits of Vice-president John Milner and the architect Theodore Jacobsen, and Allan Ramsay's portrait of Dr Richard Mead. The 'landskips' consisted of eight small round views of the Foundling Hospital itself and seven other London hospitals, painted by various artists—Gainsborough among them—and hung in the Court Room, one on each side of the four large paintings. Not all of these had been completed by 1 April 1747, but all were in place by 1751.[17]

By that time the Hospital had also acquired Hogarth's famous *March to Finchley*. On 16 March 1750 he had announced in the

* The fifteen artists were Francis Hayman, James Wills, Joseph Highmore, Thomas Hudson, Allan Ramsay, George Lambert, Samuel Scott, Peter Monamy, Richard Wilson, Samuel Wale, Edward Hateley, Thomas Carter, George Moser, Robert Taylor, and John Pine.

General Advertiser that subscribers for his copperplate engraving illustrating the guards' march to Finchley in 1746 could also obtain a chance on the original painting by paying 3s above the subscription price of 7s 6d. The drawing took place on 30 April, and on 1 May the *London Evening Post* reported:

> Yesterday Mr. Hogarth's Subscription was closed, 1843 Chances being subscribed for. The remaining Numbers from 1843 to 2000 were given by Mr. Hogarth to the Hospital for the Maintenance and Education of exposed and deserted young Children. At Two o'Clock the Box was open'd, in the Presence of a great Number of Persons of Distinction, and the fortunate Chance was drawn, No. 1941, which belongs to the said Hospital; and the same Night Mr. Hogarth deliver'd the Picture to the Governors. His Grace the Duke of Ancaster offer'd them 200 l. for it before it was taken away, but it was refus'd.[18]

The painting was hung in the Committee Room.

Hogarth also designed the Hospital's arms, the official grant of which was received early in 1747. Richard Yeo, an engraver at the Royal Mint, offered to engrave the design on a new seal for the Hospital, but more than twelve years elapsed before he kept his promise.[19] Other gifts of art poured in, among them Chevalier Andrea Casali's painting *The Adoration of the Magi*, which was completed in 1750 and installed above the altar in the chapel.[20]

To describe further the Foundling Hospital's art collection, which became still larger and more varied as the years passed, would only repeat what has already been done most impressively by Benedict Nicolson, whose *The Treasures of the Foundling Hospital* also incorporates a catalogue raisonné based on the work of John Kerslake, Deputy Keeper of the National Portrait Gallery. But perhaps something more should be said about the artists who began it. Hogarth's scheme led, as he had hoped, to a few commissions: Hayman was asked for two paintings for the chapel at Cusworth Hall, and Hogarth himself received the commission for *Paul Before Felix* from the Society of Lincoln's Inn. The exhibit also brought swarms of visitors to the Foundling Hospital and substantial contributions to its charity boxes. Of more consequence for the future of British art, the Hospital became, for lack of any other, London's art centre. The annual meetings of the artists' committee on Guy Fawkes Day, when they dined together at the Hospital at their own expense, laid the groundwork for a larger organization of artists able to hold annual exhibitions of their works. This idea, proposed at the yearly meeting of the artists' committee in 1759, resulted in the first annual exhibition of British art, held in the spring of 1760, but not at the Foundling Hospital. Eight years later these exhibitions brought about the foundation of the Royal Academy.[21] From 1760 on the Hospital ceased to be a meeting place for artists, but its collection remains 'an admirable cross-section of a particular phase in British art, unparalleled elsewhere'.[22]

The opportunity to see outstanding works by contemporary artists was not the only inducement to Londoners to visit the Foundling Hospital in the 1750s. The chapel, too, drew large numbers of people, although the dilatoriness of the workmen prevented its formal opening for regular Sunday services until 16 April 1753, when the Bishop of Worcester gave the sermon and George Frederick Handel provided the music. But, in fact, the Governors had used it for benefit concerts since 1749 and also for the christenings, which always attracted a large attendance of the curious. On these occasions four governors with white wands passed up and down the middle of the chapel after the prayers and just before the sacrament began, while a foundling boy and girl went along each row of seats with plates to receive the collection. All agreed that it was an edifying and moving sight.[23]

The first of many concerts for the benefit of the Hospital was given on 27 May 1749, when Handel 'Generously & Charitably offered a Performance of Vocal and Instrumental Musick', the proceeds to be used for finishing the chapel. Originally scheduled for 24 May, the concert was postponed to the 27th at the request of the Prince of Wales, who planned to attend.[24] The *Gentleman's Magazine* reported the event:

> Saturday 27. The P. and Prss. of Wales, with a great number of persons of quality and distinction were at the chapel of the Foundling's hospital; to hear several pieces of vocal and instrumental musick, compos'd by George Frederick Handel, Esq.; for the benefit of the foundation. 1. The musick for the late fireworks, and the anthem on the peace. 2. Select pieces from the oratorio of *Solomon*, relating to the dedication of the temple; and 3. Several pieces composed for the occasion, the words taken from scripture, and applicable to the charity, and its benefactors. There was no collection, but the tickets were at half a guinea, and the audience above a thousand.[25]

The 'anthem on the peace' was the 'Dettingen Te Deum', and the 'pieces composed for the occasion' included the 'Foundling Hospital Anthem'.

This was the beginning of Handel's long association with the

Foundling Hospital. Not only did he love children but he had also been influenced in favour of such institutions during his years at the University of Halle by Professor August Hermann Francke, whose passionate devotion to orphans had created an orphanage* that became a model for similar establishments throughout Germany.[27] Elected a Governor on 9 May 1749, Handel at first declined the honour because 'he should serve the Charity with more Pleasure in his way than being a member of the Corporation'.[28] But a year later, on 9 May 1750, he permitted the Governors to elect him. On that day he also received their thanks for his gift of an organ to be used in the chapel.[29]

Eight days earlier Handel had conducted the first of many performances of the *Messiah* that he was to give for the Hospital's benefit. The organ was not fully completed for the occasion, but the boys of the King's Chapel and the soloists sang well, and the concert proved so great a success that Handel offered to repeat it on 15 May to accomodate those who had not been able to obtain admission. The proceeds of the two performances, for which tickets were sold at half a guinea each, amounted to £969 7s.[30] Handel had written the *Messiah* in a period of twenty-four days in 1741 and had given it its first performance in Dublin on 13 April 1742 for the relief of prisoners and for the support of two hospitals.[31] Thereafter he gave five performances of the oratorio in London—three in 1743 and two in 1745—but it failed to achieve any popularity.[32] Perhaps the success of the performances at the Foundling Hospital owed something to the milieu in which they were given.

Be that as it may, the *Messiah* became an annual tradition at the Hospital, and over the years it produced substantial sums for the charity's benefit. Handel conducted the *Messiah* for the last time on 15 May 1754. Then, virtually blind, he suggested that his amanuensis, John Christopher Smith, act as organist and conductor for the annual event, but he still attended every performance. During the rehearsal on 6 April 1759, he suffered a fainting spell and just over a week later, on 14 April, he died.[33]

Including the performance of the *Messiah* given on 3 May 1759 and his first concert in 1749, Handel had earned for the Hospital with

* Although Francke had founded his pietist Orphan House at Halle in 1695 and had written an account of it, *Segensvolle Fussstapfen* in 1709, translated as *Pietas Hallensis*, the Governors did not consult this account when they were drafting their plan for operating the Hospital—a surprising omission, for the book was widely known and, in fact, provided inspiration to the great Methodist evangelist, George Whitefield, when he opened his Orphan House at Bethesda, Georgia, in 1740.

his music a net total of £6725 10s.[34] Little wonder, then, that in 1754, upon learning from the treasurer that Handel intended the *Messiah* to be performed exclusively in the Hospital's chapel, and that other persons had procured a copy of it from Ireland and were planning to perform it for their own benefit, the Governors decided to present a petition to Parliament for an act vesting all property rights in the oratorio solely in the Foundling Hospital, subject to Handel's own use of it in his lifetime. The Committee requested one of the Governors to call upon Handel and ask for his approval of the petition, but 'he found that the same did not seem agreeable to Mr. Handel for the Present',[35] and nothing more came of the proposal.* Upon his death, however, Handel bequeathed to the Hospital 'a Fair Copy of the Score and all Parts of his Oratorio call'd the Messiah'.[36]

The Governors paid tribute to their generous benefactor with a memorial concert in the chapel on 24 May 1759 under Smith's direction. The tickets for the affair were printed on mourning paper, sealed with black wax, and inscribed: 'In Grateful Memory of George Frederick Handell, Esqr., May 24, 1759, 12 o'Clock'. They sold for half a guinea each, and, anticipating a large attendance, the Governors requested that gentlemen come without swords and ladies without hoops. The program included the 'Foundling Hospital Anthem', the 'Hallelujah Chorus', the anthem 'Let Thy Hand be Strengthened', and an organ concerto performed by the blind organist, John Stanley.[37]

Performances of the *Messiah* continued to be given in the chapel every year after Handel's death until 1777, when the custom ceased. An effort to revive it was made in 1788 but failed for lack of interest on the part of the professional soloists asked to participate. Indeed, after Handel's death the annual concert never again enjoyed its former popularity. In contrast to the earlier period, the performances during the last eighteen years brought in only a little over £2000. The low point was reached in 1772 when the net proceeds amounted to £14 10s.[38] Nevertheless, the total income resulting from Handel's association with the charity had, by 1777, added up to more than £9000—no mean contribution.

Multiple attractions, therefore, drew Londoners to the Hospital where one might sometimes hear Handel's superb music, often have an opportunity to look at the children, and always be able to view the

---

* Dr Paul Henry Lang has suggested to me that no composer would agree to such a monopoly, least of all a promoter-impresario like Handel who was not a man to be pushed.

art collection. In fact, attending services at the Foundling Hospital on a Sunday morning became the fashionable thing to do, and soon there was a waiting list of persons eager to rent pews. Prior to its formal opening, the Governors had asserted in respect to the chapel that 'it will not be proper to let out any of the Pews to any particular Persons', but by 1755 they had changed their minds and were renting pews to those who applied for them at a guinea a year for each person's seat, and by 1766 they were also charging 8s a year for tickets admitting persons to seats in the galleries.[39]

The children, of course, could always be seen on Sunday mornings sitting in the chapel gallery under the watchful eyes of the matron and nurses. But from the middle of the century onward a visitor could usually see the boys on weekdays, too, at work making herring nets and twine in the ropeyard along the walls that had been built at each side of the approach to the Hospital. Or, he might find them at work in the former kitchen of the west wing, now converted into a kind of shop with a counter where the children's work was displayed and sold. If the visitor brought a proper introduction from a Governor, he or she might also be permitted to see the younger boys at work winding silk or netting purses in one of the rooms of the west wing and the girls in the east wing busy with their knitting, spinning, sewing, and mending.[40] For by the autumn of 1751, the east wing, begun in the spring of 1748, had been finished, and walls 160 yards long were being built from both wings toward Red Lion Street, with a third wall, equipped with gates, connecting them. It was along these colonnaded walls that the ropeyards were set up.* Construction of the east wing had been made possible, in large part, by the receipt of a legacy of £11,000 from the estate of Thomas Emerson, one of the Governors.[41]

So many Londoners found a visit to the Foundling Hospital an irresistible pleasure that they even came to see the children after they were in bed. This disturbed the children's sleep, and the Committee soon put an end to it by ordering that a bell be rung at 7.0 p.m. for the children to go to bed and that the wards be cleared and locked up half an hour later.[42] Regularity, the Governors believed, should mark the children's days. At mid-century, therefore, the life of the children can be described, in great measure, by reference to clock and calendar.

At 5.0 a.m. in spring and summer, at 6.0 a.m. during September, and at 7.0 a.m. in autumn and winter, the porter rang a bell at the gate

---

* The colonnades still exist, all that remains of the Foundling Hospital.

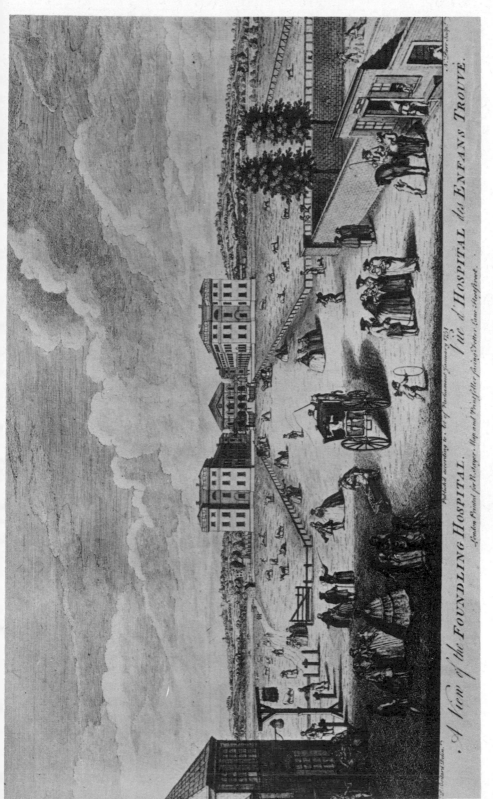

4. Perspective View of the Foundling Hospital, 1751

and around the courtyard to awaken the children. In summer, however, the younger children were permitted to sleep until six o'clock. All were allowed an hour for washing and dressing in their brown drugget uniforms trimmed in scarlet, which Hogarth had designed. Then they went to their respective duties until eight o'clock, when they sat down at the long tables in the dining rooms to breakfast on broth, gruel, or milk porridge, depending on the day of the week, for these were served in fixed rotation. Meanwhile, as soon as the children left their wards, the nurses cleaned the rooms and locked them up until bedtime, except on Sundays. On that day the children remained in the wards, emerging only for chapel service and meals.

After breakfast, a schoolmistress taught the younger children—those aged four to six—to read from hornbooks and, at intervals, supervised their play in the open air. The older boys worked under the direction of a master, dressing hemp, making twine and nets, or netting purses; the two or three strongest boys helped the gardener. At the same time the older girls were busy, under the eyes of the female members of the staff, sewing, knitting, spinning, darning, and performing all sorts of household work in the kitchen and laundry.[43] Dinner was served at noon, with a half hour allowed for the meal. It would consist of boiled mutton, beef, or pork, depending on the season, alternated with rice milk, dumplings, suet or hasty puddings, according to the day of the week, together with such vegetables as the garden might supply. Roast beef or roast pork made Sunday dinner, served at 1.30 p.m. because of the chapel service, a welcome change even though it would be followed unvaryingly by Monday's meatless meal of potatoes and other vegetables.

The afternoon's tasks continued those of the morning with time out for suitable open-air exercise, which, the Governors were convinced, would contribute to the children's health. For the girls, this might be a walk with their nurses in the fields adjoining the Hospital. For the boys, who also took their recreation under adult supervision, a game of ball might enliven the day. Always, however, at work, meals, study, or play, the boys were restricted to rooms and areas separate from those used by the girls. Supper was a slight meal: three times a week it consisted of bread alone; twice a week, bread and milk; and twice a week, bread and cheese. And so to bed at 7.0 p.m. Charter Day—17 October—released everyone from the daily routine; not only was it a holiday, but the children also enjoyed roast beef and plum pudding for dinner.

It was, on the whole, a Spartan, regimented, and supervised life, but not intentionally an unpleasant one. Its austerity arose in part from necessity and in part from the Governors' conception of the kind of lives most of the children could expect to lead when they left the Hospital. The constant supervision grew out of the Governors' desire to isolate the children from any contact with 'improper persons', such as visitors' footmen or servants, who might corrupt their morals, as well as the desire to prevent the children from begging for fruit or money from visitors. In short, the Governors ordered the children's days into a pattern that they believed would strengthen their characters and equip them for adult life.[44]

7

The General Reception:
Internal Problems, 1756–1760

IN THE EARLY 1750S approximately 150 children spent their days following the Hospital's established routine although, with the completion of the east wing, the Hospital could easily have held about four hundred. The reason for this disproportion between available space and actual population was lack of money. Many of the infants received died while at nurse in the country before reaching the age of four when they were brought back to the Hospital. It would, therefore, require the admission of a very large number of children to produce enough survivors to keep the Hospital's wards completely filled at all times. But the reception of more infants would necessitate an enlarged staff, more country nurses, more first-year clothing, increased travelling costs for the nurses coming up from the country to receive the children and take them back, greater expenses of every kind. And the Hospital had never had sufficient funds to permit the reception of children on so large a scale. Instead, the Governors found it necessary in the 1750s to limit receptions to once a month or once every two months and on those occasions to admit only twenty children, ten boys and ten girls.

Yet more than enough children were offered could the Governors have secured the means to care for them, and this resulted in disorderly scenes whenever the Committee announced a date for receiving children. As a consequence, the Governors had been obliged to change the reception procedure as early as 1742. Instead of admitting the infants of the first twenty or thirty women who fought their way to the door, they decided to use a plan proposed by Vice-president Milner:

> That all the Women who bring any Children be let into the Court Room as they come, and there set on Benches to be placed round the Room . . . . That as many White Balls as there shall be

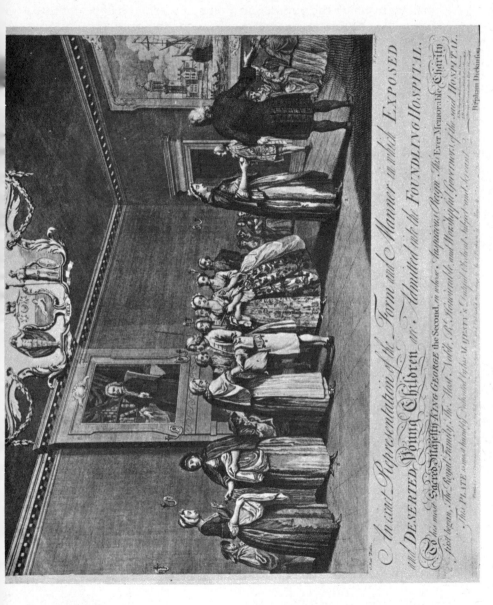

5. Admission of Children to the Foundling Hospital, 1749

Children to be taken in, with five red Balls for every Twenty Children who are to be taken in and so in Proportion for any greater or lesser number, and as many black Balls as with the white and red shall be Equal to the number of Women present, shall be put into a Bag or Box and drawn out by the Women who bring the Children. That each Woman who draws a white Ball shall be carried with her Child into the Inspecting Room in order to have the Child examined. That each Woman who draws a red Ball be carried with her Child into another Room there to remain till the Examination of the Children, whose Nurses drew white Balls is ended. That each Woman who draws a black Ball shall be immediately turned out of the Hospital with her Child. If on such Examination any of those Children are rejected but not so many as there be red Balls drawn, there shall be a second Drawing of Lotts by putting into the Bag or Box as many white Balls as there are Children wanting to make up the number ordered to be taken in, And as many black Balls as with the white will be equal to the whole number of red Balls drawn in the first Drawing. And the children whose Nurses draw those white Balls to be taken in if duly qualified, if not a third Drawing to be made in the manner with the second, and so on till the whole number be compleated. . . . The Lotts to be drawn in the Court Room in the presence of all the Women to prevent all Suspicion of Fraud or Partiality.[1]

The new balloting system, which the Committee followed until 1756, eliminated disorder but not disappointment. For example, on 15 November 1745 fifty-seven children were brought, but only eighteen could be admitted. On 23 May 1746 seventy-nine were brought, but less than a third could be received. On 16 June 1749 twenty of the eighty-three offered were taken in.[2] And this pattern continued through the early 1750s. The records show that from 1 January 1750 to December 1755, 2523 children were brought to the Hospital on the days appointed for admitting them. Of this number, only 783 were taken in; the Governors, appalled at the enormous need that they were helpless to meet, reluctantly turned away 1740. Most of these children probably came from parishes within the Bills of Mortality or from villages close to London, not because the rules of the Hospital placed any formal restrictions on a child's geographic origin but because the expense and practical difficulties of transporting a child under two months of age from remote parts of the kingdom, with no assurance of its reception by the Hospital upon arrival, would tend to discourage people from making such a journey. Nevertheless some children were brought considerable distances.[3]

As early as 1753 the Governors began to consider how they might expand their work in the face of the Hospital's limited funds. The first proposal was to apply to Parliament for an act that would compel the parishes within the Bills of Mortality to deliver to the Hospital's care as many of the parish orphans and foundlings as the Governors might demand and to pay a weekly allowance to the Hospital for the support of these children. But nothing came of this idea.[4] By 1756 the Governors had concluded that expansion could be achieved only by financial support from Parliament itself.

On 11 February 1756, therefore, the Governors approved and sealed a petition to the House of Commons, asking for its support in extending the charity.[5] On 6 April the matter came before the House, which resolved

. . . That the enabling the Hospital for the Maintenance and Education of exposed and deserted young Children, to receive all the Children which shall be offered, is the only Method to render that charitable Institution of lasting and general Utility.

. . . That, to render said Hospital of lasting and general Utility, the Assistance of Parliament is necessary.

. . . That, to render the said Hospital of general Utility and Effect, it should be enabled to appoint proper Places in all Counties, Ridings, or Divisions, of this Kingdom, for the Reception of all exposed and deserted young Children.

The Chancellor of the Exchequer then 'by His Majesty's Command, acquainted the House That his Majesty, having been informed of the State and Condition of the said Hospital, recommends it to the Consideration of the House, to make some Provision for the better carrying on so useful a Charity'.[6] On 3 May the House resolved

. . . That a Sum not exceeding Ten thousand Pounds be granted to his Majesty, towards enabling the Governors and Guardians of the Hospital for exposed and deserted young Children to receive into the said Hospital all Children, under a certain Age, to be appointed by the said Governors and Guardians, who shall be brought to the said Hospital after the First Day of June and before the 31st Day of December 1756.[7]

Probably the imminence of war with France—fighting had already broken out in North America, and the French were assembling a squadron of ships at Brest to invade England—inclined Parliament to view the Governors' application favourably, or, at least, that is what Jonas Hanway believed.[8] The notion that England was suffering a dangerous decline in population was widespread. Indeed, some put the loss since 1714 at more than a million people, blaming it on the excessive consumption of gin by the poor and the enormous consumption of men by war. For, as Jonas Hanway remarked, 'one war is come very quick on the back of another'.[9] Expansion of the Foundling Hospital, therefore, must have seemed an attractive method for repairing some of the losses in British man power and guaranteeing a supply of future soldiers and sailors for England's wars. Later in 1756 a somewhat similar apprehension about the scarcity of seamen brought into existence the Marine Society, which undertook to equip landsmen and boys for service in the Royal Navy.

We should not, however, discount the humanitarian impulse that motivated many sensitive men and women in the years from 1756 to 1758. This period also saw the founding of the Magdalen House for penitent prostitutes and the Female Orphan Asylum for homeless young girls, institutions created by men who mixed a high degree of altruism with their practical reasons. It was a time, in short, when men thought well of projects whereby, according to Joseph Massie, 'Charity, Humanity, Patriotism, and Oeconomy [might] be made to go Hand-in-Hand'.[10]

With funds thus assured by Parliament, the Governors set about preparations for the influx of children that the Hospital might now expect after 1 June. They directed their architect, Theodore Jacobsen, to prepare a receiving room at the gate, ordered twenty cradles and clothing for five hundred infants, engaged additional employees, asked the country inspectors to provide 140 nurses to come in relays to the Hospital during the first five days of June, and purchased thirty beds to accommodate those who had to spend the night before taking children back to the country for nursing. And they ordered that a notice be placed in three newspapers stating that the unlimited reception of children under two months of age would begin on 2 June. This advertisement was also printed on large sheets and posted up around London 'in all the usual places'. The chapel's Reader, the Hospital's physicians and surgeons, and the High Constable of Holborn, with an adequate number of constables, were all requested to be at the Hospital by 10.0 a.m. on 2 June. A newspaper notice also urged all Governors to attend on that day 'to assist in preserving decency and good order'.[11]

But only twenty-two members of the Committee and a few other Governors were present at the appointed time, although the beginning of the General Reception apparently created a considerable disturbance in the neighbourhood. One newspaper gave this account of the first three days:

On Wednesday last the Foundling Hospital was opened for the

reception of all children under two months old ... when 117 children were taken in. On Thursday the same business was repeated with ... the number not quite equal to the first day, amounting only to 43; one of the children had a bank note of 20 l. pinned to its side. On Friday only 19 were brought.

It is surprising the distraction this admittance occasioned. Some of the women after having delivered their children, returned and begged for them again, which could not be granted, being contrary to the rules of the house. Many men in the absence of their wives carried their children, and upon their being missed by the mothers, disturbances were raised in the streets adjacent to the hospital, which greatly diverted many of the unfeeling spectators. One man, a sober green grocer not far from Temple Bar of 60 years of age, who had a child by his maid a young virgin of 17, sent her out of the way, and trotted with great satisfaction to the hospital, thinking to get rid of all his cares; but the poor girl, coming back and missing the child, followed him, and overtook him in Red-lion-street, when, with much difficulty she got the child from him, and carried it home again, to the great entertainment of all the persons that were looking on, who gave their assistance to alleviate the distress of this poor unhappy young creature.[12]

Although the newspaper reported that 'only 19' were brought on Friday, 4 June, the total number of children received at the end of two weeks stood at 299; by 28 June, 126 more were added. In fact, the flood of infants poured in faster than the Committee could find wet nurses for them. On 7 July a letter went out to every Governor asking for assistance in locating suitable country women willing to undertake this task. Even the Bishop of Worcester was asked to help and responded by making inquiries in his diocese.[13]

Record keeping became a constant battle against confusion, and sometimes, despite the unending labours of the clerks, confusion prevailed. Nevertheless, the Governors sought in every possible way to maintain accurate information as to the whereabouts of the children at all times and to preserve all evidences of their identities. An elaborate system of books recorded baptisms and burials; when, where, with what nurse, and under whose inspection a child was placed; and when it was returned to the Hospital. Printed forms provided for a detailed description of each child's clothing and any distinguishing marks—a procedure that had, of course, been observed since 1741.

In the early days of the Hospital these descriptions frequently stated that a child was 'well dressed', 'exceedingly neat', 'very finely

No. 61.   Hatton-Garden, ~~April~~ May 8th . 1741 at 9 —— o'Clock

Letter G. a Female Child about a month old

Marks and Cloathing of the Child

Cap Holland wth scolloped edging wth a red ribbon
Biggin ~~plain~~ bordered wth plain cambrick
~~Forehead-Cloth~~
Head-Cloth a raged
Long-Stay common
~~Bibb~~ diaper
~~Frock~~
~~Upper-Coat~~
~~Petticoat~~
~~Bodice-Coat~~
~~Barrow~~
Mantle printed flowered flannell red a green
Sleeves corded dimitty
Blanket common
~~Neckcloth~~
Roller common
~~Bed~~
Waistcoat diaper
Shirt Holland wth cambrick ruffles
Clout raged
Pilch raged wollen
~~Stockings~~
~~Shoes~~

Marks on the Body.

a paper pind on the Head

6. Billet describing a Child's Clothing and Identifying Marks, 1741

dressed', or mentioned 'a fine cambrick cap with a laced border', a 'cambrick ruffled shirt', or 'a pair of white brocaded silk shoes tied with a white ribband'.[14] But after 1756 more often than not the descriptions mention ragged and dirty clothing. Some children arrived almost naked, a state of affairs that prompted the Governors to publish a notice in the daily newspapers that 'any Person who shall be detected in stripping any such Child or Children of their Clothing, or any Part thereof, shall be prosecuted with the utmost Severity, at the Expence of this Corporation'.[15]

In all periods, the tokens left with the children, whereby they might be identified should their parents ever desire to reclaim them, varied widely. Some were ingenious constructions of paper, embroidery, and ribbon; some were tags, usually metal, engraved with the child's name and date of birth. Other tokens were more commonplace: coins of all kinds, some pierced with holes or nicked in a pattern; pieces of metal similarly punched or nicked; buttons; pieces of ribbon; plain gold or base metal rings; odd earrings and studs. There was even a bottle tag marked 'Ale'. But there were also finer items: a large mother-of-pearl heart initialed E. L., a small gold locket, elaborate brooches, a carved ivory fish.*

Equally diversified were the written tokens. There were short notes—one on the back of a playing card—often including the words 'Cruel separation'. There was an officially sealed 'Extrait du Registre des Baptêmes de la Chapelle de Son Altesse Serenissime et Electorale de Baviere à Londres', certifying in Latin to the baptism of Maria Francisca Antonetta Maximiliana on 8 September 1756. There were letters, some addressed to the child, some to the Governors, all expressing grief at parting with the infant, pleading for its care, and promising to reclaim it whenever the parents could provide for it. Some parents, hoping to ensure that their child would be well cared for, offered a covert bribe: 'She is of ingenious Parents and if she comes to age, may perhaps have a plentiful Fortune when this Charitable Corporation will be gratefully rewarded', or claimed that the father was a benefactor to the Hospital. And there were short poems, usually displaying little gift for versification but sometimes expressing bitter comment on human frailty and injustice. One, for example, received on 19 May 1759, reflected on the situation of the betrayed woman:

> Hard is my Lot in deep Distress
> To have no help where Most should find

---

* Many of these tokens are on exhibition in the Court Room at the Coram Foundation's headquarters.

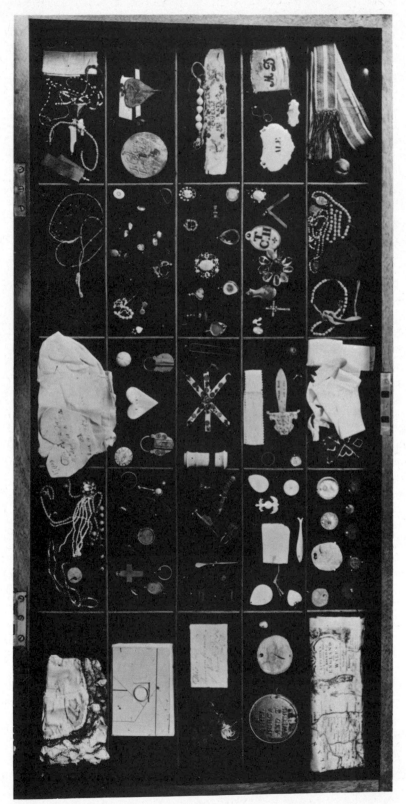

7. Tokens Received with the Children

Sure Nature meant her sacred Laws
Should men as strong as Women bind
  Regardless he, Unable I,
To keep this Image of my Heart
  'Tis Vile to Murder! hard to Starve
And Death almost to me to part
If Fortune should her favours give
That I in Better plight may Live
I'd try to have my Boy again
And Train him up the best of Men.

Another commented sadly on the human predicament, borrowing—without attribution—from Matthew Prior, who had borrowed the last line from Silenus:

But Oh! beyond Description happiest He
Who Ne'er Trust roll On Lifes tumultuous Sea;
Who with Blest Freedom from the general Doom
Exempt must never force the teeming Womb
Nor see the Sun nor Sink into the Tomb
Who Breaths must suffer. And who thinks must Mourn
And He Alone is Blest Who ne'er was born.[16]

The evidence of the tokens and the descriptions of the children's clothing, taken with a record setting forth the parishes from which the children came during the first year of the General Reception, suggest that most of them were children of the poor. Of the 1863 attributed to parishes within the Bills of Mortality, nearly 1100 came from those with a high percentage of poor residents. The poorest parishes contributed the largest numbers of children: 150 from St Giles-in-the-Fields, 100 from St James Clerkenwell, 88 from St Mary Whitechapel, 88 from St Martin-in-the-Fields, 64 from St Leonard Shoreditch. On the other hand, the forty-two parishes within the walls, an area largely occupied by respectable craftsmen and small merchants, added only 158 to the total.

The records also show that in this period the Hospital's population gained 176 from St George Hanover Square and 43 from St James Westminster. These, of course, were well-to-do parishes where large households employed many servants. Since a mistress would seldom permit a female servant to keep her illegitimate child with her, if, indeed, she did not discharge the unfortunate girl as soon as she learned of the pregnancy, it is easy to see why so many children came from these two parishes: desperate servant girls were getting rid of their bastard children in order to keep their jobs.[17] As we shall see, further evidence to support this conclusion appears in the records for the period after 1760.

The evidence of the notes and poems is more ambiguous. Taken at face value, they suggest that the women who wrote them were better educated and of higher social status than the servant girls from St George Hanover Square or the poor wretches from St Giles-in-the-Fields. But this may be a too hasty conclusion. For many of the notes and doggerel verses could have been written for illiterate servant girls by better educated upper servants, or by employers willing to keep on a good servant if only the inconvenient child could be disposed of, or even by employers' sons who had fathered some of these children. Yet there were notes and poems expressing an anguish that would seem impossible for a person other than a child's mother to simulate. These, together with the fine clothing worn by some infants and the more valuable tokens left with them, indicate that in all periods there were children admitted to the Hospital who may have been bastards but were not baseborn.

This conclusion also draws support from the fact that on 30 June 1756 the Governors resolved that 'if, after the 1st of July next, any Child should be brought to this Hospital, altho' exceeding the Age of two Months, and be under the Age of two Years, and a Sum of one hundred Pounds, or upwards, be sent therewith, to satisfy the Charge of the Maintenance and Education thereof, such Child shall be received'.[18] In the eighteenth century £100 was a considerable sum; a parent who could pay such an amount would have to be connected with a prosperous family. The first child for whose care £100 was paid was received on 3 November 1756, and from that time to 1 March 1771, the Hospital admitted seventeen such children*—twelve boys and five girls.[19]

These children, however, represented no more than a pebble in an avalanche, for children were arriving at a rate of over a hundred a week, and the Governors soon found that more employees were needed. On 26 October 1756 they decided to engage a watchman, a receiving matron, an additional porter, a clerk, two wet and two dry-nurses to reside in the Hospital, and a chief nurse and two assistant nurses for the infirmary. At the same time they ordered the purchase of thirty more beds for the country nurses, as well as twenty more cradles and additional clothing for the infants. By this time 847 children had been received.[20] Still the children continued to come,

---

* Only one of these children had died by 1771, and a list of their names bears the interesting comment: 'The mortality of one only out of 17 does not seem to be common'.

and again and again the staff had to be increased. By 1760 the Hospital and its auxiliary infirmaries were employing fourteen men and sixty-seven women. Finding wet-nurses to live in the Hospital was a constant problem, which the Governors tried to solve by asking the country inspectors to locate women for the task and, in 1759, by directing the secretary to write to all of London's lying-in hospitals in the hope of recommendations from that source.

The rapid expansion of the staff brought still other problems: the steward and matron hired subordinates without the Governors' knowledge; the matron discharged employees without the Committee's order; servants' wages were increased without official authorization; and no one made any entries in the Servants' Book from 1 July 1756 to 5 December 1757. This confusion in authority resulted in the employment of many unsuitable persons, some of whom attempted to turn the situation to their own profit. One watchman told a woman who brought a child to the Hospital's gates that she must give him a gratuity to be admitted. The porter, no more scrupulous, took a bribe of two guineas to smuggle in a child over two months of age. Other servants, working in the reception area, were more curious than venal and questioned women about the children they brought, although it was a strict rule that they might ask no questions except what parish a child came from and whether or not it had been baptized. When discovered, such employees were immediately discharged.[21]

More critical was the problem of finding enough healthy country nurses to care for so many infants, most of whom required breast-feeding and many of whom arrived in a half-starved condition. The shortage of nurses became still more acute in winter because the Governors considered it unsafe in cold weather to send the children, especially those only a few days old, on the long, slow journeys to the more remote parts of the country. The practice of sending the children all over England to be nursed did not, of course, begin in 1756. In 1752, for example, the Hospital's records show forty-one children placed in Derbyshire, fifty-eight in Yorkshire, six in Staffordshire and ten in Lincolnshire. But most were nursed much nearer to London, many of them in Chalfont, Epsom, Romford, and Staines.[23] During the first year of the General Reception, the Governors sent the 3300 children received out to be nursed in larger numbers but in a similar pattern.

Nearly all of the infants kept in the infirmary or in the Hospital in London died before the end of the year. These were the children received in so sickly a state that no attempt could be made to send them to the country. Of those nursed outside London during the year, 1141 out of 2930 died, representing a mortality rate of 39 percent, far below that of parish workhouses.[24] Country nursing, therefore, appeared to be a twofold blessing: it increased the children's chances for survival, and it relieved the pressure on the available space in the Hospital. In fact, country nursing combined with the establishment of branch hospitals beginning in 1757, about which more will be said later, provided the only way, short of an extensive building programme in London, that the Hospital could have cared for so many children.

In January 1757 the Governors, well satisfied that their work was successfully filling a major social need, decided to raise the age limit from two to six months. In June they raised the limit to one year.[25] These expansions of eligibility brought in still more children, and the need for country nurses and trustworthy inspectors grew proportionally. Governors themselves sometimes undertook the supervision of a few nurses in areas near their country homes, but, for the most part, the Committee depended on clergymen, minor gentry and substantial tradesmen. Although a few members of the aristocracy—Lady Vere, for example—acted as supervisors, instances of partician willingness to devote time and energy as well as money to the care of foundlings were rare.

What the Committee was looking for were 'ladies and gentlemen of easy fortunes & humane dispositions, conveniently situated in the country', but what they had to settle for sometimes proved to be men of small fortunes and greedy dispositions, an inevitable consequence of the inability of the Committee to know every inspector personally. Most were recommended by the less active Governors, or by friends, or by other inspectors. Some simply volunteered for the job. But no one had time to investigate thoroughly the character of every person nominated to be an inspector.

The Committee tried to induce the inactive Governors to serve as inspectors. In April 1757 a letter went out to all of them asking their help, but the response was not encouraging, and a year later the Committee was considering whether payment of an annual salary to clergymen and other reputable persons might help to secure satisfactory supervisors. They also discussed the alternative possibility of hiring full-time inspectors who would use the Hospital as their base.[27] The idea of paid inspectors under the Committee's direct control must have seemed attractive, for the Governors were learning—and painfully—that not only was it difficult to find inspectors but that 'very good Inspectors are very valuable',[28] because there were so many bad ones. Problems with inspectors fell into three categories: inattentiveness to the duties involved, exploitation of the nurses, and financial mismanagement.

Neglect of duty not only defeated the Hospital's efforts to maintain accurate records of the deaths of children in the country, but it also opened the way for fraud should payments be continued to its nurse after a child had died. Laxity also enabled nurses to obtain more than one child at a time and sometimes allowed a woman who had been refused certification of her suitability by one inspector to obtain such a certificate from another. In 1758, for example, a nurse named Martha Bury was refused a certificate by inspectors at Kingston and Richmond because she had treated badly two infants that she had formerly nursed for the Hospital—one of them, it was said, she had starved. These refusals did not discourage Martha Bury. She went to Mrs Lovibond, the inspectress at Hampton, who gave her a certificate that permitted her on 1 August to receive a child from the Hospital. Then she secured another certificate from the obliging, or forgetful, inspectress and used it on 15 August to obtain a second child. Probably no one had time to check the records on her second visit to the Hospital, and the staff simply accepted the certificate at face value. The Governors themselves did not learn of the duplication until 26 August, whereupon they immediately ordered the secretary to write to Mrs Lovibond directing her to 'enquire into the true character of Martha Bury and see that she do her duty by the Children'.[29]

Far worse than such carelessness were the instances of too great care for self-enrichment. This occurred most often where the inspector was also a shopkeeper. A man in such a position could use his dual capacity of paymaster to the nurses and seller of supplies to compel the women to buy whatever they needed from him even when they could purchase the same items elsewhere at cheaper prices. An anonymous letter, received in February 1759, described the practice:

> Many of your Country Trustees are persons in Trade & it is but too Notorious that some of them use great Oppression towards the Nurses of these deserted Innocents, refusing to pay them their due in Money—denying them Nessessarys that is wanted & that for months together—obliging them to take it out in Shop Goods, bad in quality, & at an Exorbitant price, sending up Wet Nurses to fetch the Children & then turning them over to Dry ones—& if any of the Nurses complain in the least of any of the above Hardships the Children are removed to others some of which have 3 or 4 & others that perhaps are better Housewifes cannot get one.[30]

The Governors might, perhaps, disregard an anonymous letter, but they did not ignore instances of abuse when confronted. with evidence. They promptly replaced exploiters whenever investigations established proof of their misdeeds. In 1756 they had resolved that 'no person that keeps a Chandler's shop or is of other mean occupation, shall be an Inspector', and they themselves never appointed such men. But, unknown to the Governors, otherwise exemplary inspectors sometimes did appoint a petty shopkeeper as deputy. In 1758, therefore, the Committee, in a further effort to protect the nurses, directed the receiving clerk to instruct every woman taking a child from the Hospital that she was not obliged to accept her pay otherwise than in money.[31]

Unscrupulous inspectors also exploited the nurses in another way: they deducted a fee from the women's wages before paying them. In 1758 Mr Naish of Swallowfield, for example, was taking $1\frac{1}{2}$d out of every 2s 6d payment. Other inspectors simply did not pay the nurses at all. Complaints about these practices often led to a visit by the clerk or steward to the nurses and inspector involved and frequently resulted in the removal of the nurses from the delinquent inspector's supervision.[32]

A failure to pay nurses their wages sometimes gave the Governors their first warning that an inspector had misappropriated the moneys advanced to him by the Hospital or had become bankrupt. A particularly flagrant case was that of Mr Bertie Burgh of Chertsey, who manged to obtain the supervision of 407 children and then persistently ignored requests from the secretary to render an account of the children as well as an account of the money he had drawn to pay the nurses. The matter dragged along through 1759 with Mr Burgh refusing to co-operate. The Governors then divided the children among other inspectors in the neighbourhood but still could obtain no financial accounting from Mr Burgh. Finally, in November 1760, they referred the affair to the Hospital's solicitor, Mr Plumptre. He, too, found the former inspector elusive. Although he secured numerous writs of execution against the person of Mr Burgh, the sheriff was never able to find him. Their patience exhausted, in 1763 the Governors ordered Mr Plumptre to proceed to outlaw Mr Burgh on the judgment that had been obtained against him. Only then did Mr Burgh pay his debt to the Hospital, which, with the costs of the lawsuit, amounted to £210.[33]

Not all defalcations were on this scale, but the problem of financial mismanagement by inspectors remained troublesome throughout the century. A report in 1770 described eleven accounts of inspectors as 'desperate' and two as 'dubious'—scarcely an exaggeration, for some of them had been outstanding for ten or fifteen years. One even dated back to 1749.[34] Despite efforts from time to time to collect these and similar debts, there were in 1782 still seventeen persons, four of them clergymen, who owed the Hospital a total of £690 6s 8d. On 8 May 1782 the General Court at last declared this sum 'absolutely lost' and directed the secretary to charge it off against the Hospital's capital.[35]

Although the derelictions of the bad inspectors certainly affected some children and nurses adversely and caused the Committee great concern, such men were, in fact, a minority. Most of the inspectors, who by 1759 were supervising the nursing of 5800 children,[36] performed their tasks with great unselfishness and with meticulous care of the Hospital's funds. They had no easy time of it. Their day-to-day duties included keeping correct records, supplying the nurses with clothing for the children and making sure that they brought back outgrown clothes for return to the Hospital, visiting the women often enough to be certain that they were taking proper care of the children, and paying the nurses their monthly wages as well as the 10s awarded to each nurse whose child survived for one year after she received it. And for all of this time-consuming work, the inspectors received no payment. Not surprisingly, they sometimes encountered extreme difficulty in securing proper substitutes. Mrs Burgess, an inspectress at Wrotham, who spent her winters in Southwark, wrote in January 1758 that 'she has in vain endeavoured to get several Gentlemen in the Neighborhood to assist her and also desired the Nurses to apply to them likewise, but all refused saying they would not be troubled about Bastards'.[37]

Moreover, the inspectors had constantly to guard against the failings of the nurses. The poverty of some tempted them to try to obtain more than one child at a time or to send the children, when old enough, out to beg.[38] The ignorance or carelessness of others could threaten the very lives of their nurslings. Nurse Elizabeth Booker of Plaxtol, for instance, left her two foundling children for five or six days with no one to care for them except her own young children, while she went to London. There she contracted smallpox and upon her return infected the foundlings. Luckily, both infants recovered from the disease, which the inspector pointed out 'would have been prevented if she had staid at home and took care of them'.[39] Still other nurses drank, overlaid their infants, and starved them, or, at least, they were accused of doing so, which made investigations by the inspectors necessary.[40]

The Governors, too, found the nurses a cause for concern. In the first place, they wanted only women free from 'all infectious distempers'. To make sure of this, the physicians or surgeons attending the Hospital examined them upon their arrival from the country. A female servant and the apothecary also examined them to see that they 'have good milk, that they had no breaking out, bad breath or teeth, and that they are not pregnant, and the like'.[41]

The Hospital's staff then had to make appropriate arrangements for the nurses' return journey, see to it that the women received first-year clothing for the children, as well as the few simple medicines that the Hospital supplied, and teach them how to prepare the infants' pap.[42] The Governors had also to combat public curiosity about the nurses, which proved to be a continuing problem. As early as 1747 the Committee had found it necessary to order 'That the Country Nurses do not discover their own Names or Places of Abode, or the Name or Place of Abode of any other Nurse, or the Mark of the Hospital on any of the Children, to any Person or Persons whatsoever; And if any Nurse shall presume to offend herein, such Nurse shall have her Child taken from her'. Copies of this resolution were sent to every country nurse and were posted conspicuously about the Hospital.[43] The wisdom of trying to maintain secrecy became apparent during the period of the General Reception when, on at least four occasions, someone stole a child from its nurse. Usually the abductor was a woman claiming to be the child's mother, but in one instance the kidnapper was a man.[44]

Another problem that beset the Governors was the infections that the nurses contracted from the infants. Some got the itch; the Governors compensated them with a payment of 5s. The reverse situation also occurred, and it became necessary to order that 'no Nurse bringing a Child to this Hospital which appears to have the Itch or other Infectious Distemper shall be permitted to have a Child from this Hospital'.[45]

Much worse were the occasions when infant victims of congenital syphilis infected their nurses. Dealing with such cases required great delicacy. If, indeed, the infection came from the child, the nurse deserved the sympathy and help of the Governors, and she received it. But if her husband or a lover had infected her, the Hospital owed her nothing, and the Governors had been told by no less authority than the respected Dr Cadogan that 'in the carefull examination of many persons who thought themselves infected by Children with venereal complaints, he has not found one who has been truly so'.[46]

The inspector's opinion of the woman's character and the circumstances of the case usually determined the Committee's response. But in 1758, when a nurse claimed that her foundling child had given her gonorrhea, which she, in turn, had passed on to her husband, medical opinion influenced the Governors' decision not to accept direct responsibility for her treatment despite the inspector's assurances as to the good character of both husband and wife. Mr Tomkyns, one of the Hospital's surgeons, examined both of them and pronounced that 'tho' the Pox may be contracted by suckling an Infant Child, yet a recent Clap in his opinion could not'—a view that present-day medical knowledge substantiates.* Nevertheless, since the inspector reported

> ... that the above Child had given the Woman the Itch, & upon examination finding both her and the Child not cured, the Committee ordered the Child, who is weaned, to the Infirmary, and considering not only what may be alleged for the contracting of the Venereal Disease from an infected Child, and also the Womans having the Itch, and the necessity not to alarm Wet Nurses, the Committee have desired Mr. Prior [the inspector] to manage as he thought most prudent with regard to the Cure both of the man and the woman.[47]

The consideration here, as on so many occasions, was the effect on public opinion.

On the other hand, when the Governors believed that a foundling had infected a nurse with syphilis, they arranged for her treatment and that of the child, usually at the Lock Hospital in London, although occasionally treatment was given in the Foundling Hospital's own infirmary. They also made every effort to protect the nurses from this hazard. Until the rapid influx of children from 1756 onward increased the possibility of too hasty examinations as the children arrived, only one syphilitic infant out of the 2368 children admitted in the Hospital's first fifteen years had escaped the staff's vigilance and infected its nurse.[48] Also, in this earlier period Hospital policy prescribed the rejection of any child who appeared to be infected.

But from 1756 onward the Governors no longer possessed the right to make such a choice. They could, however, place infected children with dry-nurses, thereby lessening the chance of transmitting the

---

* I am indebted to Mr Dan C. VanderMeer, Public Health Advisor, Venereal Disease Control Division, U. S. Public Health Service Center for Disease Control, Atlanta, Georgia, for verification of the fact that it would be impossible to transmit gonorrhea orally, but that congenital syphilis could be transmitted from a very young child to its nurse where the child had syphilitic lesions in the mucous membranes of its mouth. These would be teeming with spirochetes, which could readily pass through breast membranes, especially if the nurse had a crack or sore in the nipples, into the blood stream.

disease, and this they did, 'rather chusing to risque the life of the child than of the nurse'. They also established a firm rule that any child who, when received, showed any kind of eruption on any part of its body must be kept in the Hospital's infirmaries until 'the nature of such eruption can be more clearly ascertained', or until 'such eruptive distempers shall have been cured'.[49] In addition, the Committee ordered the secretary to write to all the lying-in hospitals in London, requesting that whenever these hospitals sent to the Foundling Hospital a child born of diseased parents, a note be sent along stating that fact, or if such a child was turned over to parish officials, that a similar note accompany it.[50]

The French encountered the same problem and dealt with it in much the same way. In 1736, 1750 and 1769 the Hospital of the Holy Spirit at Dijon incurred an expense of three thousand *livres* in providing treatment for nurses infected with syphilis by their foundling charges.[51] The Paris hospital also had to bear the expense of institutionalizing many of its wet-nurses who were similarly infected. And in Montpellier the promise of treatment for nurses so afflicted was actually written into the hospital's statutes.[52]

The Governors' constant care to protect the country nurses against the dangers of disease and exploitation indicates their awareness of how much they owed to these women, for greedy, stupid, or vicious nurses were, in fact, the exception rather than the rule. When we remember that thousands of women, scattered all over England, were acting as nurses during the period of the General Reception, the wonder is that no more than a hundred or so ever appear in the records as presenters of problems. Most of the women, who were usually twenty-five to thirty-five years of age, seem to have cared for the children reasonably well, at least by the standards of their communities. A few of them even taught their foundling children the alphabet, although most of the nurses were illiterate.[53] Many became extremely fond of the children and parted with them reluctantly. Some, as we shall see later, refused to give them up at all.

The children, for their part, frequently regarded these women as their mothers and, on returning to the Hospital, were homesick for the villages where they had spent their first three to five years, for they found the regimentation and confinement of the Hospital a sharp contrast to life in a country village. These tiny communities seldom contained over three hundred inhabitants whose cottages clustered together along one road with wide tracts of land stretching away on all sides. Except for the fields planted to corn (wheat), the land lay unfenced and unreclaimed—a natural playground for the village children when they were not occupied with the duties that fell traditionally to the young sons and daughters of labourers and small farmers: scaring off pigeons and crows from newly seeded fields, tending the chickens, combing wool, and collecting rushes and dipping them in tallow.

The village, in fact, offered a wider world for a child to explore than the Hospital, and the rhythm of the agricultural year offered a greater diversity of experience. Although the villagers lived an isolated life with few facilities for travel and no reason to do so, the day's work varied according to the season, and the march of the year brought parish feasts at sheep-shearing, harvest home, and Christmas, the traditional frolics of the children on May Day and Shrove Tuesday, and the annual festival held on the saint's day of the local church when gingerbread stalls, swings and roundabouts* suddenly appeared.

Moreover, the cottage that the foundling had called home was nothing like the Hospital. Most cottages in the early part of the century had clay walls, thatched roofs, low ceilings, small windows and few of them, and floors of hardened earth or of a cement-like mixture of lime, ashes, and horse dung. Usually there was only one room, although a few cottages had two. A single wide fireplace, in which the cottagers burned furze, bracken, or peat, provided the only source of heat. Light came from rushlights, water from the communal well. Sanitation was primitive or non-existent: most cottages did not possess a privy, and the villagers dumped their household waste into the street or a nearby brook. Furniture was scanty: a bedstead, table, a few stools, a clothes chest, a cradle, some sleazy bedding, and a few cooking and eating utensils.[54] Despite its austerity, the Hospital's physical facilities were luxurious by comparison. Yet they were strange and unsettling to the returning foundling who had progressed from infancy to early childhood in this simpler world, a world, nevertheless, that helped to shape his personality and the course of his future life.

* Roundabouts were merry-go-rounds, propelled by man power.

8

The General Reception:
External Problems, 1756–1760

As IF THE PROBLEMS of managing the internal affairs of the Foundling
Hospital did not cause worry enough to the Governors, they had also
to deal as best they could with problems created by persons over
whom they exercised little, if any, control. Most of the problems
stemmed from a common source: greed. In its most barefaced and
brutal form it appeared as an attempt to use the General Reception to
enrich either a parochial or a private purse.

The Poor Laws set the stage for this abuse. Since Elizabethan
times a parish had been obliged to provide for any bastard child born
within its boundaries, if the child's parents could not do so, because a
bastard did not take either his father's or his mother's settlement as
legitimate children did.[1] The Law of Settlement and Removal,
enacted by the first Restoration Parliament in 1662, did not improve
the situation, for it now followed that a male bastard's legitimate
descendants who did not acquire their own settlement in one of the
prescribed ways might also be charges someday on the poor rate of
the parish where their progenitor had been born.[2] Little wonder,
then, that parish officers hustled reluctant bridegrooms, sometimes
in chains, to the church and forced them to marry obviously pregnant
brides, especially when the bridegrooms belonged to another parish.

If parish officials could not compel a marriage, their next best
course was to force the putative father to pay for the child's support
by threatening him with jail. Since 1576 Justices of the Peace had
possessed the power to commit the parents of a bastard to prison for
nonsupport of their child,[3] but, as a practical matter, they rarely
exercised this power against the mother if she was nursing the child
and not employed. The threat of imprisonment, however, hung over
the man's head for seven years after the child's birth. If he fell into
arrears with the maintenance payments that the Justices directed him
to make, he could be locked up in jail for three months at a time. To

96

add to his vulnerability, the law, after 1733, provided that the woman's unsupported oath sufficed to establish paternity.[4] Inevitably, many a man threatened with an affiliation charge simply absconded, leaving to the parish the full burden of supporting the child.

These laws tempted unscrupulous overseers to blackmail well-to-do married men, and some women were similarly tempted. The mother of a bastard had, in fact, every inducement to perjure herself by swearing that the child's father was the wealthiest man against whom she thought she could make such a charge stick, for the wealthier the man, the larger the allowance the Justices would make. By bearing in fairly close succession three or four illegitimate children and swearing their paternity to different men, an unscrupulous woman might obtain maintenance orders against all of them and thereby receive as much as 10s to 15s a week—more than the wages of a rural labourer. She could not lose because the law required the overseers to pay her the amounts specified in the orders, whether or not they succeeded in collecting these sums. As a result, many parishes, unable to recover from the fathers even half of the ordered payments, sustained a vast expense.[5]

To parish officials eager to hold down the poor rates, and to harassed fathers of bastards, the opening of the Foundling Hospital's doors to all infants seemed like an answer to prayer: one could deposit the inconvenient child at the Hospital and be done with expense forever. The difficulty was that often the mothers did not agree. To obtain such children, therefore, parish officers and fathers, sometimes separately, sometimes in collusion, resorted to force and fraud. For the period 1758–60, the Hospital's records mention forty-two such instances that came to the Committee's knowledge. In ten of these cases, the putative father had removed the child without the mother's consent; in twelve, parish officials had taken the child; and in one, the father and the parish constable had collaborated in the deed. For the other nineteen cases, this information is lacking. But the practice was widespread: the reports of such actions came from all over England.

Some brutal parish officials broke down doors to locate children whom their mothers were trying to hide; others assaulted mothers with considerable violence when they struggled to keep their children. In 1759 the female officers of the parish workhouse of St Andrew Holborn so severely attacked a woman who had borne her child there that she spent nearly six months in St George's Hospital recovering from her injuries. The Governors of the Foundling Hospital, shocked at what they described as 'inhuman proceedings', prosecuted these officers at the Hospital's expense and obtained a conviction. The Court's sentence, however, was more lenient than either counsel for the Crown or for the Hospital approved: one month's imprisonment in the Poultry Compter, a fairly comfortable debtors' prison, and a fine of 40s each. The affair cost the Hospital £15 15s for legal charges, but the unhappy mother never saw her child again for it had died in the Foundling Hospital.[6]

More often, parish officials used threats or deception to obtain the children from their mothers or to induce the bereft women not to bring charges against them. Sometimes they claimed to have a 'special warrant' to take the woman to Bridewell or threatened to send her to Bedlam or to cut off her allowance from the parish.[7] Prolific married women who received parish aid were also subjected to such treatment in some parishes. Robert Dingley* reported a case of this kind in 1758:

Messrs. Arrowsmith & Evans, Parish Officers of Lewisham in Kent, did compulsively take away in Aprl. 1758 a Male Child from its Mother Eliz. Forrester in the absence & without the privity or consent of the Father John Forrester a Soldier of the Ist Regmt. of the 3d Battalion in the Guards—and sent sd Child as they the Parents have reason to believe to the Foundling Hospital as sd officers declared they would—. This Famely of Woman & four Children have a small allowance from the Parish & this means was used to ease the Parish & affright the Woman out of it, as they did after—when proved with child again. Mr. Forrester in Cabbage Lane behind Westminster Infirmary—he bares a good Character, helps his famely all he can but having a child every Year & much on duty, cannot maintain them without the Parishes assistence which is very scanty & that given not without reproaches & threats, so that I hope the facts being made fully to appear, sd Officers will feel the resentment of the Govrs. of the Foundling Hospital.[8]

Even after prosecutions against them had begun, parish officials sometimes continued their threatening activities. What happened during the prosecution of five parish officials of Assington, Suffolk, in 1758, for forcibly taking a child from his mother and placing him in the Foundling Hospital illustrates their methods. The Hospital's solicitor reported that not only did the vicar of the parish attempt to influence his judgment, but also

. . . that threats were made use of to Elizabeth Cooke [the mother], declaring she should be committed to Bridewell, and there flead

* Robert Dingley was a Governor and one of the founders in 1758 of the Magdalen House for Repentant Prostitutes.

alive, in order as is supposed to deter her from giving her Evidence to the Grand Jury, and to frighten her the more. This same Mr. Gurden [the vicar] did actually obtain a Warrant against the said Elizabeth Cooke from Sir Cordell Firebrace, who very unwillingly granted it. And that a Cobler at Assington . . . who is one of the Evidences for the Prosecution has been deprived of the little Business he had there on account of his having given his Testimony for Elizabeth Cooke; and this by the influence of the Parish Officers, and Mr. Gurden, the Minister there. And I overheard Mr. Gurden giving his own Account of this matter to several Gentlemen who might be supposed would be afterwards on the Grand Jury, for this was before the Grand Jury were Sworn.[9]

These parish officers eventually capitulated and agreed to return the child to his mother, to allow her 1s a week for the child's maintenance until he reached the age of seven, to drop all prosecutions against the mother, to cease harassment of all witnesses, and to acknowledge their misconduct in a public advertisement to be placed in three London newspapers as well as in the Ipswich *Journal*. Significantly, the advertisement contained the parish officers' agreement to pay personally

. . . all Costs & Charges whatever, expended by the said Corporation in order to bring the said Offenders to due shame and punishment for such inhumane treatment of a fellow Creature; such notorious Violation of the Laws of this Realm in General, and such gross imposition on the said Chairty in particular, and to deter all other Parish Officers from committing the like offence.

It added, at the end, that 'Our Expences in Defending the said Prosecution, and in all other respects, amounts to the sum of £300, and upwards'.[10]

The key to why the Governors undertook eight such prosecutions from 1758 to 1760—six of them against parish officials—appears in the phrase, 'to deter all other Parish Officers from committing the like offence', and on at least one other occasion they insisted that guilty officials place an acknowledgment of their wrongdoing in London newspapers, together with an expression of gratitude to the Governors for 'desisting from the said Prosecution which otherwise must have been our Ruin'.[11] The Governors did not, however, usually prosecute fathers for the same crime. Doubtless they thought that the deterrent effect would not be as great as in the case of parish officials and, hence, not worth the expense. They may also have considered the fact that they could sometimes recover their legal costs from parish officers but could expect scant recompense from the fathers, many of whom seem to have been men of little means. But one father whom they did prosecute was a gentleman. In addition to these prosecutions, the Governors also established a policy of restoring the children, if still alive, to their mothers—a policy that they advertised in the newspapers in 1758, adding that they would also assist in bringing to justice the persons who had wrongfully taken such children.

Many of the children, however, died either on the way to the Hospital or shortly after admission because persons who undertook to transport infants to the Hospital from distant parts of the country took no care of them along the way. The anonymous author of a contemporary pamphlet described the abuses that occurred:

> Has it not in a Great and Honourable House been publickly asserted that one man who had Charge of five Babes in Baskets, happen'd in his Journey to get overmuch Liquor, to lie all night asleep upon a Common, and to find in the morning three of his five Children he had in Charge, actually Dead?
>
> Has it not in the same Great Assembly been moreover publickly aver'd that of 8 Babes brought up out of the Country for the F. H. at one time in a Waggon, 7 Died before it reached London,—the only one that lived owing its life to this circumstance, viz. that it had a Mother so Maternally loath to part with it and commit it alone to the Carrier, that she went up on foot along with the Carrier, purely that every Now and Then she might give it the breast, and watch, and supply its other Needs occasionally &c. keeping pace with the Waggon all the way, for that purpose?
>
> Reports are current of many other precipitate Deaths of Infants, occasion'd by the like Means in their way to that Hospital. No wonder, when they are carried only as Luggage.
>
> With which kind of Luggage in two Panniers, a Man on Horseback going to London was overtaken at Highgate; and being ask'd there what he had in his Panniers, answer'd, 'I have two Children in Each; I brought them from Yorkshire for the F. H. and used to have Eight Guineas a Trip: but lately another Man has set up against me, Which has lower'd my price'.[13]

One might dismiss this account as prejudiced evidence: the tract censured the Hospital harshly on several counts, and the Hospital's treasurer, in an equally polemical bit of writing, denied that such things happened except in very few instances.[14] But the Hospital's records tend to bear out the truth of the charge and to indicate that the practice was sufficiently widespread to cause the Governors alarm. On 19 May 1759 the Subcommittee noted that

. . . the Governors are also Informed that Parish officers and other persons have under colour of sending Children to this Hospital, delivered such Children to vagrants, disorderly persons and others who for a small sum of money have undertaken to carry such Children to this Hospital tho' they were in no condition to take care of them nor to convey them safely to this Hospital whereby such Children are said to have perished for want or to have been otherwise destroyed.

Whereupon the Governors concluded that they should give notice by advertisement in the public press that 'they will, at the expence of this Corporation prosecute with the utmost Severity every such Offender who shall be principal or Accessory to any such Murther'.[15] A murder of this kind had, in fact, come to the Governors' attention as early as 1757: the father of a bastard child took it away from the woman who was caring for it and delivered it to a travelling tinker, to whom he gave a guinea to carry the child from Monmouth to the Foundling Hospital. Later the child was found drowned with a stone tied to its neck.[16] Because of such incidents, the Governors had begun in 1758 to issue receipts to every person bringing a child because 'some Persons who send Children to this Hospital may doubt whether such Children are safely delivered'.[17]

Up to 1779 a like situation existed in France where a network of midwives, intermediaries, and carters arranged for the transportation of unwanted children from the provinces to the Paris hospital. The infants were stuffed into pannier baskets tied on a donkey's back, four or five to a basket. On the journey they were given only wine for nourishment to make them sleep, and those who died, as most of them did, were tossed out along the road. Of those who survived the trip, 90 percent died within three days of their arrival at the hospital.[18]

Similarly, children brought to the Foundling Hospital by such means arrived, if at all, in a debilitated condition. Others, although coming no farther than from a London parish, had been grossly neglected and, as the treasurer wrote in 1759, 'The Children sent into the Hospital are many of them starved, and labouring under the worst of distempers, and many of them actually dying at the time of Reception'.[19] He did not exaggerate: between 9 May and 21 July 1759, for example, the Hospital received eighteen infants in a dying condition. Some did not live long enough to be carried from the reception room at the gate into the infirmary. They were, as the Subcommittee's minutes put it, 'brought into this Hospital . . . only to be buryed'.[20]

Many of the children were only a day or two old. Yet the limitations of space made it impossible to keep any but the very ill in the Hospital. Almost as soon as they came in, they had to go out again to country nurses, although both the apothecary and the matron of the nurseries agreed that sending such young infants considerable distances constituted 'a dangerous practice'. The matron pointed out to the Committee that it would benefit the children greatly to keep them in the House for a time, 'as many of them come up long Journeys to be received into the Hospital and if they are obliged to go the next day into the Country, or perhaps the same day, it must be a great deal too much for their tender frame to bear'.[21]

The exposure, starvation, disease, and general neglect that many of the children had suffered before admission, as well as the necessity for removing them to the country soon afterward, led to a high mortality rate. We can see what happened by referring to the chart in Appendix III. After its first year, the Hospital had been able to maintain, up to 24 June 1758, an overall mortality rate of approximately 45 to 52 percent in spite of the fact that it had received 7692 children in the period of twenty-seven months between 25 March 1756 and 24 June 1758. Indeed, early in 1758 the Governors had proudly compared the Hospital's mortality rate to the 59 percent recorded for children under two years old dying within the Bills of Mortality from 1728 to 1757.[22] But in the twenty-seven months from 24 June 1758 to 29 September 1760, during which the Hospital admitted 7290 children (that is, 402 less than were received in the preceding twenty-seven-month period), the mortality rate rose to 81 percent.

The records indicate, as one might expect, that the youngest children suffered the highest rate of mortality. For the entire period from 25 March 1741 to 29 September 1760, approximately 75 percent of the deaths occurred before the children reached six months of age, and 86 percent before they were a year old. But, beginning in 1756, infants under six months of age represented approximately 85 percent of the deaths, and children under one year made up 95 percent.[23]

The Governors knew only too well what was happening: from 1758 onward a weekly report of the number of deaths was given at the Committee's meetings. In 1759 the figures grew worse: week after week the secretary recorded sixty to a hundred or more deaths, and the Governors became increasingly alarmed. In April 1758 they had asked the physicians and surgeons of the Hospital to give an opinion as to the cause of so many deaths in one of the infirmaries and to recommend what they might do to prevent such losses; they also requested the Subcommittee 'to examine and report what places are most safe for the Nursing of Children, and to compare the proportion of the Numbers which have died at each place. And also to state the numbers & proportions of the Children, who have been Wet & Dry Nursed, and which have died under the care of Wet & Dry Nurses'.[24] As a result of this investigation, they concluded that the greatest mortality occurred in the areas near London,* and that the Hospital should send as many children as possible to remoter parts of the country. In November the Governors asked for a report showing how many children each nurse had cared for, how many of her charges had died, and how soon death occurred after she received them.[25]

In 1759 the Governors requested the eminent Dr Cadogan to examine all of the Hospital's nurseries and infirmaries and make recommendations. He found the wards dirty, poorly aired, full of 'ill smells', and some of them overcrowded. The Governors then laid down a set of rules to remedy these evils, and they also instructed the receiving matron to keep an exact account of all children who appeared to be in a dying condition when received.

For the most part, the Governors tended to blame the mounting mortality rate on the abuses attending the transportation of increasing numbers of children from the country to the Hospital. According to Jonas Hanway, of the first four hundred children taken in after 2 June 1756, 350 belonged to London parishes. But by 1759 the proportion had changed: from twelve in a hundred coming from the country, the percentage had risen to nearly forty-eight. Probably this change did not occur earlier because it would require some time for news of the General Reception to penetrate to the remoter areas. The Governors, hoping to reverse the trend, debated several times whether lowering the age limit to two months might prevent the transportation of children from distant parishes but never reached a decision.[26]

Undoubtedly, in 1758–60, more children than ever arrived in an extremely weak or dying state. Prior to 1756 virtually all of the children were nursed in the country, and in the 1756–58 period 89 percent were sent to country nurses. But from 1758 to 1760, only 74 percent were nursed outside the Hospital. Since the Governors were still convinced that wet-nursing in the country offered the best possible way to give a child a good start, the retention in the Hospital and its infirmaries of a quarter of the children admitted clearly

---

* The areas showing the highest mortality rates were Bow, Chertsey, Croydon, Dagenham, Epsom, Kensington, Hampstead, Knightsbridge, Lowlayton, Putney, South and West Wickham.

indicates that one in four infants was, when received, too ill to travel. This is confirmed by the data in Appendix III, which shows that 1911 children were kept in the Hospital during these years, of whom 1797 died—a mortality rate of 94 percent.

The influx of children from the country may not, however, account for all of the sick and dying children received in this period. The wretched state of women left destitute when press gangs snatched away more and more husbands for service in the Royal Navy during the Seven Years' War might explain many cases of starved babies. And the increasing numbers of prostitutes at this time* would, perhaps, account for the children found to be infected with venereal disease as well as the many who showed evidence of gross neglect and abuse.

We must also consider the cumulative effect of taking in so many children in so short a time: country nurses had to be found for them in ever greater numbers and very quickly. The dependable nurses, who had kept the mortality rate at its customary level during the first two years of the General Reception, were still caring for the children received between 1756 and 1758 and would not have been available to nurse those admitted during the last two years. Consequently, in order to find two or three thousand additional nurses for these children, the Governors, pressed for space and time, may have been forced to accept less desirable candidates than previously—women too ignorant, too careless, or too slovenly to give the children proper care. And amid the pressures and confusion, possibly the Hospital's staff sent off to country nurses infants in so precarious a state of health that they should have remained in the infirmary. Add to this the difficulty of obtaining a sufficient number of inspectors, which resulted in some inspectorates far too large for adequate supervision by a single individual, and we can see why the mortality rate for children nursed in the country from 1758 to 1760 was more than double that of the preceding two years. The Committee's minutes of 26 July 1758, in fact, tend to support these conjectures, for the Governors on that day referred to the Subcommittee the consideration of ways and means of obtaining more good inspectors and also 'more room in the Hospital, in order to give due time to examine the state of Children before they are sent into the Country'.[27]

* Saunders Welch, a Justice for Middlesex, estimated in 1758 that at least three thousand prostitutes were plying their trade within the Bills of Mortality. It is also significant that the Magdalen House for penitent prostitutes opened its doors on 10 August 1758—a public recognition of a growing social evil.

Whatever the reasons—and almost certainly no single reason can account for the sudden rise in the mortality rate that began in 1758—the Governors were deeply disturbed by the situation. Publicly, however, they did not admit how high the death toll had risen. They had good reason not to divulge the Hospital's difficulties, for it was becoming increasingly an object of considerable public criticism. Widespread knowledge of its high mortality rates could only provide its critics with additional ammunition.

Even during the years of its popularity the Hospital had always had a few critics. In 1749 someone disapproved of the institution's policy of administering baptism to all infants received on the ground that some of them might be children of 'Mahometans, Jews, or professed Infidels' and would therefore have no right to Christian baptism.[28] And in 1750 the author of *The Scandalizade*, a satirical bit of doggerel that directed its barbs against almost everyone who was anyone in London, included the Foundling Hospital, as well as Captain Coram, among its victims:

> The Hospital Foundling came out of thy Brains
> To encourage the Progress of vulgar Amours,
> The breeding of Rogues and th'increasing of Whores,
> While the Children of honest good Husbands and Wives
> Stand expos'd to Oppression and Want all their lives.[29]

In 1757 opposition of a different order appeared. Some of the country areas where the Hospital was sending its children to be nursed objected. On 15 January 1757, Rev. Thomas Trant wrote from Hemsworth in Yorkshire:

> . . . the Numbers [of children] sent down this sumer have alarmed the Country—and the farmers (several instigated by the Clergy themselves, not to say Gentlemen too) have in several Places entered into Combinations to give their milk to the Hogs, or throw it away, rather than let our Nurses have it. Nay a Dignitary, of this Neighbourhood, has thought fit to refuse a Child, when dead, Christian Burial in his Church-yard.[30]

The parish officers of Dagenham, equally inhospitable to the foundling children, threatened several nurses that if they did not return the infants to the Hospital, they would never receive any assistance from the parish should they ever need it.[31] One reason for such resentment appears in a petition to the Governors made in 1760 by the substantial residents of the parish of Farnham in Surrey. Pointing out that nearly two hundred foundlings were being nursed in their parish, they asserted:

That the Labour of this Parish is wholly taken up in the Culture and Management of a very large Plantation of Hops, in which the women are particularly useful in almost all Seasons of the Year.

That they are suffer'd to take Nurse Children without any Limitation (some having three, others four) by which they are confin'd entirely at home and contract Habits of Idleness, Drinking and the like; Add to this, that many of their Husbands are led away from their Industry into the same bad Courses, and are tempted to Live on their Wives immoderate Earnings.

That from hence, we are depriv'd of the Labour of our own Poor, who are suffer'd to live in Idleness, whilst we are oblig'd to hire others at a great Expence from distant Places to do their natural Work.

Three churchwardens, four overseers, and thirty other persons signed this document.[32] The underlying motive for such objections to the Hospital's methods was, clearly, economic self-interest, mixed in some instances, no doubt, with suspicion of any change in the settled ways of life.

Another kind of criticism also materialized in 1757 with the publication in the *London Chronicle* on 17 May of a quotation from the review of Jonas Hanway's *A Journal of Eight Days Journey* that had appeared in the May issue of the *Literary Magazine*. The anonymous author of the review had remarked:

I know not upon what Observation Mr. Hanway founds his Confidence in the Governors of the Foundling Hospital, Men of whom I have not any Knowledge, but whom I intreat to consider a little the Minds, as well as Bodies of the Children. I am inclined to believe Irreligion equally pernicious with Gin and Tea, and therefore think it not unseasonable to mention, that when, a few Months ago, I wandered through the Hospital, I found not a Child that seemed to have heard of his Creed, or the Commandments. To breed up Children in this Manner, is to rescue them from an early Grave, that they may find Employment for the Gibbet; from dying in Innocence, that they may perish by their Crimes.[33]

The charge may have contained more than a grain of truth since, as we shall see later, the Hospital's Reader was often lax in catechizing the children. Nevertheless, the indignant members of the Committee immediately ordered the Hospital's solicitor to ascertain the name of the author from the publishers of the *Literary Magazine*, the *London Chronicle*, and the *Daily Gazetteer* (which had printed the same item) and to threaten the publishers with prosecution for libel unless they printed suitable retractions. The publishers of the two newspapers, protesting that the paragraphs were inserted in their papers without their knowledge, promised to publish acknowledgments of their offense, but it required a second warning from the Hospital's solicitor before their retractions appeared in print. Jonas Hanway, however, had not waited for the Governors to act: in a letter published in the *Gazetteer* on 26 May, he not only defended himself but also denied the truth of the allegations made against the Hospital.

The Governors still did not know who had made the original charge, and when J. Richardson, publisher of the *Literary Magazine*, appeared before the Committee on 15 June, he 'denied that it was in his power to discover the Author, and that the Author would avow the truth of the said Libel'. Whereupon the Governors asked their solicitor to consult the Attorney General for advice about the propriety of suing Richardson for criminal libel. The Attorney General must have advised against it—probably to avoid unpleasant publicity for the Hospital—for the Governors took no further action. And apparently they never learned that their unknown critic was Samuel Johnson.[34]

These episodes, however, must have seemed to the Governors no more than tempests in a teapot when a paper war, as Jonas Hanway called it, broke out in 1759. It was touched off, according to Hanway, by rumours in 1758 concerning persons who made a trade of bringing children from the country to the Hospital under barbarous conditions, which 'gave a bias to the minds of many persons, and terminated in the discredit of the hospital'.[35] One of the earliest of the critical pamphlets was the work of Joseph Massie, a writer on trade, finance, and economic problems, and his three major objections set the pattern for the arguments against the Hospital that others would raise repeatedly in the next few years.[36]

In the first place, Massie asserted, the separation of parents and children, which the General Reception of legitimate as well as illegitimate children made possible, would affect adversely the welfare of society. In their old age parents would not be able to turn to their children for support, and the parish would have to supply it. Moreover, having known no parental affection or guidance, the foundlings, when grown, would probably follow their parents' example and dispose of their own children in the same way. These foundlings, as another writer put it, would grow up to form 'a set of people independent, whose breasts have never felt the filial or fraternal affection so useful to soften the heart, and humanise the brutish passions'; to turn them loose into the community, 'so hardened and unconnected', might well give rise to 'numberless mischiefs'.[37] Jonas Hanway, too, worried that children bred up in the Hospital might lack 'filial piety [which] leads to obedience to the laws of God, and supports that chain of subordination by which society is linked together'.[38]

Furthermore, commented Massie, the children's knowledge that the parents who abandoned them might have destroyed them, if the Hospital had not existed to receive them, must necessarily give these children 'such strong Ideas of most unnatural Parental Cruelty, as will not only prove incurable Wounds to the Peace of good Minds, but become a very great Encouragement to Dissoluteness and living in common'—a remark showing a sensitivity to the feelings of foundlings and the possibility of psychological damage to them not to be found elsewhere.[39]

Other writers, more concerned for the country than for the children, pointed out that the ease with which parents could rid themselves of the responsibility for supporting their children threatened the nation's productivity:

> Will Poor People work when they may have their Wants relieved without it? Wil Industry thrive, when the Principal Motives (namely their Children) which lead to it, are taken away? Wil Commerce and Manufactories flourish when, for want of these spurs to Labor, none wil Labor, in the lowest Offices, but on their own Terms? can it be expected that these Paupers wil struggle with constant Difficulties, under the severest Labor, (and which Multitudes do at present struggle with contentedly, even to the end of Life,) when they have such a Commodious Access to Ease and Relief?[40]

Massie argued, in the second place, that the existence of the Hospital encouraged immorality: 'for as People may now enjoy natural Pleasures without bearing those consequential Charges which they ought to pay, and with an Exemption from Punishment and Shame, the Consequence will be, one Sort of Increase'. The Foundling Hospital, although not a justification for having children out of wedlock, would, he believed, be so regarded by the common people.[41]

No argument appeared more often in one form or another. Some writers emphasized the protection that the Hospital's policy of secrecy afforded to sinners. This 'legal licentious Asylum for every Bastard (of every Whore, and of every Whoremonger,) under the Name of a Foundling', said one writer in a savage attack on the Hospital, conceals and protects 'from Public Infamy those who ought rather to be exposed to it . . . as Example *in Terrorem*'. It not only exempts the 'Fornicating Criminals' from all punishment, he added, 'but in its Bounty to their Bastard Infant' compensates them with 'Evil Rewards of Evil'.[42] In a more lighthearted vein, a contemporary broadside rejoiced that no woman need now fear 'to kiss and kiss again', for:

> You may go to Aldersgate-street,
> A kind Reception there you'll meet
>   Most safely to lie-in?
> No one will know my charming Fair,
> But you are gone to take the Air,
>   So return a Maid again.
>
> Because you shan't suspected be
> In staining your Virginity,
>   When that your Month is out,
> You to the Foundling House may go
> And there may leave the Child you know
>   And go take t'other Bout.[43]

Other writers who used the moral argument emphasized not the evils of secrecy but the discouragement to marriage offered by easy disposal of illegitimate children. Fewer marriages, they said, must inevitably lead to a reduction of population.[44]

Massie's third major objection was the excessive cost: 'if the Foundling-Hospital should continue to be countenanced and supported in that public and unlimited Manner which it hath been of late Years, I am humbly of Opinion, that the Charge thereof to the Public would not be so little by the end of this Century as One Million of Pounds Sterling *per Annum*'.[45] Others put the cost higher: one author prophesied that in a few years it would reach £2,000,000 and thereafter continue to mount higher and higher.[46] On the other hand, the argument ran, if the old ways were followed, the nation could trust parish officers to ferret out the fathers of bastard children and to haunt them 'like Banquo's Ghost' in order to collect payments for the support of their children.[47] Moreover, a time of war was not a time to burden the nation with avoidable expense. Nor was it proper at any time to shift the burden of caring for these children to the State and away from the poor rates, as self-interested property owners were evidently seeking to do.[48]

In addition to these major arguments, which nearly every writer put forward, a host of minor objections swarmed over the pamphlet pages: a foundling hospital was a foreign and popish notion not suitable for Englishmen; diseased children would infect healthy nurses; draining children from the countryside would affect agriculture adversely; at some time in the future bad governors might take control of the institution. A few suggested that growing up in the protected environment of the Foundling Hospital gave poor preparation for living in the world outside it—a perceptive comment that I shall explore further in a later chapter. And one writer even professed to see in the Foundling Hospital a 'Sinister Design' of a 'low liv'd Juncto' to increase the number of whores and promote general licentiousness, vice and disorder.[49]

The rise in the Hospital's mortality rate did not escape notice. Several writers commented on it as an indication that the expansion of the Hospital had failed in its purpose, which was to increase the population.[50] The *Gentleman's Magazine* in 1758 called the Hospital's mortality rate 'a matter that merits a parliamentary enquiry'.[51] And common gossip painted the picture even darker than it was: Rev. Dr Timothy Lee wrote from Ackworth in 1760 that people were saying 'that the Foundlings at Nurse in this Country died like Rotten Sheep'.[52]

Only three defenders of the Hospital participated in this pamphlet war. One was Jonas Hanway, who made only a half-hearted defense because he opposed the General Reception and agreed with the Hospital's critics that it had produced many evils. If the poor laws were executed as they should be, he believed, England would not need a foundling hospital. But since administration of those laws was left largely to 'mechanics', he conceded that the Hospital should continue its work on a limited basis, receiving only abandoned children or children of the very poor from the area covered by the Bills of Mortality. The Hospital should receive no children from the country; it should abandon its policy of secrecy; it should change its name to the Orphans Hospital to eliminate the stigmatization of the children as illegitimates; and Parliament should support it by some special tax.

Hanway denied, however, that the Hospital's mortality rates were as bad as charged. To contrast the Hospital's death rate with that of all infants included in the Bills of Mortality produced, he said, an unfair comparison. To compare similar groups, the Hospital's rate should be set over against that of infants in workhouses because one could assume that if the Hospital had not admitted the children brought there, the workhouse would have been their destiny. And workhouses had established a record of infant deaths far worse than that of the Hospital. In one workhouse, for example, out of two thousand children taken in over a twenty-eight-year period, not a child had survived. The Foundling Hospital, on the other hand, was saving some of its infants, and, Hanway calculated, every life saved represented by the age of fifty a net gain to the public of £176 10s.[53] On the whole, his appraisal of the situation appears to be realistic.*

The Hospital's second champion was Dr Robert Bolton, Dean of Carlisle, who wrote a pamphlet listing the criticisms that had come to his attention and refuting them—much to the Governors' satisfaction—point by point.[54] Unfortunately, it was not published soon enough to affect Parliament's decision to end the General Reception. A third defense of the Foundling Hospital, with some reservations about its cost, appeared in 1759 in the *Gentleman's Magazine*.[55]

Although we do not know the identities of most of the Hospital's critics, we can gather some general impressions of their values from this outpouring of pamphlets. First of all, these men were strongly sympathetic to commercial enterprise. They believed in the subordination of the poor in order that a large body of people might always be available to serve the nation's interests—the nation's interests being defined as the economic prosperity of all its people, although in practice the interests served were, for the most part, those of the upper orders of society. The pamphleteers, therefore, measured the value of a life by its potential productivity, not by its intrinsic worth as a human soul. They could and did weigh children's lives in the balance against the costs of preserving them. Such calculations, however, indicate something more than the writers' commercial concerns: they also reflect an increasing tendency to make use of scientific—or what men believed to be scientific—evidence and to advance secular rather than religious arguments to support one's position.

In the second place, these men, despite all their professed concern about sexual morality, in fact applied a double standard: if a man would pay for his carnal pleasures by supporting his bastards or marrying their mother to take her off the hands of the parish, his peccadillos could be passed over with a tolerant smile. Only when his folly imposed expense on the community did it become reprehensible. Immorality, obviously, did not lie in the act itself so much as in the consequent cost to taxpayers.

Not every reader shared the pamphleteers' views, of course, but they were sufficiently commonplace that persons with more tender

---

* Hanway, more than any other pamphleteer, could base his comments on knowledge of the facts: during 1758 and 1759 he attended Committee and Subcommittee meetings constantly and participated actively in making day-to-day decisions affecting the operation of the Hospital.

sensibilities would not have been surprised or greatly shocked by them. And even those who disagreed with the writers' priorities would not have questioned their sincerity. Almost everyone had friends or relatives who held similar opinions, for these men typified a strain in eighteenth-century English society of hardnosed conservatism that distrusted human nature and valued money more than men.

How greatly this spate of criticism affected the thinking of Parliament we do not know. Apparently the first doubts about the Hospital appeared in 1758 when scandals began to be noised about concerning persons who made a business of transporting children to the Hospital. Nevertheless, the Commons granted £40,000 that year to continue the Hospital's work 'notwithstanding many members of the house were not convinced that good would result'.[56] In 1759 Parliament remained divided in its sentiments. Although the absurdity of bringing children long distances from the country to the Hospital only to take them back to the country for nursing was becoming increasingly apparent, still 'everybody meant well', and the 'old path being now so well trodden', Parliament granted £20,000 to the Hospital on 8 February and added £30,000 more on 29 March.[57] But shortly afterward the Members' dissatisfaction with the situation found expression in resolutions adopted on 3 May 1759:

> Resolved . . . that the appointing, by the Governors and Guardians of the Hospital for the Maintenance and Education of exposed and deserted young Children, Places in the several Counties, Ridings, or Divisions, in this Kingdom, for the First Reception of exposed and deserted young Children, would be attended with many evil Consequences.
>
> Resolved . . . that the conveying of Children from the Country to the Hospital for exposed and deserted young Children in London, is attended with many evil Consequences, and ought to be prevented.

As soon as these resolutions were agreed to by the House, it was 'Ordered, That a Bill be brought in pursuant to the last of the said Resolutions'.[58]

Parliament probably did not pass these resolutions solely because of the abuses attending the General Reception, for only a few weeks later a committee appointed to consider the state of the poor and the poor laws offered a series of resolutions that recommended dismantling the existing system of poor relief and placing the poor in need of assistance, including children, in district workhouses under the management of officials appointed specifically for that task and subject to Parliament's control. Before the House could consider these resolutions, Parliament was prorogued,[59] but they indicate the thinking of some Members at that time: they were no longer willing to entrust poor relief either to private charities or to parochial officers.

Other considerations, too, must have affected the Members' attitude toward the Foundling Hospital. Not only had no one anticipated the abuses that the General Reception would occasion, but also no one had expected that so many children would be brought to the Hospital. Said Jonas Hanway: 'It was hardly thought that any more children would be sent to the hospital than such as had been usually exposed in streets and at peoples doors, . . . or died in parish workhouses, where their mothers had deserted them'.[60] Having in mind the Hospital's experience from 1750 through 1755, Parliament and the Governors probably looked for no more than five hundred children a year, whereas children had been arriving since 2 June 1756 at an average rate of approximately three hundred a month, with no indication of a slackening in numbers as time went by.

This influx of children had its parallel across the Channel a few years later when the number of children cared for by the Paris foundling hospital, which had slowly grown from 5302 in 1740 to 6018 in 1767, suddenly increased by 4616 in the next six years to 10,634 in 1772. The rise in numbers coincided roughly with the onset of deteriorating economic conditions in the provinces, a fact suggesting that most of the children brought to the Paris hospital in this six-year period were the legitimate offspring of parents driven by want to desperate measures.[61] Similar stress undoubtedly moved English parents, especially those in rural areas, to send their children to the Foundling Hospital in the late 1750s. From 1756 to 1758 wheat was scarce, and a cattle plague had reduced the meat supply. Crop failures in 1756–57 had brought on conditions approaching starvation in some regions, accompanied by a fall in the wages of labourers.[62]

Yet to most Members of Parliament the outpouring of children did not imply the existence of enormous economic and social need. Instead, it confirmed what they had always suspected: the poor were lazy, irresponsible, and without moral standards. Why, then, should Parliament spend such large sums to help people who obviously were not trying to help themselves? For the consequence of the vast influx of children was that Parliament had already spent £130,000 on the project and could see the cost mounting year by year—from £30,000 in 1757 to £50,000 in 1759. Anyone would realize that the original estimate of a cost never exceeding £110,000 a year[63] must fall far short long before a decline in the Hospital's population through apprenticing its children could bring about a reduction in costs.

Meanwhile, England had been at war for four years, and no one knew when the war would end or how much it would cost. Was this a time to issue a blank check to a scheme that seemed not only to be subject to great abuse but also to be failing in its primary objective, which was to preserve lives and thereby increase the population? Parliament did not find it an easy question to answer.

In December 1759 Parliament asked the Governors for additional information and resolved itself into a committee of the whole to consider the state of the Hospital but came to no conclusions. The King's intervention, however, produced an additional grant to the Hospital of £5000 on 20 December. In January the Commons continued its investigation. The House asked for mortality figures, estimates of expenses for 1760, and the appearance before it of any solicitors employed by the Hospital to prosecute persons charged with taking children away from their mothers by force or fraud, or with sending children to the Hospital under the care of improper persons. Alarmed, the Governors ordered the treasurer on 2 February to present additional favourable data to the House and also 'to lay the said Accounts before such particular Members of the House of Commons as he shall imagine most proper to lay before that House to the best advantage for their information that no prejudice may arise to this Corporation from any misapprehended imagination of the Publick Money having been unnecessarily squandered away in improperly expensive Buildings'.[64]

But the Governors' efforts proved futile. On 8 February 1760, the Commons passed, without division, resolutions terminating its support of the General Reception after 25 March. Faced with the termination of support, the Governors had no choice but to stop receiving children after 25 March. Accordingly, they ordered that notice of the end of the General Reception be placed weekly in the newspapers, be circulated by the General Post Office to all church-wardens, overseers, and port masters, and be posted up at the Hospital's gates. Many rushed to beat the deadline: from 12 March to 24 March the Hospital admitted 308 children. On 25 March 1760 the last child received was baptized: they named her Kitty Finis.[65]

9

The Aftermath:
Parliament Withdraws, 1760–1771

PARLIAMENT DID NOT, of course, set the Foundling Hospital adrift to care for its 6857 children with no resources save the benefactions of the charitable. Recognizing its responsibility to the children taken in by its order, the Commons granted to the Hospital on 31 March 1760 the sum of £44,157 10s and on 28 April voted an additional £3127 10s to the Hospital. Payment came less promptly. The Hospital received nothing until 17 July, and then payment was made only after a pitiful plea to the Commissioners of the Treasury reciting that a previous request on 23 April had been ignored; that, as a consequence, the Governors had been forced to use the Hospital's invested legacies, amounting to £20,500; and that now no funds remained to pay the country nurses or to purchase supplies for the Hospital. To this appeal the Treasury responded with an installment of £10,000. Further payments arrived with equal snaillike slowness, the final one of £3127 10s not coming in until 28 February 1761.[1]

The following year saw a repetition of the Treasury's foot-dragging. In June the treasurer wrote to Dr Lee:

> I have this day to ans. Bills sold to the last 500 anns. we have left. I am to sell the last on Thursday which will produce between 4 & 500 l. Our Govrs. have for sometime supported the Hospital by their own private Money. The Government owes us 44,000 l. & have not pd. a farthing of the Parliamty Grant for this Year. . . . The Treasury have promised Paymt from day to day for Mos. past. I have got the Kings Warrt. & Sign Manual but can get no Money.[2]

And so the pattern was set: early each year the Governors would submit their estimate of expenses for that year; Parliament would grant the sum requested; then would follow repeated memorials to the Commissioners of the Treasury begging for payment and months of waiting for the money to trickle in while the treasurer and

Governors scrambled about for funds to meet the daily bills, sometimes being compelled to borrow substantial sums for the purpose.[3]

As the years passed and the Members of Parliament saw the total cost of their experiment mounting steadily higher, they became increasingly reluctant to continue the annual grants and impatient to be done with the whole affair. Although the amount of Parliament's grant decreased each year, reflecting the reduction by death and apprenticeships in the number of children supported, nevertheless by the end of 1764, it had cost the country £346,632 10s to care for these children.[4]

In March 1765 the Commons appointed a committee to consider the state of the Hospital and to make recommendations for the future support and employment of the children. After examining a great quantity of information supplied by the treasurer of the Hospital at the committee's request, its members recommended, and on 26 March the Commons passed, a series of resolutions condemning the education of foundling children by the Hospital for its tendency to make them unfit for useful and laborious employment; asserting that the Hospital should apprentice its children 'with all Convenient Speed' at age seven or earlier with a fee of not less than £5 nor more than £10 each; and recommending the sale of the branch hospitals in the country as soon as possible. The moneys so received, the resolutions stated, should be used for the care of the children and for apprentice fees.[5]

The Governors learned of Parliament's action with shock and dismay on 3 April.[6] By the end of May, the General Court had met ten times to plan a strategy for combatting this threat to the Hospital's methods and to its property, for in 1765 the Foundling Hospital owned three of the six branch hospitals that it was operating.[7] The Governors decided that their best course was to present a petition to Parliament opposing the bill then being drafted to carry out the resolutions, and they devoted many of their meetings to its preparation. Haste was imperative, they thought, for 'we suppose if the Bill is brought in this Session it will be hurried thro' the house as fast as possible, to prevent our being heard. This new method is called Smugling a bill and is oft Successful'.[8]

Strangely enough, the Governors found an opponent in their midst: Jonas Hanway, whom the treasurer described as 'the projector of this new Scheme of Destruction'.[9] Not only did Hanway make 'several abusive speeches' but he also voted against presenting the petition to Parliament—the only Governor to do so.[10] Whether Hanway fully deserved the treasurer's characterization cannot be said. We know that he had written a pamphlet, which, he says, was printed in 1764 'at the instance of a Member of the House of Commons'. This pamphlet recommended 'the giving of money with Children, agreeable to the established Custom of this Country, in similar cases; with a view to have a Choice of Masters, particularly in the Country', such fee to be paid 'toward supporting the Child from the age of 6, 7 or 8 to 11, 12, or 13'. Such a practice would, he argued, 'exonerate the Public of £30 or 40. Expence on the Child, by a well-timed Application of £10 or 12'. The children, he believed, could 'be taught in the hands of the Nurses, all that they need know'. What a child needed to know he defined as the ability 'to read and say his Prayers'. He made it clear, however, that the Governors must select the masters for these young children carefully and exercise continuing supervision over them through the country inspectors.[11] In a sense, his plan bore some resemblance to a system of paid foster care terminating when the child was able to be of real service to its master. At the same time it would also reduce the population, and therefore the costs, of the country hospitals. There is no indication, however, that Hanway was recommending a forced sale of the Hospital's property outside London. But his ideas about early apprenticing of the children and the payment of fees with them bear strong resemblance to the resolutions subsequently adopted by the Commons and may well have influenced to some degree the thinking of the Parliamentary committee that presented them.

The other Governors saw the matter very differently. Their petition asserted that the education and training given to the children in the Hospital made them such desirable apprentices that the best masters and mistresses took them readily at a proper age without any fee. Boys under ten or twelve years of age, they alleged, were unfit for sea service, husbandry, and most manufactures; small girls were, similarly, unequal to the laborious household service that families with no other servants would expect, and these were the households that most often took the girls. The Governors expressed their fear, moreover, that most of the people willing to burden themselves with the care of such young children would be indigent persons tempted by the fee, who, when they had spent the money, would be obliged to seek parish help for both themselves and the children, thereby injuring the whole community and bringing public censure upon the Governors.

These fears were well founded. William Bailey had reported in 1758 in his *Treatise on the Better Employment, and more Comfortable Support, of the Poor in Workhouses* that 'Many of those who take Parish Apprentices are so inhuman, as to regard only the pecuniary

Consideration; and having once received that, they, by ill Usage and undue Severity, often drive the poor Creatures from them; and so leave them in a more destitute Condition, at a riper Age for Mischief, than they were in when first they became the Care of the Parish Officers'.[12] And the Governors, too, when later they were obliged to relax their standards, encountered instances of this sort.

The Governors also protested in their petition that they had purchased the branch hospital with funds derived from charitable contributions and not with the moneys granted by Parliament. They claimed a right, therefore, to 'enjoy their Franchises, Rights and Priviledges as also their freeholds and Estates in as free, ample and secure a manner as any other Bodies Politick or Corporate within this Realm'.[13] With their petition the Governors presented a printed case describing the physical care given to the children, their employment in the hospitals, their education, and their religious training. It offered proof that the Governors had not used any part of Parliament's grants to purchase the branch hospitals and concluded with the comment:

> That their [the Governors'] Conduct has been attended with many beneficial Consequences to the Publick, and without any Prejudices suggested, much less proved: They Might have expected a milder Treatment than a Bill of Pains and Penalties to seize their Franchises and confiscate their Estates, especially at a Time when the farther Care of this Charity was recommended to Parliament by the best of Kings, who had done this Charity the great Honour of enquiring into its Management, and declaring himself its Patron* and Protector.[14]

In addition, the Governors retained counsel to argue against the proposed bill; they urged all Governors who were Members of Parliament to attend when the petition was presented; and they sought the assistance of the Duke of Bedford, who promised his aid.[15]

The bill to carry out the resolutions already passed by the Commons was given a first reading and then dropped, yielding, undoubtedly, to the cumulative pressure exerted against it by the Hospital's counsel, the Governors who were Members, the Duke of Bedford, and the King, whose brothers had visited the Hospital and had expressed their approval of it.[16] By the end of May the crisis had passed; Parliament had granted £38,000 for the care of the children for the year 1765; and once more the Governors were plying the

---

* George III declared himself the Hospital's patron on 22 December 1760.

Treasury with repeated requests for payment.[17] But they could not mistake the trend of Parliament's thinking.

The following year saw a repetition of the events of 1765: another Parliamentary committee to investigate the state of the Hospital, a revival of the same resolutions, another bill, another protest from the Governors, a recommendation from the King for further care of the charity, and, once more, the dropping of the bill after its first reading, followed by a grant of £33,892 10s for 1766.[18] The next year, ignoring the Governors' estimate that the cost of maintaining the children for 1767 would amount to £31,387 10s, Parliament reduced its grant to £28,000, but added a special allowance of £1500 to pay apprentice fees. The Governors could consider themselves fortunate, for in April the Commons had contemplated a reduction to £20,000, prompting the Governors to hold an evening meeting to prepare a petition (never presented) against such an action. 'I suppose', the Hospital's treasurer wrote bitterly to Dr Lee, 'Mr Charles Townshend [Chancellor of the Exchequer] calls this Oeconomy. However this reduces us to a necessity of placing out as many of the Children who are in our Hospitals as we can do with safety to them'.[19]

Each year thereafter the Commons followed the same course: a penurious grant for maintenance of the children accompanied by an increasingly larger grant to be used only for payment of apprentice fees. Parliament had found an effective, if indirect, way to bring about the desired termination of its experiment in caring for the nation's foundlings. Thomas Bradshaw, one of the secretaries of the Treasury, spelled it out plainly to the Hospital's secretary in the summer of 1768. It was the opinion of the Duke of Grafton and also of Lord North, Bradshaw told him, 'that it would be pleasing to the Public that they should be exonerated from the Expence of Maintaining the Children of this Hospital as soon as possible, and therefore recommend to the Committee to continue giving apprentice fees with the children'.[20]

The opinion of Grafton, then First Lord of the Treasury, and North, Chancellor of the Exchequer, probably did reflect public feeling accurately: since 1765 England had been suffering through a period of severe economic depression and social unrest marked by unemployment, food riots, bad weather, harvests so poor that distillers were prohibited from using grain, and a great decrease in overseas trade that continued until 1770.[21] Under such conditions the use of public funds to support foundlings in what many people would consider luxury could hardly be popular.

By 1 January 1770 the Governors had apprenticed over four thousand children. For the care of the remaining 965 foundlings they asked Parliament to grant the Hospital £9650 for 1770, pointing out that the necessity of transporting many of these children from the country hospitals to London would incur additional expense. They also requested at least £4000 to pay apprentice fees for these children, whom they described as the 'refuse of the whole number received', but the Commons allowed them only £3500 for the purpose.[22]

On 15 April 1771, Parliament decided to be done with foundlings forever: it granted the Hospital £2970 to support the remaining 396 children during 1771, provided for a final subsidy of £27,030 to defray the expense of all future care of these children, and resolved that 'no further Sum or Sums of Money be hereafter issued, for the Maintenance and Education of such Children as were received into the said Hospital, on or before the said 25th Day of March 1760'.[23] Payment was made, of course, with the customary slowness.

And so Parliament's participation in the affairs of the Foundling Hospital ended. The total of its grants had amounted to £548,796 16s. Or, to put it another way, it had cost Parliament approximately £102 for each child that lived to an age when it could be apprenticed. According to Jonas Hanway's calculations, the value to the community of each such child's work in the course of its productive life could be set at a minimum of £265.[24] Considering that, without the Hospital's care, few of these children would have survived their first year and that most of those who did so would probably have become parasites upon society rather than productive citizens, it would seem that, from a purely economic point of view, Parliament had made a good investment. But, apparently, few Members thought of it in that way. From the Commons' obvious eagerness to be done with foundlings, which the willingness to apprentice them at age seven or younger indicates, we must conclude that Parliament regarded the whole affair as an expensive mistake for which the remedy was to cut costs as quickly as possible. And such a judgment on their part would not be unreasonable.

In the first place, the Commons had tried an experiment unprecedented in English experience. Never before had Parliament considered that the central government rather than the local parish might undertake the responsibility of rescuing abandoned infants, using a private charity as its agent. Lacking the kinds of statistical and sociological data that today we would think indispensable before launching such a project, no one could have predicted the enormity of the need that the Hospital would be called upon to meet. And no one could have foreseen the abuses that the undertaking would generate. When the results proved disappointing, the Members believed the experiment to be a failure, and, like most of us, they wanted to put failure behind them. Instead, for ten years they had to pay for what they thought of as a mistake. We should not wonder, then, that they paid reluctantly and sought means of escape.

Moreover, in eighteenth-century England no one thought it odd for very young children to be gainfully employed. In 1726 Daniel Defoe noted with approval that in the hillside villages near Halifax 'hardly any thing above four Years old, but its Hands are sufficient to it self'.[25] And Arthur Young, writing in 1768, mentioned girls aged seven and eight employed at Sudbury in weaving ship-flags, and boys of the same age near Winchester earning 3d a day at farm work, while at Witney both boys and girls seven to eight years old received 1s 6d to 1s 8d a week for quilling* and cornering for the weavers.[26] When so many children of the labouring poor were contributing toward their own support at seven or younger, why, then, an eighteenth-century Englishman might logically ask, should foundlings be given more education and be maintained in greater comfort than these children enjoyed for an additional three or four years at public expense? And, finally, there may well have lurked in the recesses of the collective mind of Parliament the old prejudice: children of sin surely should not receive greater privileges than the legitimate children of decent people.

Be that as it may, the pressures applied by Parliament, culminating in the discontinuance of all assistance, compelled the Governors to two expedients. One of these was the disposal of the branch hospitals, which they had established under the authorization given by Parliament in 1756. Obviously, the Hospital in London could never house all the children taken in from 1756 to 1760 when they became old enough to be removed from their nurses' homes. It was considered healthier to care for them outside London, and certainly it was cheaper, not only because food cost less and wages were lower but also because strategic location of the branch institutions reduced transportation expense. Moreover, the Governors saw an advantage in making the work of the Hospital known in various parts of the country and interesting local gentlemen in it since such a course would educate the public to the benefits of the enterprise and, they hoped, gain widespread approval for it.[27]

The Governors, therefore, had set up branches in Ackworth, Yorkshire, in 1757; in Shrewsbury in 1758; in Aylesbury in 1759; in Westerham, Kent, in 1760; in Chester in 1762; and in Barnet, Hertfordshire, in the same year. They purchased the properties at

---

* Quilling was the winding of thread or yarn on the bobbins that fitted inside the weavers' shuttles.

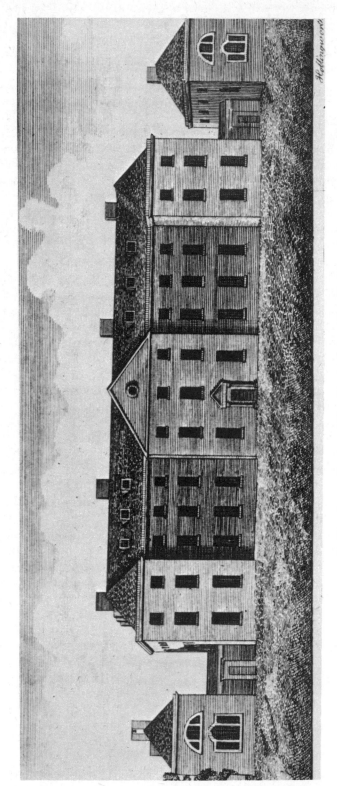

8. Northeast Front of the Shrewsbury Branch Hospital

Ackworth, Shrewsbury, and Aylesbury and leased those at Westerham and Barnet. The hospital at Chester was loaned to the Governors for three years by the Trustees of the Chester Blue Coat Charity School. The day-to-day management of each branch hospital rested with a committee of local gentlemen, who were elected Governors, but the General Committee or General Court in London decided all matters of general policy. Children were admitted only in London. From there they were sent to nurses in the country and when they were three to five years old, the Hospital's caravan transported them in groups to the nearest branch hospital.

The Governors closed down the Aylesbury hospital in 1767 and sold it in 1770. The Barnet branch was discontinued in 1768, followed by the branches in Chester and Westerham in 1769. The Shrewsbury hospital closed in 1772, but the Governors made no disposition of it until 1780 when they leased it for a term of three years to His Majesty's Commissioners for Taking Care of Sick and Wounded Seamen and for Exchange of Prisoners of War, to be used for the reception of French prisoners. In 1783 it was sold to the churchwardens and overseers of the poor of the several parishes within the Town of Shrewsbury and became a workhouse. The Ackworth hospital, which in the course of its fifteen-year-existence cared for 2664 children, did not close until 1773. The Governors sold off part of the land in 1776, but the building remained empty until the Trustees for the Society of Quakers leased it in 1778 and finally purchased it in 1786. Both the Ackworth and Shrewsbury properties were sold at a great loss.[28]

This bare outline of the acquisition and disposal of the six country hospitals does not, of course, tell their story, a story that properly belongs to another book and would add little to our central concern, the Hospital in London. It is sufficient to say here that the work of caring for the children taken in during the General Reception could not have gone forward without the country hospitals.

10

The Aftermath:
Disposing of the Children,
1760–1771

THE OTHER EXPEDIENT forced upon the Governors was, of course, the disposal of the children as rapidly as possible. One means open to the Committee was to return children to their parents. All through the Hospital's existence the Governors had received applications from parents who wanted to reclaim their children, the earliest request being recorded on 24 November 1742. After satisfying themselves that the applicant was, in fact, the child's parent, the Governors, before allowing the child to leave the Hospital, had usually required the applicant to pay for its care and to post security for its future maintenance. This some parents had not been able to do.

In 1764 the Governors decided to abandon these requirements, thereby enabling more parents to reclaim their children. This new policy they advertised in all the principal London newspapers. The only conditions they now insisted upon were satisfactory proof of a right to claim the child, which the applicants could meet by describing its clothes or the tokens sent with it or by producing the receipt given for it, and adequate evidence that the applicants were 'of such Character, and in such a Condition to Maintain' their child. The advertisement brought results: in 1764 forty-nine children were reclaimed by their parents, often unwed mothers. This was by far the greatest number of children ever claimed in any single year, for no more than three or four children were given back to their parents in any year from 1742 to 1777 except for the period 1757–60, when some twenty mothers a year applied for the return of children taken from them by force or fraud and placed in the Hospital. From 1764 onward, however, the Governors took the precaution in many cases of apprenticing the child claimed to its mother, her husband, or another relative, if they believed it to be illegitimate, in order to provide it with a settlement.[1]

But returning children to their parents effected only a very small reduction in the Hospital's population, and the Governors, therefore, found it necessary to apprentice the children at earlier ages and more speedily than they might otherwise have considered advisable. Three considerations determined their methods: the law of the land; the regulations contained in the Act of Parliament of 1740 that had confirmed and enlarged the powers granted in the Hospital's charter; and the precedents and policies established by the Governors from the beginning.

The law governing the apprenticing of children, known as the Statute of Artificers, was enacted in 1562 and changed very little until 1813. Subject to restrictions on certain trades, a child could be bound by indentures of apprenticeship to a husbandman or to a tradesman whom he would be obliged to serve until he reached the age of twenty-four. During this period the master had the duty of instructing the apprentice in the former's 'art, mystery or manual occupation'. And the Statute permitted no one to practice any trade without having served an apprenticeship of at least seven years.[2] Another act in 1601 made further provision for apprenticing pauper children: it authorized parish officials to apprentice pauper boys to age twenty-four and pauper girls to age twenty-one unless such girls married earlier.[3] The act of Parliament that enlarged the Governors' powers in 1740 granted them similar authority to apprentice the foundlings.[4] In 1767 an act relating to parish poor children within the Bills of Mortality allowed London boys as well as girls to be apprenticed to age twenty-one, but, in fact, the Governors had been apprenticing the Hospital's boys to age twenty-one in many instances since 1760, when the Solicitor General advised them that the act of Parliament gave them a discretionary power to do so.[5]

In addition to these legal restrictions, the Governors had gradually developed their own policies, beginning in 1749 when, on 13 December, Elizabeth Rich, a widow of Fishmongers Alley, Southwark, asked for a girl apprentice. Her application gave rise to three decisions, all significant for the future: first, that the Governors would never give money with any child apprenticed from the Hospital; second, that they would always gather information concerning the character and circumstances of anyone applying for an apprentice by inquiry to the minister and churchwardens of the applicant's parish; and, third, that the Committee would inform Mrs Rich that, in the Governors' opinion, all of the children were at that time too young to be apprenticed, the oldest of them having not yet reached nine years of age.[6]

By 1751 the Governors began to consider the matter of apprenticing the foundlings more urgent. Some of the children were now more than ten years old, and the Governors believed that the boys should be placed out at eleven, or twelve at the latest. Accordingly, they sent a letter to the Directors of the East India Company, asking them to recommend to their captains the taking of a few boys from the Hospital to serve on their ships, but the Directors replied that the manning of East India ships was controlled entirely by the owners from whom they hired their merchantmen.[7]

Although the Governors had always considered the boys of the Hospital destined for sea service, as it turned out the first child to be apprenticed was taken by Stephen Beckingham, one of the Governors, who executed indentures on 7 August 1751 for John Bowles, the fifth child received by the Hospital.[8] In 1752 five more children found masters, three boys being apprenticed to ships' captains and two girls to household service, and this pattern prevailed until the beginning of the General Reception. Up to 5 May 1756, of the first fifty-nine children apprenticed, twenty-three girls were put into household service; twenty-nine boys were sent into sea service; four boys were bound to husbandry and one boy to a bookbinder in London. As we have already noted, Stephen Beckingham took one boy, probably as a gardener or household servant. Most of these fifty-eight children at the time of apprenticing were between ten and twelve years of age; seven were younger, twelve older. The remaining child in this group, Charles Dilke, aged seven, was chosen on 4 June 1755 by Richard Shrapnell, the executor of the will of Lewin Cholmley of Stoke Newington, to be the beneficiary of a provision of Cholmley's will that directed his executor to select a boy not exceeding ten years of age from the Foundling Hospital and to use Cholmley's residuary estate as a trust fund to educate and maintain that boy.[9] During these years some requests for children were denied when it appeared to the Governors that the applicants proposed to take the child out of the country or did not contemplate a formal apprenticeship.[10]

Little by little, their increasing experience with apprenticing led the Governors to establish other practices to benefit the children, one of the earliest of which was the incorporation in the indentures of an agreement on the master's part to pay a male apprentice £5 a year during the last three years of his apprenticeship. From 1752 onward the Governors almost always made such agreements with boys' masters. Other policies that came into effect during these years included a resolution not to place boys out as livery servants; a resolution not to place a child with the keeper of a public house; and a resolution that all children might be apprenticed only to Protestants. The Governors also instituted a policy of keeping some control over the children after apprenticing them: a master who wished to transfer his apprentice to another person was expected first to obtain the Committee's permission.[11] We need not, I think, strain too much to see in these early policies of the Governors the beginnings of some of the practices followed by twentieth-century social workers when placing children in foster care. For they, too, try to put a child with a family of the same religion as his own; they investigate carefully the foster parents' character and financial situation before allowing them to take the child; and they continue their supervision and control over the child after placement.

The Governors also drew up and had printed a set of instructions, which the children learned to read so 'that the same may be fully imprinted on their minds before they leave this House'. The instructions not only gave the children good moral advice but also informed them of their rights as apprentices.[12] The ceremony, in which the Committee called before it the child who was about to be apprenticed, admonished him to conduct himself properly in his new life, presented him with the pasteboard folder containing the 'Instructions to Apprentices',* and then handed him over to his master, constituted for the foundlings the rite of passage from childhood into the adult world of work. For most of them no more solemn occasion, except marriage, would mark their lives.

Although the Governors endeavoured to adhere to their basic principles, the pressures applied by Parliament from 1765 onward necessitated some modifications of both policy and methods to deal with the dramatic increase in the number of children apprenticed each year. Moreover, the Governors had to abandon their preference for placing boys in the sea service because the merchant marine could scarcely absorb the large number of boys discharged from the Royal Navy after the end of the war in 1763 and needed none from other sources. The Governors, therefore, had to apprentice most of the boys to artisans and tradesmen in a wide variety of occupations. For the most part, those who took boys from the Hospital came from the lower ranks: peruke makers, cheesemongers, butchers, comb-makers, blacksmiths, farriers, bakers, weavers, feltmakers, file-smiths, papermakers, tailors, ropers, tallow chandlers, cork cutters, shoemakers. Some boys were taken by gentlemen (often Governors or their friends) to serve as gardeners, and the country hospitals apprenticed large numbers of the boys to local farmers to learn husbandry.

* See Appendix IV for a copy of the form of indentures used by the Hospital and also a copy of the 'Instructions to Apprentices'.

Only a handful received the opportunity to acquire skills by which they might later expect, as journeymen, to earn above-average incomes. These fortunate few included a boy apprenticed to a gentleman to be employed in his counting house; a few boys apprenticed to apothecaries (who would have charged anyone other than the Foundling Hospital an apprentice fee of £100 to £200); two boys apprenticed to a goldsmith (a craft that often demanded as much as £300 with an apprentice); one boy apprenticed to a cabinet maker; and one to a surgeon. This boy's prospects and those of the goldsmith's apprentices were best of all, for after serving their apprenticeships, they might, with a bit of luck, earn as much as £50 a year.[13] Nearly all of the girls went out as household servants, although a few were bound to milliners, mantua makers, makers of necklaces, and the like, to learn these trades.

The pressure to dispose of the children as quickly as possible also induced the Governors to act favourably upon applications from manufacturers for groups of children to work in their industries, although relatively few such requests were received in this period. The first mass apprenticing occurred in 1760–61 when John Arbuthnot, a calico printer of Ravensbury, Surrey, took sixteen girls to work for him and learn his trade. No complaints against him appear in the records until completion of the apprenticeships, when some of the girls charged that he had not given them the new clothing specified in their indentures.[14] The twenty-four children placed with Felix Ehrliholtzer, an embroiderer and tambour worker of Plaistow, Essex, in 1766 also seem to have fared well. Jonas Hanway visited them in 1771 and found them clean and in good health. Moreover, Ehrliholtzer was willing to hire the girls as skilled workers upon completion of their service. The Governors were so well satisfied with this master that in 1773 they agreed to apprentice six more girls to him.[15]

Other mass apprenticings did not turn out so successfully. What happened to some of the twenty-one girls apprenticed in 1767–68 to Job Wyatt, a wood screw maker of Tatenhill, Stafford, will be discussed later. What happened to the children apprenticed in 1765 to Martin Brown, a clothier of Holbeck, Yorkshire, to be employed in his woollen manufactory, was great suffering, the consequence of a decline in their master's business. Brown wrote to Jonas Hanway on 30 March 1768 that twenty-two out of seventy-four children had died in one year and that he wanted to be relieved of responsibility for twenty of the girls. The Committee at once ordered that a visitor from the Ackworth hospital investigate the matter, and so noxious did he find the apprentices' situation that the Governors decided to remove the remaining children to the Ackworth hospital temporarily and to arrange for a magistrate to discharge them from their apprenticeships. They also instructed the Ackworth hospital to assist the parish officials in placing the children out in new apprenticeships 'that no extraordinary Burthen may fall on their Parish by this unfortunate accident', for by reason of their apprenticeship to Brown, the children had all acquired settlements in his parish and, therefore, possessed a claim upon it, rather than upon the Hospital, for aid.[16]

A surprisingly large number of children were apprenticed to the husbands of the nurses who had cared for them since infancy. The strength of the affection that grew up in the intimate relationship between nurse and child made many nurses reluctant to part with the children when the time came for them to return to the Hospital. Often, the Hospital's clerk reported in 1759, the nurses showed 'the most lively sorrow in parting with them'.[17] The foster fathers, too, became fond of the children nursed by their wives, and the records tell of one man who travelled from Yately in Hampshire to London solely to visit the child that had passed from infancy to childhood in his home.[18]

It is not difficult to understand the feelings of these foster parents. Quite apart from any consideration of the help that another pair of hands might provide in a country labourer's household, there existed the strong psychological bond forged between the woman and the child she had nursed at her breast, especially if—and it was not uncommon—none of her own children survived infancy. Both the man and his wife, having watched the child's development, having taught it to walk and talk and to become part of a family, would not find it easy to cast off and forget the responsibility that had been theirs. As the fox observed so wisely to the little prince, 'c'est le temps que tu as perdu pour ta rose qui fait ta rose si importante . . . . Tu deviens responsable pour toujours de ce que tu as apprivoisé'.[19]

As a consequence of this bond between foundling and foster family, 'I find', wrote the treasurer in 1761, 'the Nurses who have brot up our Children acquire so great an affection for them that they would frequently maintain them at their own expence rather than part with them, but we don't often accept these offers for fear of being a burthen on poor familys or on Parishes which may be inconvenient to them'.[20] When the Governors did accept such offers, they were confronted with a legal problem, the only solution for which was to apprentice the child to the nurse's husband, for common law made no provision for adoption, which was not authorized by statute in Great Britain until 1926.[21] To effect an adoption in the eighteenth century required an act of Parliament. But if the Governors allowed the children to remain with their nurses without any legal ties, these children would never acquire a settlement. Lacking a settlement, they and their descendants would experience great difficulty in obtaining parish aid should they ever need it. The only method, then, by which these foundling children could gain a settlement in a parish for themselves and their progeny was by serving a formal apprentice-ship of at least forty days in that parish. The formalities of apprenticeship, therefore, became imperative to ensure a child's future security, even though the nurses and their husbands were, for the most part, taking the child out of affection. Apprenticeship in these situations provided the legal basis for what was, emotionally, an adoption.

In deciding upon applications for apprenticeships of this kind, the Governors had two principal concerns: could the nurse and her husband provide properly for the child? and how would the proposed apprenticeship affect the parish in which they lived?[22] The usual procedure was to require a certificate from the minister and churchwardens of the parish involved, stating that the person proposing to take the foundling as an apprentice had a legal settlement, that he was 'in such Circumstances as not likely to become burthensome to the Parish', and that the parishioners did not object to the proposed apprenticeship. The Hospital's local inspector was also asked whether or not he recommended the applicant. If the proposed apprenticeship seemed a desirable one, the Governors frequently allowed the nurse 12d or 18d a week to support the child and send it to school for a year before executing the indentures, especially when the child was only six or seven years old.[23]

From the child's point of view, the foundling was often as reluctant to part with the only mother he had ever known as she might be to part with him. Runaways of children to their former nurses were not uncommon, although few ran away from the Hospital itself, probably because it offered scant opportunity for escape. Also, the excitement of living in a new environment and making new friends among other foundlings may have provided for many a countervailing force against homesickness, at least for a time. The urge to run came most often when the child found himself apprenticed and was unable or unwilling, for one reason or another, to adapt himself to his new situation. Certainly, it could not have been easy for a child who had spent his early childhood in a country village, followed by a few sheltered years in an institutional milieu, to adjust to the very different way of life of a tradesman's household.

So often did such unhappy children return to their nurses that by the 1770s the Governors automatically assumed that a missing child would turn up at his old home. Their first act, therefore, upon learning of a runaway, was to direct the secretary to write to the Hospital's inspector or a clergyman living in that neighbourhood, asking him to watch for the child.[24] They had also taken the precaution of sending a printed notice to all inspectors and former inspectors to advise them of the Hospital's policy in such situations: it would allow no payments to nurses for the care of runaway children, for the law required them to give notice to a child's master of his whereabouts; otherwise they ran the risk of prosecution for unlawfully detaining an apprentice. The notice also advised inspectors to inform the overseers of the poor of a runaway child's presence in the parish, so that these officials could take appropriate action. But, the notice concluded, 'should it plainly appear to any Inspector that a child has been improperly treated by its Master or Mistress, the Governors of the Hospital will be very thankful for an immediate Notice thereof, in order to procure proper redress or such punishment as the law may direct'.[25]

Some of the children contrived to travel considerable distances: one girl, for example, made her way from her master's residence in the London suburb of Islington to her former nurse's home at Yately in Hampshire. Another child ran away from his master, a tailor in North Dalton, Yorkshire, and appeared at the home of his former nurse in Luton, Bedford.[26] Upon being returned to their masters, for it was the Governors' policy to return the child in nearly all cases, some determined children would run away again and again. One boy ran away at least four times from his London master to his old home at Newbury. Such persistence finally convinced the Governors that they should try to find another master for the boy in his old neighbourhood.[27]

Not only did the runaways present problems for the Governors, but also they frequently imposed a burden upon the families where they sought refuge. Many a poor nurse could not afford to feed an extra mouth. One woman with seven children, for example, had no means of supporting her large family save her husband's labour and her own, for having no settlement in the parish where they lived, they could obtain no help from parish officials. She notified the boy's master when a former nursling appeared at her cottage, but he, accusing the boy of stealing, refused to take him back and had the boy's indentures formally cancelled by the justices of the peace. The Committee, in this case, felt morally, if not legally, constrained to take the boy back and to pay the nurse a guinea for her expense in keeping him.[28] In addition to the expense, the Committee also had to find a new master for the boy and, meanwhile, keep him isolated from the other children, for the Governors did not, as a rule, permit a child who came back to the Hospital after being apprenticed—some runaways returned to the Hospital—to associate with the other foundlings during the usually short period of their stay.[29]

The reasons for this policy of segregation do not appear in the records. But we may speculate that one reason might have been to prevent children who had been abused by brutal masters from terrifying the other children with tales of their own experiences, thereby building up a fear of apprenticeship in the minds of the children still too young to be placed out. For, despite great efforts on the part of the Governors to find good masters for the Hospital's children, there were too few persons available to conduct proper investigations of prospective masters when so many apprenticings were taking place in so short a period. The apprenticeship records for 1760–70 show what happened in response to Parliament's coercion:[30]

Year	Number of children apprenticed
1760	42
1761	47
1762	39
1763	37
1764	93
1765	253
1766	256
1767	479
1768	1176
1769	1430
1770	555

Obviously, the Governors could devote more time and personal attention to locating suitable masters when they were placing out children at an average rate of eighteen a year, as they did up to 1760, than time and human resources would permit when the number of placements mounted to 1430 in 1769.

True, some children were placed out directly from the Ackworth and Shrewsbury branches, but the majority were apprenticed from London, where all preliminary investigations and follow-up visits after apprenticing had to be made by a handful of active Governors and by the steward and schoolmaster, who could give only part of their time to these duties. And from 1770 to 1773 only the schoolmaster made such inquiries in addition to those made by the

Governors. In 1773 the task, still on a part-time basis, was delegated to the clerk. These employees, of course, travelled about London on foot and, when making follow-up visits, were expected to see only two or three children in a day.[31]

Yet how else could the Governors have undertaken such investigations and visits? Even if they had considered hiring a person to devote his entire time to the task, thereby creating a position for which no precedent existed anywhere, how could they find a person as well qualified as a trusted member of their own staff? No one except a Governor or a subordinate officer of the institution, persons thoroughly familiar with the Committee's point of view, would understand what the Hospital expected of the masters with whom it placed its children. The only solution to the problem that occured to the Committee was to encourage greater participation in such work by the less active Governors, but probably no more than a dozen of them were ever willing to sacrifice their leisure for these activities.* We should not wonder, then, that some children found themselves apprenticed to brutal masters, and some masters acquired lazy, dishonest, or impudent apprentices.

When masters complained, the Governors usually tried to reconcile the parties. They would ask the master to bring his apprentice before the Committee, reprimand the child for his misdeeds, and urge the master to 'make some farther Trial'. If the arrangement still proved unworkable, the Governors encouraged the master to find another person willing to take the child and co-operated in transferring the indentures. But some children demonstrated such intractability that they were passed from master to master several times. In 1765 when a watchmaker sought to assign his foundling apprentice, Clarissa Harlowe, to a milkman, no place could be found on her indentures to inscribe the transfer because the great number of previous assignments had used up all of the available space.[32]

On the other hand, when the children complained of their masters, or others complained on their behalf, sometimes anonymously, the Governors took even greater interest in the matter. First, they looked into the truth of the charges. One of the Governors might make discreet inquiries, or the Committee might summon the master to appear before it and to bring his apprentice with him, so that both might be examined. Then the Committee took appropriate action.

* Today the average caseload of a social worker at the Thomas Coram Foundation for Children is 25. It would, therefore, by today's standards, require a minimum of 160 caseworkers to place and supervise the four thousand children whom the Hospital had apprenticed by 1 January 1770.

Many complaints concerned masters who failed to feed or clothe their apprentices decently or who forced them to live under filthy conditions. Some masters disappeared, leaving the child to fend for itself, often by begging from neighbours. Some neglected their duty to teach their apprentices a trade; others taught them to steal. And some masters overworked, beat, tortured, and starved the children.[33] All of these forms of abuse were inflicted on Elizabeth Owen. Apprenticed at the age of ten to Joshua Fox of Carlton, Yorkshire, she was turned over by him to his son-in-law and daughter, John and Hannah Walker. In the course of the next two years, the Walkers frequently compelled her to work at spinning from six o'clock one morning until three o'clock the following morning while confined naked in one room and not allowed to go to the privy. When she could contain herself no longer and dirtied the room, they beat her for it with a birch rod, a whip, or a thick walking stick, sometimes until she could neither sit down nor lie on her back. Once on a winter's night they forced her to bathe in the river amid floating ice. She was given no more than two meals a day, had once been held so close to the fire by her mistress that her face was burnt, and had had so many injuries inflicted upon her left arm, including a dislocated wrist, that she could no longer stretch it out. When the matter came to their attention, the Governors immediately undertook a prosecution against master and mistress.[34]

Some masters committed sexual assaults upon their young female apprentices. Sarah Drew, for instance, reported at a Subcommittee meeting that her master, Job Wyatt (the wood screw maker of Tatenhill mentioned earlier), had 'attempted to debauch her at Eleven Years of Age and completed it afterwards and continued the same ill Usage till Xmas last & beat her if she refus'd to submit to his Will. That she likewise was inform'd her Master had also debauch'd several other Apprentices amongst whom were Mary Johnson Mary Rise and Ann Beauchamp who often talk'd of it to her'.[35] The Governors immediately ordered that an application be presented to the local magistrates for the discharge from their apprenticeships of all girls bound by the Hospital to Job Wyatt and that new masters be found for them.[36]

And some masters even murdered their apprentices. William Butterworth, a weaver of Manchester, killed his apprentice, Jemima Dixon, by inches. From 1 February to 10 April 1771, he starved her, slapped and kicked her, and beat her with a weaver's shuttle, a leather strap, a brush, and a stick, sometimes kneeling on her back to do so. According to the testimony of another apprentice, Butterworth 'punch'd or kick'd her on the Belly with his foot and broke her Belly that she could neither hold her stool or Urine, & that she had a Cloth put under her at Nights tied on with some bandage & that when she foul'd the bed in the night he Wm. Butterworth made her bring the excrements down stairs in the Morning & stood over her & made her eat it, & that he did so several times'.[37] Upon trial, Butterworth was found guilty of murder, but the judge reprieved him. The outraged Committee protested to the Secretary of State but were told that subsequent to the reprieve, Butterworth had applied for and obtained a pardon, and that a pardon could not be set aside.[38]

Mary Jones was more fortunate. She was bound in 1765 to James Brownrigg, a painter in Fetter Lane. His wife began immediately not only to whip the girl severely but also to plunge her head repeatedly into a pail of water. One Sunday morning while the Brownriggs slept, Mary made her escape and fled to the Foundling Hospital with an eye so badly injured that for a time it was feared that she might lose it. The Governors haled Brownrigg before the Chamberlain of London and obtained the girl's discharge from her master. Two years later Mrs Brownrigg killed another apprentice, an eleven-year-old parish child, by a succession of beatings, following upon almost two years of assorted tortures that had reduced the girl, according to the surgeon who examined her, to 'all one wound from her head to her toes'. Mrs Brownrigg was tried at Guildhall, convicted of murder, and executed at Tyburn on 14 September 1767.[39] The exploitation of child labourers obviously did not begin in the 'dark, satanic mills' of the Industrial Revolution.

The Governors tried to deal effectively with any improper treatment of apprenticed foundlings that came to their attention. After the death of Jemima Dixon, they petitioned the Secretary of State, asking that examples be made of persons committing crimes against these children. At a considerable expense for legal fees, they prosecuted persons who had injured the children, and sometimes they succeeded in collecting damages from the wrongdoers; these sums they always invested for the child's benefit. They took into the Hospital's infirmary children who were seriously ill or injured and arranged for their medical care. They found new masters for abandoned and mistreated children when, for one reason or another, such children were not eligible for parish aid. And they remonstrated with numerous masters who welched on their agreements in the indentures of apprenticeship and refused to give their apprentices new clothing upon completion of their service or to pay the boys for their last three years' work. The Governors also tried to prevent ill treatment of the Hospital's children not only by visiting as many of them as possible but also by withholding payment of part of the apprentice fee until the second or third year and then paying the balance only after they had satisfied themselves that the apprentice was well situated.[40] Of their deep and continuing concern for the children's welfare there can be no doubt.

How many of the Hospital's children suffered neglect or abuse at the hands of their masters in spite of the Governors' efforts we cannot determine with any certainty. The records for this period mention less than a hundred such instances, which would seem to be a very small percentage of more than four thousand apprenticeships. But how many unreported cases of abuse may have existed it is impossible to know.

For good or ill, however, apprenticeship offered the only gateway to adult independence open to the foundlings. It insured their future by giving them a settlement and—theoretically, at least—by teaching them a trade. At its worst, it was a system conducive to exploitation and semislavery, in which masters profited from cheap labour, gave little instruction in return, and, as we have seen, abused their apprentices brutally. At its best, however, it was an excellent and practical system of imparting skills, which were taught in a one-to-one relationship; moreover, it was a system designed to encourage pride and satisfaction in one's work because the worker learned to perform every step leading to the finished product. It was also a system well fitted to maintain social stability by passing on the traditional ways of doing things, thereby discouraging innovation and upward mobility.

11

New Methods, Old Objectives,
1760–1799

AFTER THE RECEPTION of Kitty Finis on 24 March 1760, the Hospital took in no more foundlings until 1763 for lack of private funds to support them. The purchase and fitting out of the country hospitals had used up much of the capital accumulated over the years, chiefly from legacies, and benefactions of all kinds had dwindled into insignificance during the period of the General Reception. If Parliament was supporting the Hospital, many people reasoned, it did not need private charity. In 1760, therefore, the Governors had the will but not the wealth to take up again the philanthropic role that the institution had played from 1741 to 1756.

The Hospital did, however, receive a handful of children—twenty-six, to be exact—before 1763. These were the orphans of soldiers who died for England in the Seven Years' War. Dr Richard Brocklesby, an army physician, first suggested the indiscriminate reception of soldiers' children to the Committee in 1759, but at that time the Governors reluctantly concluded that 'the present Circumstances and Powers in this Corporation do not enable them to comply with so charitable a Request, however agreeable to their inclinations'.[1]

But on 7 May 1760 the Committee, at the request of Lord Barrington, the Secretary of War, recommended to the General Court that the Hospital take in the orphans of soldiers who died abroad during the war when such children had no ascertainable settlement. The General Court concurred with this recommendation at its annual meeting and ordered the immediate reception of six children, ranging in age from four to twelve, whose fathers had been killed in the Battle of Minden. On 30 December 1761 the General Court acted to include orphans of sailors dying in the service of the Royal Navy, but, in fact, none were received. In all, the Hospital took in thirty-four children of military men during and immediately after the war.[2]

Later in the century when war broke out with France in 1793, the Hospital again undertook to care for the orphans and fatherless children of soldiers and sailors. Acting upon the Committee's recommendation, the General Court resolved at a special meeting on 29 January 1794:

> ... that it is the opinion of this meeting that the admitting into this Hospital the exposed and necessitous children of soldiers and seamen who are, have been, or shall be employed in the service of their country during the present War, will be productive of considerable advantages to the public by holding out an encouragement to those brave and meritorious subjects engaged in the public service and securing an object of great importance to the community at all times but particularly at the present, vizt.: The preserving the lives of and training up in Habits of Industry, Virtue, and Religion, Infants in the Inferior Classes of Society who might otherwise be Exposed to Poverty, Disease, Idleness and Vice . . . .
>
> Resolved that in the reception of such children the usual limitation of age to one year be extended to five years.[3]

The first of these children entered the Hospital on 19 February.

As soon as the Governors' patriotic intention came to public notice through publicity in the newspapers, a few contributions for the support of these children began to arrive. The first such contribution, in fact, was a £10 note sent to the editor of the *True Briton* to be forwarded to the Hospital before the Court had passed its resolution. The United Society for the Relief of the Widows and Children of Seamen, Soldiers, Marines and Militia Men Who May Die or Be Killed in Actual Service During the Present War not only recommended children to the Hospital's care but also solicited contributions to a separate fund established for the children's maintenance in the Hospital. But the fund received few contributions. There was a better response in Canterbury where subscriptions totalled £106 1s before the end of the year.

By October 1796, however, the total contributions amounted to only about £150, forcing the Governors to inform the War Office that they could not accept six soliders' orphans recommended by that Office without financial assistance because the Hospital's own funds could support no more than 350 children, and only one vacancy remained to make up that number. The Secretary of War responded with an immediate contribution of £100 and a few days later arranged for the payment to the Hospital of £300 for the care of the six orphans. A month later the Governors learned from Sir Richard

King of the plight of another orphan whose father had died of yellow
fever in the West Indies* and whose mother, having gone aboard the
Amphion to inquire about her husband, was killed when the ship blew
up. No funds were available, but the Committee voted to take the boy
in, and the treasurer engaged to pay for the child's board himself until
a vacancy occurred.[4]

Unlike soldiers' orphans dependent upon charity were the children
admitted upon payment of £100, a practice that began in 1756 and
continued throughout the century (it was terminated by the General
Court on 21 January 1801). These children represented a very small
percentage of the Hospital's population at any time. Only seventy-
five such children entered the Hospital between 1756 and 1799, that
is, an average of less than two a year. In some years there were none,
and only once did the annual total exceed four: in 1799 the Hospital
took in six. Of the seventy-four for whom a record of sex was found,
forty-two were boys; thirty-two were girls. No data indicates why the
scales tipped in favour of boys, but there are at least two possible
explanations: it might signify the preference of a society still largely
patriarchal for guaranteeing the preservation of males, or it might
indicate no more than the fact that boys outnumber girls at birth. Be
that as it may, the payment that assured the child's immediate
admission bought him no preferential treatment thereafter: not until
1798 did the Committee resolve to try to find 'a more favorable
situation or trade' when apprenticing a child received with a money
payment.[5]

Soldiers' children and those received with money, however,
formed special cases. Different considerations and procedures govern-
ed the admission of other children, which began once more when
the General Court on 11 May 1763 authorized the reception of not
more than one hundred London children to be maintained by private
funds. Very quickly the Governors replaced the pre-1756 scheme of
drawing lots by mothers whose identities remained carefully con-
cealed with a new system of petitioning that required each mother to
divulge in writing her name and circumstances. A Governor or an
employee of the Hospital—the secretary, steward, or clerk—then
investigated the truth of the petitioner's story, unless a person of high
status had recommended her.

Not all of the children received under the new method were
illegitimate: some were children of widows, or of women deserted
by their husbands, or of men whose wives had died in childbirth, all
of whom destitution had forced to part with their children. The

* The parents of many of the soldiers' children received by the Hospital
died of yellow fever in the West Indies.

Hospital still took in abandoned infants, of course, the petition on their behalf usually being made by the persons who found them. Frequently one of the Governors, Lady Vere or Lady Betty Germain, or officials of other charities recommended worthy cases. Robert Dingley, for example, applied in 1766 for the admission of three children born to women in the Magdalen House. A few were children born to victims of rape. One orphan, four years of age, having been left at its mother's death with 'some poor Irish Papists' was received so that it would not 'be educated in the Popish Religion'. And a few persons still left children at the Hospital's gates.[6]

But most applications that resulted in admissions came from destitute, unmarried women seduced by lovers under a promise of marriage and then deserted when they became pregnant. These applicants usually asserted that they could avoid disgrace and find employment if they were not burdened with the care of a child. Mary Cole's petition on 7 December 1768 typifies many:

> The most humble Petition of Mary Cole, seduc'd & reduc'd and the Person who is the Cause of my Misfortunes has deceiv'd me and is gone abroad, by the best Intelligence I can have. He made me a promise of Marriage, with many Vows and Protestations, before I unhappily yielded to his Solicitations, by which I am now brought to this Miserable Condition, depriv'd of the Esteem and regard of my friends, and relations, destitute of many Necessaries, Supported only thro' small Donations, and Benefactions of a few charitable Persons, who have Compassion towards me in my unhappy Condition; Having no dependance (when able to work) but my daily Labour, and not able to provide for my Child. Therefore, I humbly pray your Honours will have pity upon my unfortunate Case, and take my Child under your Protection, which will be means of preserving us both, for which Act of great Charity I shall ever in Duty be bound to pray. I am
>
> your Honours most unworthy and poor
distress'd hble. Servt.
Mary Cole.[7]

Usually the petitions came from servant girls, who signed with a mark or with a crude signature the plea written for them by a more literate friend. Most often the father was also a servant. In France, too, the parents of most illegitimate children came from the lower ranks of society. The mothers were often country girls living away from their families while employed in towns as servants, textile workers, or casual labourers. The fathers were usually fellow workers, soldiers, or in cities such as Strasbourg, students. But many servant girls bore bastard children as a consequence of rape or seduction by their employers or by sons of the house.[8]

Over the years the petitions to the Foundling Hospital's Governors varied little. In the 1780s a number of women stated that their husbands or lovers had been pressed into the Navy, and the investigator's very brief reports in this period say little more than 'a good character; in great distress'. In the 1790s Mr Atchison, the schoolmaster, wrote much more detailed reports, but his remarks and the basic pattern of the petitions only demonstrated how little conditions and attitudes had changed in thirty years.[9]

The number of children that the Governors were able to receive fluctuated from year to year, depending upon the Hospital's financial resources. After the Hospital had received the first one hundred, authorized in 1763 and completed in 1764, it took in only four during 1765. In 1767 the General Court increased the total by thirty. Fifty more were added in 1768, and by 1770 the number dependent on private charity reached two hundred.

But, once again, the Governors found themselves in their old predicament: more children were being offered to the Hospital than its funds could support. To solve the dilemma, at least partially, the Committee devised a procedure of notifying all applicants whom the Governors had interviewed and whose petitions had been investigated and approved to assemble with their children in the Hospital's Chapel on a stated Saturday. The women then drew lots in the presence of the Governors and other spectators to determine which children the Hospital would admit at once and which would have to await another chance at a later date. In especially needy cases, the Governors often made an allowance of 2s 6d a week to a woman, after approval of her petition, to keep herself and her child alive until the next reception day. They also gave similar support to women who drew black balls until the succeeding admission date.

In 1772 the Governors decided to add another hundred children to the total maintained by non-governmental funds, since these had now been augmented by the sale of the Aylesbury hospital. At the same time, although they lowered the age at reception from eight to six months, they expanded the geographical area from which children might come to include those born 'in or within 5 miles of the Bills of Mortality'. Authorization for fifty more children was given by the General Court on 29 December 1773; for sixty more on 11 May 1774; and for another hundred on 25 January 1775. In 1776 the Court directed that the reception of children continue indefinitely at the rate of ten a month. As a result of this resolution, 120 children a year entered the Hospital through 1782, when, for financial reasons, the

Governors found it necessary to cut back to sixty a year. By 1785 they had to curtail the number again, this time to ten children quarterly. On 27 December 1786 the General Court was finally forced to reduce the number of children to ten a year because of the Hospital's increasing deficits. Not until 1792 did the Hospital have sufficient funds to permit enlargement of the annual number of children received. During this five-year period the Governors could do no more than try to decrease the total number of children supported to 350 and hold it at or below that number. But as the development of the Hospital's estate in the 1790s gradually improved its income, expansion of its population again became possible, so that on 1 January 1800 the number finally reached four hundred.[10]

Over the years some unusual admissions took place: several sets of twins; a mulatto child and also the child of Black Peggy, a Negro girl; a child whose criminal parents were being transported to Botany Bay; one or two children of insane mothers; and a child 'dropt on the Stairs leading to the Parliament House', whom the Commons asked its Speaker to recommend to the Hospital's mercy.[11]

A happy aspect of this period was the decline in infant mortality. Beginning three weeks after the end of the General Reception, the number of infant deaths dropped dramatically—from eighty-five in the week of 9–16 April 1760 to fifteen the following week. And thereafter the number remained consistently low except during epidemics of smallpox or measles. On 3 May 1797 the treasurer reported that of the 1684 children received from 1771 to that date, 482 had died under the age of twelve months—an infant mortality rate of 28.6 percent. But, he added, in the ten years from 1787 to 1797 the death rate for babies had been only one in six.[12] In France, on the other hand, the transportation of foundling infants from the provinces to Paris during the 1770s resulted in a mortality rate for these children of 80 percent. Later in the century, because of the deprivations occasioned by a constant state of war, the mortality among infant foundlings in Paris reached 95 percent by 1797.[13]

In contrast to the Foundling Hospital's favourable mortality rate for infants, its overall death rate rose steadily, probably because, as the years passed, the Governors kept the children in the Hospital longer before apprenticing them. For the thirty-five year period from 1760 to 1795 the chance that a child would live to be apprenticed was only 46 percent, which was approximately the same chance it had between 1741 and 1756.[14] The hazards of growing up had changed little in the course of the century.

Far more remarkable than the change in a foundling's life expectancy was the shift in the Governors' concept of the Hospital's purpose. Yet the shift came about so gradually and as such an inevitable outgrowth of the system of maternal petitioning in use after 1763 that they did not recognize the change at once. In fact, the first hint of an additional purpose—the primary purpose of saving infant lives never changed—does not appear in the records until 1795. Then we find the Committee ordering

> . . . that in all future enquiry into the merits of any petition for the admission of children into this Hospital, that it be always enquired whether in a recommendation to this charity from the mistress of a servant, whether if the child is received in consequence of such recommendation, the Mistress or any other proper person will take the Petitioner into service again.[15]

In short, the Governors wanted to know whether the reception of the child would also secure respectable employment for the mother, thereby commencing her rehabilitation.

By 1797 the duality of purpose was recognized. In the words of a statement prepared by the treasurer:

> The Foundling Hospital has Two Objects to preserve and educate Infants otherwise exposed to perish, and to restore the mothers to a course of Industry and Virtue so that almost every Act of the Charity is attended with a double Benefit, the preservation of the Child and of the Parent. In this respect the Governors have great reason to be satisfied for in Course of the preceding Year . . . not less than 50 unfortunate Women have been preserved from Vice and Despair . . . . and it is deserving of observation that no Instance has come to the Knowledge of the Committee of any Woman so relieved, who has not been thereby saved from what she would in all probability have been involved in a Course of Vice and Prostitution.[16]

When Captain Coram formulated his plan for a foundling hospital, he undoubtedly expected to benefit the mothers as well as the children to the extent that providing a refuge for their children would prevent the women from becoming murderesses, but the idea of taking more positive steps to rehabilitate them certainly played no part in his scheme, nor did such a thought occur to anyone else until after the General Reception. Even then no one set forth the rehabilitation of the mothers as a goal and designed methods to accomplish it. Rather, the goal came into existence as an accidental product of the new methods used after 1763 because the petitioning process gave the Governors exact knowledge about the situation of each mother; this enabled them to see for the first time how often the burden of an illegitimate child precluded such women from obtaining employment and turned them to prostitution as a means of survival. By the end of the century, then, what had occurred was a gradual development of something very like individual casework, directed as much toward providing constructive help for the unfortunate woman as for her child. And this dual objective, in fact, still guides the policies of the Hospital's present-day successor, the Thomas Coram Foundation for Children.

From 1760 to the end of the century, the Hospital admitted over two thousand children.[18] This number included all the categories that we have already discussed plus one other: parish children. The commitment of these children to the care of the Foundling Hospital resulted directly from the enactment by Parliament in 1767 of the Act for the Better Regulation of the Parish Poor Children, often referred to as the Hanway Act. It took effect on 1 July 1767 and applied to 'the seventeen parishes without the Walls of London; the twenty-three parishes of Middlesex and Surrey, being within the Bills of Mortality, and the Liberty of the Tower of London; and the ten parishes within the City and Liberty of Westminster'.[19]

This Act was the direct outcome of Jonas Hanway's agitation for better care of pauper infants coming under the jurisdiction of parish officials. As early as 1757* he had become interested in the conditions under which parish workhouses cared for children and, according to his earliest biographer (who was also his secretary for many years), 'alone and unassisted, he explored the then miserable and unhealthy habitations of the parish poor in these crowded cities, exposed his tender lungs to the pestilential air of the workhouse sick-wards, and procured a complete account of the interior management of every workhouse in and near the metropolis'.[20] His numerous accounts of the deplorable conditions that he had observed—conditions that produced a mortality rate of 60 to 90 percent or more in children under age four—combined with his personal solicitations, led, first, to an act passed by Parliament in 1762. This act required every London parish to maintain annual registers of pauper children received, discharged, and deceased—records that provided the statistical ammunition for Hanway's continuing battle to secure decent care for parish infants and laid the foundation for the Hanway

---

* Hanway, a bachelor, after his retirement from the Russia trade in 1750, devoted most of his time to philanthropic causes. He was the principal mover in establishing the Marine Society in 1756 and, jointly with his former partner, Robert Dingley, promoted the establishment in 1758 of the Magdalen House for penitent prostitutes.

Act of 1767, which the poor called the 'act for keeping children alive'.[21]

Although the act was generally known by Hanway's name and he was its principal promoter, the Governors of the Foundling Hospital gave him every encouragement and assistance in securing its passage. Apparently they were willing to overlook their recent disagreement with him when his proposals promised an opportunity to enlarge the Hospital's work and to secure additional revenue in doing so. For acting upon Hanway's representations, the General Court appointed a select committee on 14 May 1766 to 'consider of the best means of rendering this Hospital more useful to the Publick in regard to the infant Poor within the Bills of Mortality'. This committee met several times and agreed upon a plan whereby parish officials, except those of parishes within the walls of the City of London, would be forced to turn over the care of all illegitimate children, orphans, or foundlings to the Governors of the Foundling Hospital and to pay the Hospital for their care; at the same time parishes would give outdoor relief to mothers of legitimate children to enable them to support their children without being obliged to enter a workhouse. Taylor White, the treasurer, then drafted a proposed bill to carry out the committee's ideas and presented it to the General Court on 25 June. Pleased with the bill, the Court continued the life of the select committee for the purpose of prosecuting the design.

From that point on, with Sir Charles Whitworth (who was both a Governor and a Member of Parliament) acting as intermediary, the select committee worked with the Parliamentary committee appointed to consider the state of the infant poor within the Bills of Mortality. Together they settled on a compromise bill that gave parish officials an alternative to placing infant paupers in the Foundling Hospital but did follow the Governors' recommendation that parish boys not be bound to apprenticeships beyond the age of twenty-one.[22]

As soon as Parliament passed the act, officials of many parishes began negotiations with the Governors to take their pauper children. The Hospital's neighbouring parishes, St Andrew Holborn and St George the Martyr, were the first to agree to the Hospital's terms: an entrance fee of 20s to cover the cost of clothing the child, transporting it to the country, and burying it if it should die; and 12s 6d a month in advance for the child's care.[23] The monthly charge amounted to £7 10s per year, the sum that Parliament was paying for the support of the children taken in during the General Reception.

In the last half of 1767 the Hospital received 179 parish children of whom only twenty-six had died by 13 January 1768—a mortality rate of 14.5 percent, which represented a sharp contrast with the infant mortality rate in parish workhouses. The following year the Hospital took in seventy-three more parish children. But, in the words of the treasurer, 'it not being made compulsive on the Parishes to send their Children the numbers yet sent are not great, many Parishes yet rather being unwilling [sic] that their Children should die than pay for the keeping them alive'.[24]

In fact, some parishes proved to be most unwilling to pay for the care of their poor children after sending them to the Hospital. For example, the officers of the squalid parish of St Leonard Shoreditch asked the Hospital to return all of that parish's children on 30 August 1769. When the Governors refused to comply on the ground that the Hanway Act and their agreement with the parish prohibited removal of the children under the age of six unless they were claimed by their parents, the parish officials began systematically to withdraw a child or two at a time, always asserting that the children were 'being demanded by their parents'. At the same time, they stopped paying for the children's care. By the summer of 1770 the parish owed the Hospital £124 5s, and the Governors were finally compelled to threaten the parish officers with legal action in order to collect the debt.[25] St Leonard Shoreditch behaved no better toward the children—presumably older children—that it maintained in its workhouse: in 1774 the parish officers admitted that their building was so small that they had to put thirty-nine children into three beds.[26]

But St Leonard's was not the only parish delinquent in its payments. St Giles-in-the-Fields fell sixteen months behind in 1772 and paid up only after repeated threats from the Hospital's solicitor. Other parishes did little better. In November 1774 ten parishes owed the Hospital a total of £455 7s 9d for the care of sixty-six children, and once more threats of prosecution were required to produce payment. Less than a year later fifteen parishes were in arrears for the care of 133 children, with unpaid charges ranging from £4 12s to £305 4s 4d. And intermittent difficulty in obtaining compensation from the parishes continued throughout the rest of the century: in 1793 St Olave Southwark had been indebted to the Hospital for £92 18s for over three years. On the other hand, some parishes paid quite willingly 3s 6d a week to maintain their pauper children in the Hospital beyond the age of six years until they were old enough to be apprenticed.[27]

At first, the Governors, undiscouraged by the difficulties with St Leonard Shoreditch in 1769, thought that increasing the number of parish children received would be a good thing. The Hospital had been paid £1377 16s 4d for the care of such children for the year 1770 and by that time had taken in 337 of these children.[28] But this number, the Governors realized, represented only about 11 percent of the 3023 foundlings and bastard children born in the parishes covered by the Hanway Act during the four years from 1767 through 1770.[29] With the cessation of all Parliamentary support imminent, it seemed desirable to the Governors to put pressure on the parishes to turn over all their pauper infants to the Hospital: the moneys paid by the parishes for the care of such children would enable the Governors to keep open the Ackworth and Shrewsbury hospitals in addition to carrying on a much needed humanitarian enterprise.

In the summer of 1771, therefore, the Governors gave long and serious consideration—even to the point of drafting a tentative bill—to a plan for seeking from Parliament legislation that would extend the Hanway Act by compelling parishes to send all their pauper children to the Foundling Hospital and to maintain them there until the age of ten. Hanway, however, vigorously dissented, perhaps because he saw the proposal as a criticism of the effectiveness of 'his' act. But his opposition accomplished nothing: the Governors thanked him politely for his views and went ahead with their plans.[30] In the end, nothing came of the idea. Apparently, the Governors did not succeed in enlisting any Parliamentary support for such a piece of compulsory legislation, or, perhaps, as more and more parishes became dilatory in making their payments, the Governors' enthusiasm for the idea faded away.

By the 1780s increased costs had necessitated a higher rate, and the Hospital was charging parishes £9 a year for each child, on which, if all went well, the Hospital might realize a profit of 6s 1½d while the child was at nurse in the country and 19s 8d while the child resided in the Hospital. Since the average number of parish children cared for by the Hospital during these years was approximately fifty, it is evident that, although the Hospital was making little profit from it, this part of its work, at least, imposed no additional burden upon the charity of the institution's benefactors.[31] By the end of the century the Governors were apparently no longer eager to receive these children, for on 30 March 1796 they resolved to admit no more than a hundred parish children and in July raised the rate for their care to 4s 6d a week each.[32] This change probably made little difference to the parishes, for the records indicate that very few parishes ever utilized the alternative of sending their pauper children to the Foundling

Hospital as authorized by the Hanway Act. Evidently many parish officials ignored the law or made their own arrangements for country nursing.

Although the categories of children taken in and the manner of their reception changed a great deal after 1760, daily life in the Hospital differed little, except in details, from earlier years. Clock and calendar still ruled the children's days, as we can see from the treasurer's description written in 1799:

> At the age of four years the children are returned to the hospital. They are then . . . placed in the schools; where they are gradually accustomed to regular and early habits of order and attention; the lesser children being occasionally let out to play, during the school hours. They rise at six o'clock in summer, and at daylight in winter; part of them being employed before breakfast in dressing the little children, in cleaning about the house, and the boys in working a forcing pump, which supplies all the wards, and every part of the hospital, abundantly with water. At half past seven they breakfast, and at half after eight go into school, where they continue, the boys till twelve, and the girls a little later. At one o'clock they dine; and return to school at two, and stay there till five in summer, and in winter till dusk; except on Saturdays, when they have a half holiday. They are also instructed . . . in their catechism; and are occasionally employed in and about the house during play hours. At six o'clock in the evening they sup, and at eight go to bed.[33]

By the end of the century the children were spending a somewhat greater part of their time in the classroom. Also, twice a week for an hour they were taught to sing the Foundling hymns and anthems. But part of their training was still devoted to working with their hands. Now, however, instead of making twine and fish-nets or netting purses, the older boys spun worsted yarn or assisted the gardener, while the younger boys learned to knit stockings. Sewing still formed the girls' primary occupation: they sewed not only for the Hospital's own needs but also for people who paid to have shirts or other items made for them. Recreation, like all other aspects of their lives, was still closely supervised, but now the children could also count on immersion in the Cold Bath once a week, which some of the children looked upon as recreation but which the Hospital's staff regarded as a prescription to strengthen young bodies.[34]

Some changes in apprenticing practices also took place in the last quarter of the century. Most of them tended to increase the Governors' continuing control over the apprenticed child. Although, by custom, masters had from the beginning sought the Governors' consent to the transfer of an apprentice to another person, the refusal of a master in 1787 to honour this convention awakened the Governors to the fact that they possessed no legal means to prevent such occurrences: nothing in the indentures prevented a master from disposing of his apprentice in any way he chose. To remedy this defect, the Governors directed the Hospital's solicitor to draft a clause to be added to all indentures whereby the master must agree not to assign his apprentice to anyone 'without the consent & approbation of the said Governors & Guardians in writing for that purpose first had & obtained'. Once more the Hospital had anticipated public policy, for in 1792 Parliament forbade the transfer of pauper apprentices without the prior consent of the parish officers.[35]

The Governors tightened their control of apprenticeships again in 1791 by adding to the indentures another clause that required the master to give notice in writing to the Hospital before complaining of his apprentice to a magistrate, so that a representative of the Hospital might attend at the time of the child's examination.[36] Moreover, the Committee was able to investigate prospective masters far more thoroughly and to follow up apprenticeships far more efficiently during the twenty-five years from 1775 to 1799, when the number of children bound out averaged less than thirty a year, than the Governors had found it possible to do in the aftermath of the General Reception. In 1791, for example, the schoolmaster visited eighty-four apprenticed children.[37]

During the last quarter of the century the reports of the steward concerning prospective masters show that considerable efforts were also made to ascertain every applicant's background, financial stability, and family situation, and that neighbourhoods, too, were examined for potential harm to the child's morals. The unfavourable report on Joseph Eley, a hosier of 62 Lower East Smithfield, who applied for a female apprentice in 1785, typifies many such reports and indicates the closeness of inquiry:

> The Petitioner has not been set up in business above 2 or 3 months so that his Neighbours know nothing of him, he was before Shopman to a Hosier. He lives in a very small low rented house in East Smithfield among Seamen & the place thereabouts is of very ill repute for loose Women of the lowest Class. The persons referr'd to in the Petition give him the Character of an industrious Man but his Wife has been upon the Town & in the Magdalen since then, & her being married, she has been upon the Town again, & is of a very light Character now.[38]

As a consequence of such thoroughness, we find in the records fewer accounts of mistreated apprentices. But when instances did come to the Governors' attention—when they learned, for example, in 1780 that Judith Davis had been 'inhumanely beaten with a knotted whip Cord'—they moved as quickly as ever to take legal action on a child's behalf.[39] They also stood ready to help the apprenticed children in other ways. One boy complained to the Committee that his master, a silk dyer, was simply using him to perform menial tasks and had failed to teach him his trade; at the Committee's direction, the schoolmaster found the boy a new master (another silk dyer).[40] And on more than one occasion the Committee consulted the child's wishes in respect to a contemplated transfer of his indentures when the proposal did not arise because of his misconduct.[41]

Often, however, the transfers came about because of masters' dissatisfaction with their apprentices, although the records seldom specify the nature of their complaints against the children beyond 'much misconduct' or 'bad behaviour'. Occasionally we find a charge of theft lodged against a child. The Committee usually responded to the masters' charges by reprimanding the children—sometimes threatening a boy with being sent to sea—and by extracting promises of better behaviour. If this proved ineffective, the Committee assisted the master in arranging a transfer of his apprentice, often to sea service, which the Governors seem to have regarded as a cure for all disciplinary problems involving boys.[42] When girls gave evidence of being unmanageable, no such convenient remedy was available until the last two years of the century when the Governors hit upon the scheme of sending them, with an apprentice fee, to Samuel Oldknow, the great cotton manufacturer at Mellor, who bore the reputation of being an exceptionally humane employer. Oldknow soon put an end to this solution. On 14 June 1799 he wrote to the Hospital: 'Indeed the plan is altogether wrong to take young women apprentices such as from their refractory ungovernable tempers nobody else like to manage and I wish to be understood that unless I have an offer of four girls under twelve for one above—I do not wish to receive another offer'.[43]

A report prepared by the schoolmaster in 1798 indicated that out of 252 children then apprenticed, thirty-six were either 'not free from blame, but requiring judicious management' or had 'turned out ill', a failure rate of 14.3 percent.[44] Perhaps the rate was equally high, or higher, in previous years, but unfortunately no earlier survey was made, and, therefore, no basis for comparison exists. In 1805, however, the schoolmaster reported that out of fifty-three boys still apprenticed, four had been sent to sea for misconduct, three were 'complained of for misbehaviour but have promised amendment', and fourteen 'have absconded and gone to Sea', a failure rate of 40 percent.[45]

To this I must add my impression that the records for the last quarter of the century indicate the receipt of more complaints from masters proportionately than in earlier years. But why this should be so is hard to explain: the records offer no information except a statement in 1800 that many of the children in the latter part of their apprenticeships, 'finding they are working for victuals and clothes only, become dissatisfied and wish to get into other services from which they are to receive wages'.[46] Perhaps this indicates that the apprenticed foundlings, aware that many of their contemporaries were no longer being required to serve apprenticeships before practicing a trade, resented their own restricted positions. Beyond that hint I can only speculate. Perhaps masters had become more demanding. The treasurer reported in 1799 that the Hospital frequently placed boys with London shopkeepers who expected them to be able to write and keep accounts.[47] Perhaps, as we shall discuss in a later chapter, the very degree of education that masters now required of their apprentices actually militated against harmonious master-apprentice relationships, especially during the years of war at the end of the century when uneasiness permeated all of British society. Or perhaps no change actually occurred, but better follow-up procedures and more precise record-keeping have simply produced a general impression of increased difficulties with the apprenticed children.

Be that as it may, the majority of apprenticeships obviously turned out reasonably well, and the Governors used every means they could contrive to ensure their success. In addition to keeping an eye on the children while apprenticed—the girls being visited by the matron, the boys by the schoolmaster—the Governors revived in 1794 a custom, followed in the 1760s, of giving a gratuity to apprentices whose masters testified to their good behaviour upon completion of their service. From the masters' letters of recommendation we can deduce that the qualities desired were honesty, sobriety, and diligence.[48] In 1800 the Governors decided to add to the Instructions given to the children when they were placed out a paragraph stating:

And as a Proof that we still Interest ourselves in your future conduct, you are further to take notice (as an encouragement for you to follow the advice here given you) that if at the expiration of the term for which you are bound, you shall produce Testimonials to the Satisfaction of the Committee of your Regularity, Diligence and good behaviour during the above time you shall receive such pecuniary reward not exceeding the sum of five guineas as the Committee shall think you entitled to, together with a Certificate under the Seal of the Corporation as a mark of their approbation which you may retain and bear as a standing memorial of your good behaviour.[49]

Although the Governors seem to have experienced difficulties in the 1780s in finding masters who would take apprentices without fees—on at least four occasions the Committee resorted to advertising in the newspapers the availability of children for apprenticing—nevertheless they remained opposed to placing groups of girls with manufacturers. Probably this opposition sprang from an unsatisfactory incident in 1777 when the Governors discovered that twenty-five girls apprenticed to a mill at Stockport not only were scantily clothed but also spent all their time tying bobbins of silk as they broke and so learned no occupation by which to earn a living on reaching maturity. And this had occurred despite the owner's promise to teach the girls to sew and do household work.[50]

But in 1792, impressed by the secretary's report of his visit to the Cuckney Mills, operated by Messrs Toplis & Co., worsted manufacturers of Nottinghamshire, the Committee decided to apprentice to this firm twenty-five boys and ten girls over six years of age. The firm agreed to instruct the children in reading, writing and accounts; to send them to church every Sunday; to allow a local representative of the Hospital to visit the children from time to time and report his observations to the Committee; and either to find suitable masters for the children at age fourteen or to employ them in the firm's own business. The Cuckney Mills were already employing parish children, and, according to the secretary, their work was easy and not injurious to their health, and they were well treated in every respect.[51]

The secretary's observations were confirmed by the enthusiastic report of Joseph Moser describing his visit to the Cuckney Mills in April 1797. The children who came from various London parishes, from the Foundling Hospital, and from other charities appeared, he said, healthy and clean. They were neatly dressed in uniforms, the boys in 'a coat of brown mixed cloth, a green waistcoat, leather breeches, and good hats, shoes, and stockings', the girls in 'gowns of blue and white Manchester check, blue petticoats, and white beaver or felt hats, black stockings, and very good shoes'. The children's living quarters seemed also extremely neat and clean, and their food consisted of meat pies, suet puddings and brown bread. The mills were employing about four hundred children at the time of this visit, some of the boys working on the night shift, for the owners kept the machines in operation twenty-four hours a day. Nevertheless, said Moser, proper attention was being given to the education and religious training of all the children. And he contrasted the treatment of these children with the hardships endured by those employed in another mill in Yorkshire that he had visited earlier.[52]

But every Eden holds its serpent: by the spring of 1798 Messrs Toplis & Co. had fallen into bankruptcy, and the children were thrown upon a parish quite incapable of supporting so many of them. Through the prompt efforts of the Hospital's local representative, the Rev. Mr Hume, and the Committee, the Hospital's children were quickly transferred to apprenticeships with farmers and tradesmen or sent into sea service. Because of the humanitarianism and watchfulness of the Governors on this and other occasions, nearly all of the foundlings escaped the hardships suffered by the many pauper children who were sent by the cartload from London workhouses to the Lancashire and Yorkshire mills, where most of them were badly housed and fed and grossly overworked.[53]

Watchfulness, of course, was the key word in every situation where the children lived outside the Hospital's walls. In the last quarter of the century the Governors were also supervising the country nurses more closely than ever, no longer depending solely upon local inspectors but, in addition, sending a member of the Hospital's staff frequently to visit the nurses unannounced. Afterward, 'a written report is made by such visitor of the state of health and condition of each particular child by name', and this report was read at the next meeting of the Committee.[54] In the 1780s and 1790s such visitation became practicable because the children were being nursed in fewer places and much nearer to London than they were during the years of the General Reception. By 1794 the Hospital was placing its infants out to nurse in only five counties: Essex, Hertfordshire, Hampshire, Kent and Surrey.[55] A number of nurses still asked to keep the children they had cared for, and the Governors usually granted the requests and apprenticed the children to the nurses' husbands.

Most of the old problems with irresponsible inspectors and negligent nurses disappeared after the General Reception. The nurses who remained in the Hospital's service were well tested—one woman nursed a succession of its children over a period of twenty-seven years—and those added to its list had to come with high recommendations. The cost of nursing rose, however, and by 1795 the Governors found that a good nurse expected to receive 3s a week.[56] They paid willingly, for their old objectives of preserving infant lives and raising healthy children able to become self-sufficient and productive citizens never changed however much the Governors endeavoured to adapt their methods to changing conditions or sought better ways to achieve their goals.

12

Financial Security Achieved,
1771–1799

ALTHOUGH THE COST OF NURSING rose in the 1790s, the Hospital could pay its nurses 3s a week in 1795 with less strain than such payments would have imposed at any earlier period of its existence as a private charity, for in the last decade of the century its land proved to be its financial salvation. Until that time the Hospital's property had largely retained its rural character. Commercial activity near the Hospital had, in fact, decreased: after 1759 the Governors ceased renting the buildings at Powis Wells and had converted them, as well as the Coach and Horses Alehouse, into infirmaries.

But with the ending of Parliamentary support, the Governors began to think about other means of providing income for the institution. As early as 30 May 1770 the treasurer had recommended that, in addition to finding tenants for the Lamb Alehouse, the Coach and Horses, and the Powis Wells buildings, the Governors consider a plan to let a part of the Hospital's lands on building leases.[1] The proposal remained 'in contemplation' until 1775 when the General Court on 29 March resolved:

> . . . that the General Committee be empowered to receive proposals, treat, and agree for letting on one or more building Lease or Leases, for any Term not exceeding 99 years, the House & Garden called the Coach & Horses and also the land on the South Side of the Hospitals private Road leading to Grays Inn Lane from Lambs Conduit Street belonging to this Hospital; and that Plans of the said Land be made out by the Surveyor.[2]

But nothing came of this resolution except the execution on 15 April 1778 of a ninety-nine-year lease of the Coach and Horses building and adjoining land to William Harrison, one of the Governors, at a peppercorn rent for the first two years and £23 a year thereafter. The lease also required him to tear down the old building and to erect on the leased property, at a cost of about £3000, three houses to front upon Lamb's Conduit Street.[3] A year later the Governors let for ninety-nine years at £25 a year to John Kingston, one of their number, a small piece of ground at the northeast corner of Queen Square, on which he agreed to build a house at a cost of at least £2000. Because twenty-two residents of Queen Square signed a petition against this building project, claiming that it would 'deprive them of the Prospect wch they now enjoy' and, therefore, would lessen the value of their houses, the Governors required Mr Kingston to covenant, under penalty of £1000, that the front of his building would not project beyond the line of the other houses on the east side of the Square and that he would erect no building whatsoever on the land at the north end of the Square.[4]

From time to time a few additional proposals for taking small pieces of land on building leases came in, but they were not accepted: many of the Governors preferred to maintain the Hospital's rural situation, even though its isolation kept it vulnerable to thefts. That the area was still a dangerous one cannot be doubted: in 1784 the proprietor of the Blue Lyon in Gray's Inn Lane asked for and received permission to erect a watch box on the east wall of the Hospital's property near his place of refreshment and to station an armed guard there for the protection of his patrons.[5]

In the 1780s, however, the Governors' worries about the Hospital's financial problems resurrected the idea of devising a plan for the orderly development of the estate, with the expectation that the rents from building leases would rescue the Hospital from its difficulties. In March 1787 the General Court finally authorized such a scheme, and the Committee went so far as to advertise in the daily papers for persons interested in submitting designs for subdividing the estate.

But already the idea of developing the Hospital's lands was under attack. In April an anonymous pamphlet (almost certainly written by John Holliday, one of the Governors) appeared in opposition. It argued, first, that the erection of houses on the estate would thwart the original intention of the Earl of Salisbury who, the writer alleged, had been willing to sell his land only as a site for a hospital and for no other purpose; second, that with proper management and reduction in the number of children cared for—especially parish children who, he claimed, represented a financial loss to the institution—no real financial difficulties would exist; and, finally, that surrounding the Hospital with other buildings would cause deterioration in the healthy climate of the area and increase the number of deaths among the children.[6]

These arguments apparently carried weight with some of the Governors, for in June the General Court rescinded its previous resolution, stating

> . . . that it is the opinion of this Court that to erect any building on the lands belonging to this Hospital on which no buildings are already erected, by which a free & open circulation of wholsome air is now enjoyed by the children in the said Hospital, would be detrimental to their Health, and contrary to the original Institution of the Charity.[7]

But the October General Court resolved not to confirm this resolution, and in December the Court decided to develop the area south of the private road built some years before to connect the Hospital with Gray's Inn Lane.

Meanwhile, John Holliday and Dr Stephen White, the son of the former treasurer, Taylor White, were duelling with pamphlets, White contending for development of the Hospital's lands in imitation of the Portland and Bedford estates to the west, and Holliday disparaging the arguments of the 'learned divine' and reiterating his former assertions. He also added the objection that development was impractical because the Hospital lacked access to the west and north and possessed only a challengeable right to use Lamb's Conduit Street.[8]

The seesawing of policy, brought about by the disagreements among the Governors, came to an end when twenty-seven opponents of development, led by Holliday, petitioned Lord North, the president, to call a special General Court on 21 April 1788 to consider the propriety of granting leases of the Hospital's lands. The extraordinary attendance of ninety Governors, including seven members of the nobility who hardly ever attended meetings, testified to the importance of the issue. The outcome was a resolution—but one not passed unanimously—supporting the previous decision to proceed with development of the Hospital's estate.[9]

After this meeting the Governors did not waver. They quickly recognized the validity of Holliday's argument that lack of access to the west would handicap any development of that part of the estate and directed the treasurer to approach the Duke of Bedford with the suggestion that the opening of new streets to connect the Hospital's property with the Duke's private road (now Woburn Place) might benefit both estates. The Duke agreed to the proposal in 1794, thereby making possible the construction of Guilford, Bernard, and Great Coram Streets and Tavistock Place.

By that time a Building Committee of five Governors, appointed

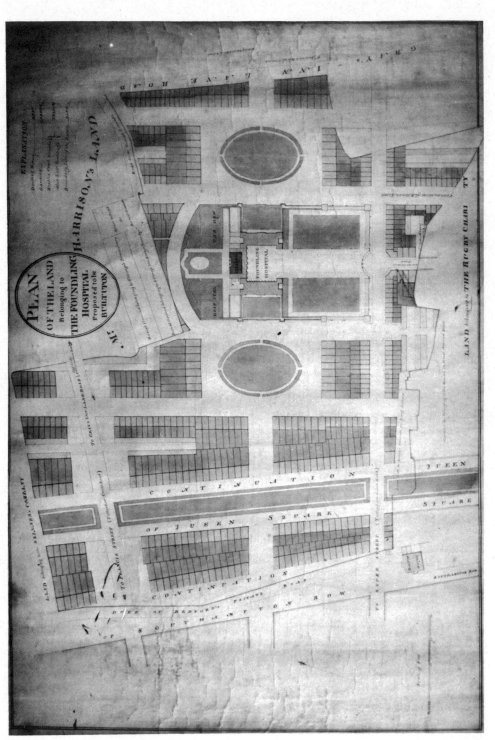

9. Merryweather's Building Plan for the Foundling Estate, 1792

on 30 June 1790, had been long at work, preparing plans and receiving proposals from prospective tenants. In December they submitted to the General Court the plan of Samuel Pepys Cockerell, the Hospital's architect, for laying out in building lots the lands east and southeast of the Hospital, together with Cockerell's statement of the principles that should govern the development of the estate. These, he said, were: first, to leave ample space around the Hospital itself and to surround it with buildings that would enhance its character; second, to attract speculative builders by allowing the erection of all grades of houses from first class to those renting for £25 per annum, provided that the location of the latter did not diminish the desirability of the former; third, to mesh the boundaries of the new development harmoniously with the adjoining built-up area, so that traffic between the two might flow smoothly; and fourth, to devise a plan capable of execution in parts, each complete in itself. Calculated at the lowest rate, Cockerell believed, the rents from the whole estate should amount to at least £4000 a year.[10]

The Governors, for the most part, followed Cockerell's principles, although they did not adopt his design for laying out the estate. Instead, they decided to develop first the lands west of the Hospital, and in March 1792 they selected the plan submitted by Thomas Merryweather, their own secretary. His plan provided for the extension of Queen Square to the Hospital's northern boundary and for the creation of two new squares east and west of the Hospital, connected by a semicircular street north of the institution's buildings. This street was never built, nor was Queen Square ever extended northward, but the two squares—Brunswick and Mecklenburgh—became the central features of the development that followed. True to Cockerell's first principle, however, the Governors reserved nine acres surrounding the Hospital for its own use.[11] By the end of the year the anticipated rents from the new leases granted on the western part of the estate, when added to those from the few earlier leases of lands fronting on Guilford and Lamb's Conduit Streets, amounted to £949 19s per annum.

The Building Committee had also contracted with James Burton for the sale of clay from the west field for making brick. He agreed to pay 2s 6d per thousand bricks and to manufacture them at the northwest corner of the estate in order to prevent smoke pollution in the area of the Hospital.[12] From this beginning Burton very quickly became the chief speculative builder on the estate. In all, he built 586 houses, commencing with those on the west side of Lansdowne Place. Brunswick Square, which he once proposed naming Rockingham Square in tribute to the Duke of Portland, who became the Hospital's president in 1793, was largely Burton's creation. Not only did he build the houses on its south and west sides, but in 1796 he also enclosed the square with 'good cast Iron Palisadoes 5 feet high' and laid out its walks and gardens. The Hospital shared part of the expense in order to 'give great Chearfulness and appearance of success to the Whole Plan ... and by so much contribute to the earlier letting of the Ground on the North side of the Square and at a better Rent'.[13]

By 1797, however, the war with France had brought building activity almost to a stop, partly because of scarcities of materials and partly because of difficulties in obtaining credit. The Governors, therefore, found it advisable to extend Burton's contract so as to permit a year's delay in finishing the houses then under construction and a similar delay in beginning the payment of rents. Very wisely, the Governors also promoted the development of their lands by using a portion of the Hospital's capital to assist builders with loans on the security of the buildings and through purchases of the profit rents.[14]

The development of the estate inevitably created new problems. There were legal snarls to untangle in order to obtain an undisputable right to the use of the part of Lamb's Conduit Street that ran across lands belonging to the Trustees of the Rugby School.[15] There were prolonged negotiations with Henry Doughty, an adjoining landowner, for the exchange of small pieces of property at the southeast corner of the estate to enable the Hospital to extend Guilford Street to Gray's Inn Lane.[16] There was even a lawsuit against the Hospital in 1792, brought in the Court of Chancery by the Attorney General for an injunction to restrain the Hospital from granting any further building leases. The Attorney General's case, based on information supplied by Edward G. Lind, one of the disgruntled Governors, made use of essentially the same arguments Holliday had advanced four years earlier. Lind probably had more at heart than the children's health: he was now occupying the house that John Kingston had built at the northeast corner of Queen Square upon the land leased to him by the Governors in 1789, and, we may presume, wanted to preserve his view of the distant hills of Highgate and Hampstead. The case was heard on 23 and 24 January 1793, and the Court, unimpressed by the plaintiff's arguments, did not even call upon the Hospital's counsel for his defense before refusing to grant the injunction. It took six years, however, for the Governors to collect £105 from Lind to reimburse the Hospital for a part of the legal expenses that his complaint to the Attorney General had caused.[17]

Another kind of legal difficulty arose from the Governors' desire to restrict commercial activity on the estate. To achieve this end a clause that required occupants of buildings to obtain a license from the Governors before opening a shop or public house was written into all leases. In 1797 the Governors tightened their control still further by adding a new clause designed to limit a tenant's right to assign such a license to another person.

Moreover, the Governors tried to confine commerce to one place by designating for occupancy as shops the buildings in the narrow street lying north of Guilford Street and west of Grenville Street, known as the Colonnade. Even there they ruled out any activities likely to prove objectionable. A tallow chandler, for example, was allowed to open a shop but 'no melting [was] to be permitted on the Premises'. What could happen when such restrictions were ignored was related by Henry Layton, a carpenter who had built three houses in Millman Street on building leases and then sublet them to respectable tenants. In September 1797 he asked for the Governors' assistance, telling them that

> . . . a most daring and unbecoming Nuisance has crept in, viz, a Person openly carrying on at the corner of the said respectable Street, night and Day (Sunday not excepted) the Business of Oyster opener, and dealer in Fish, throwing the Shells and putrid Fish in contempt and defiance about the Inhabitants Doors to the great loss of your Petitioner, whose Tenants already threaten to leave his Premises if the above Nuisance is not removed.

All this had come about because the proprietor of a public house allowed the fishmonger to place his stand on the pavement in front of the door to the publican's establishment.[18]

In addition to the legal problems, there was also the problem of making certain that the builders on the estate did not employ sleazy materials and shoddy workmanship. The Governors had good reason to be watchful, for walls had collapsed and cellars had caved in. And in 1796 a member of the Building Committee detected the use of poorly made bricks and scrimping on timbers despite weekly inspections by the Hospital's architect, Cockerell. Even Burton, to whom the Governors granted so many leases, was not faultless: in 1796 the Governors found it necessary to direct him to take down the front and back walls of four houses that he was building in Guilford Street because of his failure to use proper bricks. Yet the Governors realized that if they insisted on too high a standard of construction, especially when builders were suffering from war-time shortages, they might discourage speculative builders from taking leases on the estate at all.[19] Their dilemma was how to find a middle course between so great a demand for perfection as to scare off speculative builders and so little care for the quality of building as to produce houses that would rapidly become slums, and they never arrived at a wholly satisfactory solution.

There was also the continuing problem of trying to ensure order and safety in the area, for increasing urbanization had not discouraged robbery or vandalism. In fact, the presence of the Hospital's new stuccoed wall along Lansdowne Place and Guilford Street seemed actually to invite attack by writers of indecent graffiti, so much so that in 1794 the Governors considered protecting the walls with an iron railing. In 1796 they stationed a constable at the Hospital's gates to deal with vagrants and disorderly persons. They also discussed whether a watch box at the south-west corner of the wall might provide additional protection.[20] More serious was the ever present possibility that persons going out in the evening might be robbed in their own neighbourhood. In 1792 a gentleman returning from Highgate to Holborn lost his watch and three guineas to four footpads who accosted him in Gray's Inn Lane at the corner of the Hospital's property.[21] The Governors, of course, could do little to prevent such incidents despite their concern for the estate's reputation: the hazard was not peculiar to that part of London but rather was a risk taken by any person who ventured into a little-travelled spot, especially at night.

Finally there was the problem of collecting rents from slow-paying or, occasionally, bankrupt tenants. One of the Hospital's tenants who became bankrupt owed more than two years' rent, amounting to £47 5s. In October 1797 the Governors found it necessary to send notices to a large number of tenants, giving them a month in which to pay their arrears or face legal action. The threat elicited payments from twenty-seven tenants. But this did not end the problem of rent delinquencies, for in April 1798 the Hospital's tenants were still £1585 11s 1d in arrears.[22]

In spite of the many difficulties, however, the venture into estate development proved to be doubly successful. In the short run, the rentals quickly produced a substantial increase in the Hospital's income (by 1799 they amounted to £3045 12s 4d a year) thereby permitting the Hospital to increase the number of children taken in. Over the long term, the results of the Governors' decision to develop the estate proved even more impressive. By the middle of the nineteenth century the annual ground rentals equalled the original purchase price of the entire property. By 1893, when many of the ninety-nine-year leases were expiring, the rentals amounted to £13,628, and by 1908 they had reached £25,000 a year. By 1926, when the estate was sold, the annual rentals had risen to £42,000, and

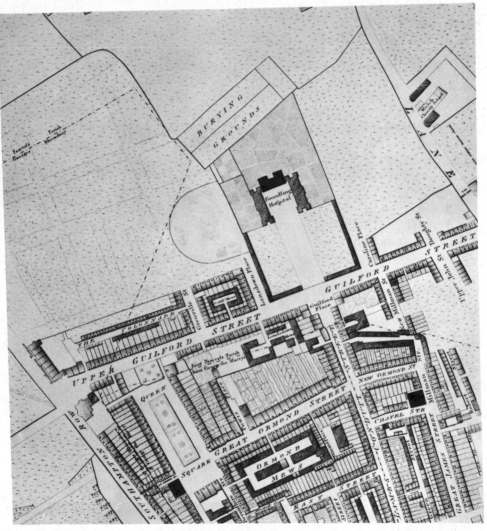

10. Section of Horwood's 1799 Map of London showing the Foundling Hospital Estate

the sale of the property in that year for £1,650,000 assured the continuance of the institution's work with children down to the present day.[23] Thus, the wise use of the Hospital's land guaranteed its survival in comfortable security.

The greater part of the estate's development still lay ahead in 1799, but even then a visitor to that part of London would have found it very different from what his grandfather might have seen in 1742 when the Hospital acquired its fifty-six acres from the Earl of Salisbury. The Hospital's own buildings, of course, dominated the area and were joined to the city on the south and west by paved streets: Guilford, Millman, Grenville, and Lamb's Conduit Streets, Guilford Place, Lansdowne Place, a portion of Caroline Place (now Mecklenburgh Place), and portions of Bernard and Doughty Streets. All of these streets by 1799 were solidly built up with architecturally undistinguished, four-storey houses, constructed of cream-coloured bricks, topped with slate roofs, and ornamented externally only by brick arches framing the doors, simple fanlights, and, in some cases, bay windows or French windows opening onto iron balconies. The observer of 1799 would discover, too, that the south side of Brunswick Square had been completed, although some of the houses remained unoccupied, and that Guilford Street now ran without interruption from Southampton Row to Gray's Inn Lane.

The rest of the land to the west he would find open: the lines of Tavistock Place, Great Coram and Bernard Streets, as well as those of the streets that would eventually connect them, had been laid out, but that was all. Proceeding along the Hospital's north and east boundaries, the end-of-the-century visitor, like his grandfather, would still have walked through open fields, for in 1799 Mecklenburgh Square, originally proposed to be called Coram Square, existed only on paper. Nevertheless, the estate was well on its way to urbanization.[24]

But not only had the Hospital's estate taken on a new appearance, the Hospital, too, had changed in the course of the century. Without ever losing sight of its original commission to extend protection to deserted infants, the institution's methods for achieving its ends had moved, as we have seen, nearer to modern ideas of casework with children. Yet some things had not changed at all: a week before Christmas 1799 a baby girl was found abandoned at the Hospital's gates.[25]

PART III

The Consequences

The adoption of an helpless unprotected infant, the watching over its progress to maturity, and the fitting it to be useful to itself and others here, and to attain eternal happiness hereafter,—these are no common or ordinary acts of beneficence.

Thomas Bernard, *Reports of the Society for Bettering the Condition and Increasing the Comforts of the Poor*, IV, 1803.

13

Managing the Institution

THE FOUNDATION ON WHICH the administrative structure of the Foundling Hospital rested consisted of its large body of Governors. The Royal Charter had appointed 375 of them; others were added by election at General Courts. From time to time a few were elected because of special services to the institution, but most became eligible by pledging an annual contribution of five guineas or by making a gift to the Hospital of at least £50 (reduced in 1772 to £30). So large an amount—more than double the twenty guineas required to become a life governor of the Magdalen House—ensured that the life Governors would all be men of substance.

There was, of course, no provision for electing a woman Governor regardless of how large a donation she might give. But the clause in the Parliamentary Act of 1740 that eliminated any requirement for a Governor or officer of the Hospital 'to take the sacrament of the Lord's supper, or any oath or oaths whatsoever'[1] as a prerequisite to election did open the ranks of the Governors to men holding a diversity of religious and political views. And throughout the century, the Governors were a heterogeneous lot. Among them at almost any time one might find clergymen, merchants, naval and military officers, lawyers, doctors, bankers, artists, musicians, country gentlemen, and peers of the realm. In personality and background they ranged from the hard-working, serious but sometimes eccentric, Anglican philanthropist, Jonas Hanway, a man of modest means, to the inordinately wealthy, but patriotic and generous, Jewish merchant, Sampson Gideon; from the parsimonious treasurer, George Whatley, who melted down the sealing wax from incoming letters for re-use, to the learned physician, botanist, and collector, Sir Hans Sloane; from the earnest Evangelical banker, Henry Thornton, to the notorious politician and publisher of the *North Briton*, John Wilkes, who, it is said, once attended a General

Court 'in a gay and rather fantastic dress attended by a couple of dogs' and 'sat much observed',[2] which was scarcely surprising.

That disagreements did not occur often among such dissimilar men can be accounted for chiefly by the fact that most of the Governors rarely attended meetings. As Jonas Hanway put it, 'many people give money, who will not give anything else',[3] least of all their time. The day-to-day direction of the Hospital's affairs lay in the hands of the fifty members of the General Committee, whom the Governors elected each year at the annual meeting, and who met every Wednesday to transact the Hospital's business. One might, therefore, have expected that the rest of the Governors could find time to attend the four quarterly Courts in March, June, September, and December, and the annual meeting in May.

But such an expectation was seldom realized. Unless some controversy, such as the debate engendered by the proposal to develop the Hospital's estate, engaged the Governors' interest, or unless the Governors were filling an important post—morning preacher, apothecary, surgeon, organist, treasurer—for which there were rival candidates, attendance at quarterly and annual Courts averaged considerably less than fifty. In fact, the seven Governors who attended the March quarterly Court in 1766 could not hold a meeting for lack of a quorum. And it was not unusual for the attendance at annual meetings to number less than thirty even though the occasion was always marked by a lavish dinner and an edifying procession around the table of the children singing hymns. Even when elections or controversial issues aroused greater interest, the attendance seldom reached a hundred. The largest meeting after the first in 1739 occurred in 1791: 140 Governors turned out to vote on the two candidates for the office of treasurer.[4]

Attendance at the weekly Committee meetings was no better. The first few meetings saw twenty-two to thirty-one Governors present, but thereafter during 1740, 1741, and 1742 nine to twelve was the average, and by October 1740 one meeting had already been adjourned for want of a quorum. This pattern did not change throughout the century: in the mid-sixties the average attendance was eight or nine; in the nineties, ten to twelve.

The Subcommittee, which, beginning in 1748, met every Saturday morning to audit bills and take care of any other pressing matters, by mid-century often consisted of only two or three Governors. In the seventies the usual attendance was four to six. By 1794 the minutes indicate that the Subcommittee had not met for some time, and intermittent neglect of such meetings seems to have continued during the rest of the century.

Both at the beginning of the Hospital's operations and in the last decade of the century, the Governors attempted to establish daily visiting committees, but such efforts did not last long. Special committees, of course, were appointed from time to time for various purposes, e.g., the Building Committee in the 1790s, but they usually consisted of Governors who attended General Committee meetings regularly. It is apparent, then, that throughout the century, the Governors left the day-to-day running of the institution in the hands of a very small group of men even though a considerable number of them felt their responsibilities strongly enough to attend when any major issue had to be decided.[5]

Few of this small group of active Governors were members of the nobility, although such men were often named to the General Committee. Up to the spring of 1740 apparently the novelty of the enterprise had engaged the attention of the Dukes of Montagu, Portland, and Richmond, the Earls of Chesterfield, Cholmondeley, Findlater, and Abercorn, Viscount Torrington, and Lords Gower, de la Warr, Lovel, and Vere Beauclerk, as well as that of the Duke of Bedford, the president, who presided over half a dozen meetings. The interest of the Earls of Abercorn and Findlater and that of Lord Vere Beauclerk and his wife continued for some years, but that of the others dropped markedly from 1740 onward. For the most part, those who guided the affairs of the Hospital in its first three years were men whom we would today characterize as substantial, middle-class citizens. In addition to Captain Coram, there were the vice-presidents, John Milner, Martin Folkes, an antiquary, Peter Burrell and William Fawkener, both merchants. And there were also Taylor White, a barrister; the banker, Sir Joseph Hankey; the architect, Theodore Jacobsen; Peter Sainthill, a surgeon; James Vernon; Lewis Way; John Waple, who was accountant general for the Court of Chancery; Alexander Hume Campbell, the Lord Register of Scotland; and a group of physicians that included Dr Benjamin Avery, Sir Hans Sloane, and Dr Robert Nesbitt, who attended over seventy-five meetings in the first three years.

Essentially the same pattern persisted through the rest of the century. From 1758 to 1765 Jonas Hanway and George Whatley dominated the Subcommittee, often being the only Governors present. In the 1770s William Harrison and Thomas Nugent joined Whatley in regular attendance at such meetings, and these men plus a few others were still faithfully attending them in the 1780s. By the end of the century others had replaced them, but the circle of active Governors still included no members of the nobility. It did, however, include a few medical men and Taylor White's son, the Reverend

Dr Stephen White, who also served as treasurer from 1791 to 1795.

This brings us to a characteristic of the whole body of Governors that explains, at least in part, the feeling of continuity that we sense in the policies of the Hospital: there was a considerable continuity of family representation among its Governors. Over the century their number embraced not only Taylor White and his son, Stephen, but also his son, Taylor White, Jr, as well as several generations of Heathcotes, Hoares, Hankeys, Meads, Milners, Nesbitts, Burrells, Plumptres, and Thorntons.

Continuity also characterized the officers of the Hospital. In addition to the long term of office of Taylor White, who became treasurer in 1745 and served for twenty-seven years, another treasurer, George Whatley, served for twelve years from 1779 to 1791. Many of the vice-presidents, of whom there were six at any one time, performed their duties for equally long terms. Lord Vere Beauclerk, for example, served from 1739 to 1756 and again from 1758 to 1767, and the deeply religious Earl of Dartmouth served from 1755 to 1802. Jonas Hanway was a vice-president for fiteen years until his death. Even the institution's secretaries provided continuity. There were only five in the eighteenth century, and two, Harman Verelst, the first secretary, and Thomas Collingwood, served for fifteen and thirty-two years respectively.[6]

As Boswells of the institution, all of its secretaries and treasurers kept meticulously detailed records, to which the Governors frequently referred for data and precedents on which to base their decisions. Thus, these records—an unacknowledged recognition of the importance of the past to the future—also promoted continuity. But, as we have seen and shall see, continuity never barred innovation.

Another characteristic of many of the Governors, both active and passive, was their tendency to have more than one charitable or civic interest. Dr Avery served as a trustee of Guy's Hospital and also of Dr Williams's Library. James Vernon was one of Dr Bray's Associates and a Trustee for the Colony of Georgia. We have already noted Hanway's many philanthropic concerns, several of which his fellow Governor, Robert Dingley, also shared. The Thorntons—John, who acted as treasurer of both the Magdalen House and the Marine Society, and his son Henry—had multiple philanthropic interests, and this was equally true of Sir Joseph Hankey, Sampson Gideon, Henry Hoare, Nathaniel Cholmley, and the Earl of Dartmouth, to name only a few. But as a final example, consider the activities of Thomas Bernard, the retired solicitor who held the office of treasurer at the end of the century. He helped to found the Society for Bettering the Condition and Increasing the Comforts of the Poor, worked for the establishment of the Royal Institution and the School for the Indigent Blind, and was the prime mover in opening a free chapel for the poor in the notorious Seven Dials neighbourhood.[7]

So far as possible the Governors tried to exclude self-interest in their relationships with the Hospital. The By-laws adopted in 1740 provided that:

> No Committee shall Contract for or Purchase any thing what-soever for use of the Hospital, in which any Governor and Guardian has any Property, Interest, or Concern (Land or Houses only excepted). Nor shall the General Court or Committee Elect any Governor and Guardian of the Hospital into any Place or Office of this Corporation to which any Salary shall be annexed.[8]

And in 1792 the General Court resolved:

> . . . that the following addition be made to the fourth By Law of this Corporation, vizt. And in all cases where any debate or controversy shall arise concerning any matter wherein the private interest of any Governor of this Hospital shall interfere with the interest of this Corporation, such Governor, or Governors, shall have no right to debate or vote, but shall (after having stated his or their case) withdraw until the matter is determined.[9]

Except for the actions of Mr Lind in trying to prevent the development of the estate, the Governors seem to have kept steadfastly to these resolutions.

Not only were the Governors determined to avoid evil, they were equally intent upon shunning any appearance of it. Because the Hospital had been a controversial project at its inception and had stirred up public discussion, much of it hostile, during the General Reception, the Governors became unusually sensitive to any rumour of scandal or unfavourable notice in the newspapers and sought constantly to present the Hospital in the best possible light. For example, in 1745, they ordered the following advertisement to be published in the *Daily Advertiser and London Courant* and in the *General Evening Post*:

> Whereas, It has been industriously reported That many of the Children in this Hospital have died, and That others of them are dangerously Ill, by eating of Milk since the Distemper has been amongst the Cows: This is therefore to assure the Publick That the said Report is intirely false and groundless; For that the Children

are in perfect Health, and that there has not one died in the House since the 27th of February last. They have eat no Milk, nor has any been used in the said Hospital for six Weeks past.

By Order of the Committee.[10]

But from time to time gossip, which ranged from charges that the Governors were deliberately breeding up the children in ignorance so that they would become better servants to stories alleging that the inoculation of the foundlings against smallpox caused them to suffer from scrofula and other diseases, forced the Governors into combat. They also had to worry about reports that they showed special preference in admitting children; that nurses forcibly drugged children while transporting them to the country hospitals; that members of the Committee had abetted a defaulting steward in his acts and had aided him in escaping from his sureties; that the Governors did not give proper regard to the character and circumstances of persons to whom they apprenticed the foundlings, so that many of them had been bound to infamous persons; or that the porter had rudely turned away persons seeking to attend services in the chapel. And the years did not lessen the propensity of Londoners to spread malicious tales about the institution: in 1799 the circulation of a story that the children were ill cared for by their country nurses brought about the Governors' decision to display the children newly returned from the country 'in a conspicuous situation' in the chapel during the following Sunday's services.[11]

The Governors fought back with such weapons as they could command to offset gossip with favourable news. They frequently gave to the newspapers what we would today call a press release whenever unusually large sums turned up in the charity boxes, or when the Hospital received anonymous benefactions, or when inquiries seeking advice came in from foreign institutions, or on any other occasion when the Hospital's activities could be portrayed in an advantageous light.[12] They published Dr William Cadogan's treatise, *An Essay upon Nursing, and the Management of Children From their Birth to Three Years of Age*, in 1748. In 1749 they sent four framed pictures of the Hospital to Ralph Allen at Bath, asking him to hang one in each of the Great Rooms, one in the Pump Room, and one in the Coffee House. In the same year they ordered the steward and messenger to take two of the boys with them whenever they went out on the Hospital's business, thereby letting the general public see some of the children. Encouraging inspection of the children and visitation of the art collection by fashionable London society, and making sure that the boys worked on their fish nets in public view, served the same purpose.

They held public baptismal services for newly admitted infants, either at the Sunday morning services or following Sunday evening prayer. They directed the Reader in 1784 to hold services in the chapel every morning during Passion Week to show the public their attention to the children's religious training. And in the 1760s the Governors even considered for a time the advantages that might accrue if they were to change the institution's name from Foundling Hospital to Orphan Hospital because of 'the general notions of the common people that the name Foundling carrys with it the Idea of contempt, and that of Orphan of compassion'. Their object in all of these efforts was, as the minutes recorded in 1772, 'to give the world just impressions of the Humanity and Utility of this Charitable Foundation', but otherwise, as the secretary once put it, to avoid making 'too much noise'. A public relations expert today would, I suppose, say that the Governors endeavoured to maintain a low profile for the Hospital except when it could show a favourable one.[13]

The Governors did not always act wisely or harmoniously—on occasion some of them were as blinded by petty vanity or as resentful of the ideas of newcomers as the rest of mankind—but their disagreements most often arose from honest differences of opinion about what was best for the Hospital. And usually they based their judgments on practical knowledge of business affairs and public psychology, on past experience, and, most of all, on humanitarian concern for the welfare of the children under their care.

In the eighteenth century the concept of an executive director, of course, still lay in the future. But, in practice, the Hospital's treasurer performed that function because he was the only Governor who lived at the Hospital. Occupying the spacious separate quarters at the south end of the east wing, he inevitably became more involved in the daily routines of the institution and was more often called upon to resolve minor problems on his own initiative than the rest of the Governors. This did not, however, prevent any of the treasurers from pursuing other interests. Taylor White, a barrister with a large practice on the Northern Circuit, had necessarily to be away from London during sessions of court. Sir Charles Whitworth, his successor, was a Member of Parliament and spent considerable time on legislative matters. And Thomas Bernard, although retired from his profession, was kept busy by his many philanthropic interests. In short, no one regarded the office of treasurer as a full-time job, but, in fact, all of the treasurers devoted many hours to their duties at the

Hospital. Bernard, it is said, even went so far as to sit at the head of the boys' table at dinner every day while his wife presided over the girls.[14]

The presidents, on the other hand, did little more than lend the prestige of their names to clothe the institution in respectability and preside at Courts on occasions of great moment. Over the century only three men held this office: the Duke of Bedford (1739–1771), Lord North (1771–1793), and the Duke of Portland (1793–1809). After 1758 the Hospital also enjoyed the prestige of the King's protection: George II became the institution's patron in 1758, and George III followed his grandfather's example two months after his accession to the throne.[15]

Women, as we have seen, played no part in the governing of the Hospital, although the Governors welcomed their legacies and benefactions and sought their aid as country inspectors. They always gave serious consideration to the opinions of the inspectresses and of the Governors' wives who visited the Hospital and frequently followed their advice.[16] But even this small degree of participation—and it was small indeed, for few women ever offered suggestions—lessened in the last half of the century. After 1757 the minutes do not mention the receipt of any feminine advice about the management of the Hospital. In an age that produced such extraordinary women as Lady Mary Wortley Montagu, Hannah More, Mary Wollstonecraft, and Selina, Countess of Huntingdon, it is surprising to find that none of them interested themselves in the affairs of the Hospital. Perhaps these women were too busy with their other concerns. Perhaps some women turned their humanitarian impulses toward charities that could be pursued under the aegis of the Church because of increasingly refined notions about the propriety of respectable women devoting time to an institution that had become the centre of so much criticism during the General Reception. Perhaps the ebb and flow of fashions in charities dictated the interests of others. Or perhaps later generations of Governors, preferring to keep matters in their own hands, discouraged feminine advice. However it was, I can only speculate on the reasons, for the records offer no solid evidence.

But if women had nothing to do with making policy, they had everything to do with carrying it out as it affected the physical care of the children. The Hospital employed wet and dry nurses, schoolmistresses, coatmakers, cooks, kitchen servants, laundresses, housemaids, and, during the years of the General Reception, a washer of the dead. The number varied from time to time. During the General Reception, the female employees of the Hospital numbered sixty-six; in the early 1770s the number averaged twenty-four; by 1788 it had risen to thirty-three; and it continued close to that level until at least 1795.[17]

Presiding over the women was the matron, the only woman among the ranks of subordinate officers, a group that also included the steward, apothecary, schoolmaster, clerk, and secretary. One would like to know more about these women, but the records afford few glimpses of them. One, at least, came from a very respectable background: Elizabeth Leicester, who became matron in 1759, was the daughter of an army captain and the sister of a Prebendary of Peterborough. Some of the others seem to have been strong-minded women: Mrs Leicester's predecessor, Susan French, resigned because the Governors refused to give her an increase in salary and the power to discharge nurses and female servants 'on a Minutes warning'. And in 1775 the Governors discharged Mrs Farrer because she flatly declined to sit in the centre front of the chapel gallery during the Sunday services. On the other hand, Jemima Jones, who served as matron in the early 1790s, appears to have been a weaker woman, unable to obtain obedience and respect from the other female employees or to work harmoniously with members of the staff—her particular bête noire being the apothecary, Mr McClellan. Her successor, Mrs Johnson, liked him no better and once drenched him with a pail of water.[18]

Robert McClellan officiated as the Hospital's resident apothecary for forty-two years and undoubtedly in the later part of his life, vexed by gout and age, became crotchety and set in his ways. He was, Lievesley tells us, sometimes vulgar in his speech: on one occasion, probably to annoy Mrs Johnson, he picked up a turkey drumstick at dinner and, showing it to the matron, said to her, 'It reminds me of a Clyster Pipe'.* Yet this same man wrote several hymns, which were set to music by Dr Cooke and used in the chapel, and having received four guineas for a cantata** that he composed, he gave the money to the chapel. Certainly, the Governors thought well of him: upon his retirement in 1797, they voted him a resolution of thanks and a gratuity of £50, which equalled a year's salary.[19]

McClellan was not the only employee whom the Governors rewarded for faithful service. A number of instances of gifts to employees leaving the Hospital's service because of old age or illness appear in the records. To one aged nurse who had no relatives or friends to help her the Governors gave a pension of £5 per annum. In 1755 they paid the cost of an attendant for a steward, who had been

* A clyster pipe was an instrument for administering an enema.
** The cantata was *The Redbreast*, set to music by John Stanley in 1784.

175

admitted to the Charter House as a pensioner, because his infirmities made constant care necessary. They continued to employ a spinning mistress, too old and feeble to do much work, at a guinea a year because she had nowhere else to go. A schoolmistress who became ill was sent into the country to regain her health at the Hospital's expense, and on several other occasions when employees fell sick, the Governors arranged for their care in hospitals. They gave a brewer who was badly scalded in the course of his work two guineas for his loss of time, and the widow of a messenger received £4 from the Committee to help her pay the debts resulting from his long illness. Moreover, in 1770 when the Governors found it necessary to discharge a number of nurses and servants to reduce expenses, they gave those discharged a month's wages plus a gratuity of five shillings.[20] From all of this we might conclude that the Governors were assisting their employees with an early form of old-age, unemployment, and workmen's compensation benefits. But such a conclusion would not be warranted because the employees possessed no rights to any such payments. What was given to them was given out of charitable consideration of individual cases. It, therefore, tells us more about the Governors' humanitarianism and paternalistic sense of responsibility for their staff than it does about their social progressiveness.

What the Governors expected in return for kindly consideration was, first of all, that their employees have had the smallpox, be Protestant, and, beginning in 1746 (probably as a reaction to the Forty-Five) take the Oaths of Allegiance, Supremacy, and Abjuration. But, of more importance, they demanded absolute subordination and obedience, together with a willingness to live largely cut off from contact with the outside world, for they required most of the employees to live in the Hospital. Female employees were not allowed to go outside the gates without permission from the matron, and such absences, in 1760 at least, were limited to one day a month. Even the secretary, matron, and other minor officers could not absent themselves from the Hospital without the approval of the treasurer, Committee, or Subcommittee. No resident of the Hospital might stay out later than nine o'clock in the evening in winter and ten o'clock in summer without authorization from the treasurer, nor were any of them privileged to frequent the alehouses near the Hospital. In fact, they were forbidden to drink 'spirituous Liquors' at all or to gamble. And the Governors discouraged visitors calling upon nurses and servants by laying down a rule that all visits had to take place in the servants' hall. No perquisites were allowed, and the

Governors made clear to all from the start of their employment that they could be discharged without notice.

Such restrictions could hardly have accorded with the natural desires of a group, most of whom were single and under forty years of age, for the Governors had established a firm policy of engaging no employee over that age, except a steward, matron, or chief nurse, for whom they set an age limit of fifty. Undoubtedly, the enforced intimacy of so small a community accounts for some of the quarrels among the employees that from time to time disturbed the peace and quiet that the Governors were at all times trying to maintain.[21]

Certainly, so monastic a life proved intolerable to many of the employees. Of the 380 female servants and nurses employed between 1758 and 1771, 129 quit and two left to be married—a voluntary resignation rate of 34 percent. A few left or were discharged because of illness, and wet nurses were dismissed when their services were not needed. Four died while in the Hospital's service, and many dismissals are unexplained. But where explanations appear in the records, the most common reasons for dismissal seem to have been inability to do the work; quarrelsome, abusive, or disobedient behaviour; offending the matron; ill treatment of the children; drunkenness; and moral misconduct, which included 'lying out o'nights'. Seventeen percent of the women suffered dismissal for such reasons, which would indicate some degree of chafing under the strictness of the Hospital's discipline, a premise also supported by the fact that the term of employment for many of the women lasted less than a year.

For the male employees, which included, in addition to the minor officers already mentioned, a messenger, one or more clerks, a gardener, brewer and baker, porter, and watchmen, the records indicate a similar situation. From 1760 to 1771 forty-two men were employed. Fourteen of them quit, and one steward absconded with over £600 of the Hospital's funds—a voluntary termination rate of 35.7 percent. One man was dismissed for violently beating a boy, one for laziness, three for drunkenness, and seven for unstated reasons. Eight of the men remained in the Hospital's service a year or less.[22]

It is apparent, then, that during the period of the General Reception and its aftermath, the Hospital experienced a substantial turnover in its staff, and the number of voluntary resignations suggests a considerable degree of dissatisfaction on the part of the employees. Whether isolation from outside contacts was the principal cause for such dissatisfaction cannot be said. Possibly some employees thought the work too arduous for the salaries paid, for in 1780 the matron advised the Subcommittee that she could not secure laundry maids at the former salaries of £6 and £8 a year to replace two who were dismissed, and that salaries of £8 and £10 would have to be paid in order to attract servants of good character. And in 1784 the Committee, recognizing in its minutes that the nurses of the boys' wards were very incompetent, added that the 'wages paid them is not sufficient to procure proper Servants'.

On the other hand, although the subordinate officers could take almost no independent action, could make no purchases, order no work performed by outside workmen, nor hire or discharge any employee without the Governors' authorization, nevertheless a number of them evidently found their situation comfortable, enjoying the privileges of private rooms and meals served at a separate table, and stayed on for many years. We have already noted the long service of the apothecary, Robert McClellan, and of several secretaries. One of the schoolmasters also reinforced the stability of the staff: Robert Atchison, who despite his poor vision, taught the boys for nearly forty years.[23] Thus, the thread of continuity in personnel, as well as in policy, tied the years together.

14

Money, Money, Money

THE GETTING AND SPENDING of money formed, necessarily, one of the Governors' primary concerns: it was the engine that moved all other activities. And getting it in sufficient quantities remained a problem throughout the century. The principal sources, other than Parliament's grants, were legacies, gifts, annual or special subscriptions, income from investments, and rents. Lesser sums came in from the children's work, tolls charged for use of the Hospital's private road, sale of gravel taken from its lands, and the like.

The Committee at its first meeting on 29 November 1739 recognized the priority of fund raising: its first instruction to the treasurer was 'to apply to the Executors or Trustees of Persons who have left or shall leave Legacies to this Charity to receive the same'. This action soon brought about the payment from the estate of Josiah Wordsworth of £500, a sum that he had bequeathed in 1732 contingent upon the coming into existence of an institution to care for foundlings. It also resulted in the discovery of several similar bequests, the collection of which, however, required lawsuits or prolonged negotiations to extract payment from reluctant fiduciaries. But some executors paid willingly even when not legally obligated to do so. In 1741, for example, John Dekewer, the executor of the estate of Benjamin Devinck, honoured the deceased man's request to give the Hospital £50 out of his estate even though his will did not mention this request. And in 1742 the widow and daughters of Samuel Holden consented to give the Hospital £2000 out of Holden's residuary estate, which he had designated for unspecified charitable purposes, because they held 'a favorable opinion of this charity'. Another legacy that was promptly paid came from across the Atlantic: a bequest of £100 from Charles Pym, who died in 1741, a resident of the Island of St Christopher.[1]

The legacy from Charles Pym headed a parade of benefactions

from other parts of the world, indicating that news of the Hospital's activities had circulated widely, probably because of the number of merchants among the Governors. Donations arrived from Germany, Jamaica, Antigua, Virginia, and Madras. From Bengal came two unusual gifts: £200 in 1754 from the Masonic Lodge at Calcutta, accompanied by a request to use the money, if possible, for the benefit of Masons' children, and in 1764 a legacy under the will of Omychund, a black merchant of Calcutta. This legacy provided for the deposit of 37,500 rupees in trust with the East India Company, which was to remit interest of 1500 rupees annually to the Hospital and the same amount to the Magdalen House. But the executor never turned over the principal to the East India Company, although he remitted the interest—the Hospital's share totaled £1501 1s 10d—more or less regularly until 1776. After that the Hospital received no more payments from Omychund's estate.[2]

A number of the Governors also remembered the Hospital in their wills, one of the most unusual of such bequests being that of Sir Charles Whitworth, a former treasurer, who gave £100 to the Hospital in 1778 with the direction that 'the interest whereof to be annually laid out in purchasing cakes to be distributed to the Children and Persons of the House every New Years Day in the Morning after Breakfast, in like manner as I have caused to be done every year during the time I have had the Honor of being Treasurer'.[3] And the faithful apothecary, Robert McClellan, continued to have the Hospital's interests at heart even after his retirement. When his will was proved in May 1799, the Governors learned that he had left the Hospital £100 in 3 percent stock.[4]

The Governors made every effort to ensure that they would be informed immediately of any bequest. As early as 1741 they resolved 'That circular Letters be sent to the proper Officers of each Diocess in the Country, to search for Legacies left to this Hospital, to give Notice thereof to the Secretary, by sending him a Certified Copy of each Clause, . . . and for which Ten Shillings and six pence shall be paid by this Corporation'.[5] When necessary, they took legal action to collect such legacies. Nevertheless, many were never received. A report prepared by the treasurer in 1821 indicates that fifty-three legacies made to the Hospital in the eighteenth century had not been paid. Of these, twenty-nine had depended upon a contingency that had not occurred, two were invalid because they violated the Mortmain Act,* and one testator had died insolvent in the Fleet Prison. The report did not state the reason for non-payment of the

* The Mortmain Act, 9 Geo. II, c. 36, forbade the giving of lands to charities.

other twenty-one.[6] But we can surmise what happened to the legacy of £20 left to the Hospital by Henry Jacomb: in 1783 the Governors were advised that Mr Jacomb at the time of his death had been 'indebted upon bond to the amount of many hundred pounds; that there is a possibility on the conclusion of a law suit, whenever it may happen, which has now lasted above 40 years, that some effects may come'.[7] Apparently nothing remained for the legatees when the lawsuit finally ended.*

The unpaid legacies, however, represented only 15 percent of the 349 testamentary gifts made to the Hospital during the course of the century,[8] while those that were paid formed the largest source of the Hospital's revenue, exclusive of the funds received from Parliament, up to 1771. In the period from 1739 to 1756, legacies made up 36.73 percent of the Hospital's income, averaging £2324 a year, and from 1757 to 1771 they constituted 51.63 percent of its non-Parliamentary revenue, averaging £2140 a year. From 1772 onward, although legacies remained important, income from investments and rents superseded this source of funds, which from 1772 to 1789 averaged only £1518 a year. Whether this occurred as a long-range effect of bad publicity during the General Reception or as the more immediate consequence of periods of economic depression in 1765–69, 1773–75, and 1778–81 cannot be said with any certainty,[9] since wills may reflect either states of mind or states of the economy or both as they existed when the wills were drawn up. But, as we shall see later from an analysis of general benefactions, there is reason to think that the falling off in legacies after 1771 most likely resulted from public disenchantment with the Hospital during the General Reception.

We can be more certain, however, of the proportionate representation of the sexes among those who did make bequests to the Hospital. Its Legacy Book shows that in the course of the century 58 women and 291 men remembered the Hospital in their wills.[10] Women, therefore, made up only 16.6 percent of the whole, a fact suggesting either that far fewer women than men favoured the idea of a foundling hospital or that, for the most part, men controlled the purse strings. The latter explanation receives support from a comparison with the subscriptions made by women to other mid-eighteenth-century charities, such as the Marine Society and the Magdalen House. An analysis of subscribers to these charities during their first few years of existence shows that women constituted only 5 percent of the contributors to the Marine Society and

*Perhaps this lawsuit was the model for *Jarndyce and Jarndyce,* of *Bleak House* fame.

24 percent of the benefactors of the Magdalen House.[11] On the other hand, a substantial number of women who possessed funds of their own gave generously both to the Magdalen House and to the Foundling Hospital.

Among those who contributed to the Hospital were several of the Lady Petitioners: the Duchesses of Richmond, Bedford, and Somerset each subscribed ten guineas a year; the Countess of Burlington donated at least ten guineas; the Duchess of Manchester and the Countesses of Huntingdon and Albemarle subscribed to the fund for building the chapel; and the Countess of Harold (after 1736, Countess Gower), as one of the executors of the estate of her father, the sixth Earl of Thanet, arranged for the payment to the Hospital of £500 out of funds designated by the Earl in his will for charitable uses.[12] Lady Betty Germain was a regular and extremely generous benefactress: not only did she pay an annual subscription of ten guineas, but she also gave £500 to the building fund in 1741, subscribed for the building of the chapel, and provided for a further gift to the Hospital of £1000 from her estate. And Princess Augusta continued to make an annual gift of £30 for more than twenty years in addition to her contribution of £50 to the fund for building the chapel. Indeed, at least twenty women subscribed for this purpose, largely due to the solicitations of Lady Vere Beauclerk.[13] But after the deaths of the women who had been the Hospital's benefactresses from the beginning, we find nothing in the records to indicate that later generations of aristocratic women followed their example, a circumstance that parallels the waning of feminine interest in the management of the Hospital during the second half of the century and also furnishes another indicator of the institution's loss of popularity.

The pattern of general benefactions, annual subscriptions, benefactions for the chapel, and donations slipped into the charity boxes, as charted in Appendix V, demonstrates still more vividly how public opinion affected the Hospital's finances. The immediate response at the beginning, when the Hospital was seeking funds to start its work and to establish a permanent home, was an outpouring of contributions never duplicated during the rest of the century. By 25 March 1742 the Governors had received £9157 2s in general benefactions, £740 13s in annual subscriptions, and £170 8s 7d from the charity boxes, making in all £10,068 3s 7d collected in little more than two years. Yet this occurred during a period of financial depression. When the Hospital settled down into a steady routine, contributions dropped off: during the next two years they totaled only £1899 11s in spite of the fact that these were years of prosperity.

But when the move from Hatton Garden to Lamb's Conduit Fields had been accomplished, and people began flocking to visit the Hospital's new building, contributions started to rise, especially those deposited in the charity boxes. From 25 March 1746 to the beginning of the General Reception—a period that saw the construction and opening of the chapel and the east wing, the establishment of the Hospital's art collection, and annual performances of the *Messiah*—benefactions continued at a high level, with fluctuations paralleling rather closely those of the economy. Beginning in 1757, however, the Hospital's revenues from all forms of charitable gifts other than legacies dropped dramatically—from £2674 13s in 1756 to a low of £299 16s 11d in 1765—and remained at a consistently low level until 1772. Yet these fifteen years witnessed periods of prosperity from 1757 to 1761, in 1764, and during 1771 and 1772. Obviously, Parliament's support was acting as a countervailing force to inhibit private charity.

We can also observe the effect on the Hospital's revenues of the public criticism that began in 1758. In that year charitable contributions other than legacies amounted to £1230 11s; in the following year the total was £979 7s 11d, and by 1760 it had dropped to £765 19s 9d. Only once up to 1772 did it exceed this sum: in 1764 the total was £830 8s 9d. But in 1773, by which time most people were aware that Parliament had terminated all grants to the Hospital, general benefactions rose substantially—from £222 18s in 1772 to £855 5s 4d in 1773 and £929 4s 11d in 1774—and this happened in spite of the fact that 1773 and 1774 were years of economic depression. The level of giving then dropped again and did not exceed the 1773–74 amounts until the mid-1780s when the chapel's musical programmes once more drew Londoners back to the Hospital. During these years, however, the pattern of general benefactions tended, for the most part, to parallel economic fluctuations, although the level of giving never rose again to its pre-1756 heights.[14] It therefore seems safe to say that the Hospital's charitable revenues rose and fell on the tides of public interest and approval and not in response to movements of the economy, except for periods when the Hospital's activities were inviting sustained interest or, conversely, when the Hospital was attracting very little attention. This pattern of contributions, one that responded not so much to the push and pull of economic fluctuations as to the ups and downs of public opinion, reflected, of course, the status of the Hospital's benefactors: most of them possessed sufficient wealth to carry them comfortably through periods of general financial adversity. Such men would not be forced by the condition of the economy to withdraw their support of an institution but could follow their inclinations, a fact that the Governors obviously realized, for their sensitivity to all forms of publicity demonstrated a keen understanding of how those inclinations might be affected.

Some gifts received by the Governors were designated for the children rather than for the Hospital, the earliest of these being a quantity of fine old linen, two coral necklaces, and two corals set in silver sent to the Hospital by an unknown benefactor in April 1741 with a note stating that they were presents for the infants, Thomas and Eunice Coram. Some donors did not name individual children but specified a use. Peter Wilbraham, for example, in 1759 gave the Hospital £15 in trust, the interest to be used 'in buying a shirt and shift for two boys and two girls, and in buying four boys a book each'.

Legacies to foundlings probably sprang from sentimental attachments or even stronger emotional ties. Among such gifts were those of Thomas Strode and his wife, Hester. He left £20 to a boy named for him, and she left £20 to Hester Yargrove, one of the girls. And Thomas Peach of Dingley bequeathed £50 to a boy named Thomas Dingley to whom he had stood godfather. Although the *Annual Register* reported erroneously in 1766 that 'a boy, bred up in the Foundling-hospital, has been lately left the sum of 8000l. and a girl 1000 l. by their supposed father, of which the directors are appointed the trustees', two large legacies were, in fact, given to children in the course of the century. In 1770 Edward Meinzies, captain of the privateer, *King of Prussia*, died in the East Indies, leaving £1000 under his will to a boy reputed to be his son. By an examination of the billets, the Governors ascertained the identity of the boy, who had already been apprenticed to a cabinet maker, and then requested the executors to hold both the principal and interest in trust until the boy came of age. The other major legacy to a child was the provision made under the will of Lewin Cholmley, described in an earlier chapter, which benefited Charles Dilke.[15]

The Governors did not, of course, sit back and wait for benefactions to arrive. By various means they sought out gifts for the Hospital: subscription books left with the steward and publicized in the press; parchment rolls placed in the hands of Governors willing to undertake the task of soliciting annual subscriptions; charity boxes fastened up in the Hospital and, in the early years, also entrusted to the proprietor of the Crown and Anchor Tavern; charity sermons, which usually produced handsome collections; and solicitation of the King's bounty, an effort that brought the Hospital a gift of £2000 in

1749 and, in 1754, £1000* as a fund to defray the expenses of conducting services in the chapel.[16] They also raised funds in every other way that they could think of: they sold hymnbooks for use in the chapel; they collected tolls for use of the Hospital's private road into Gray's Inn Lane until it was closed off in 1797; they sold gravel to builders of turnpike roads and clay for brickmaking to builders on the Hospital's estate; and, from the beginning, they invested immediately any surplus funds, even for short periods, in interest-bearing securities.[17]

Some of these methods produced relatively small sums, but the Governors could not afford to ignore any source of income. From 1747 onward they even turned the work of the children to account. The first income-producing occupation of the boys was winding silk; the girls' work in the early years saved expense rather than earned money, for their employment consisted of sewing and knitting articles for use in the Hospital. The Governors soon concluded, however, that winding silk was too effeminate an occupation for the older boys and decided to employ them in dressing hemp and in making twine, rope, and herring nets, which the Committee considered suitable occupations, 'being laborious and to be performed in the open Air, and in every respect consistent with their Destination to Navigation and Husbandry'. This decision led to the fitting up of a ropewalk under the arcades where the boys could work in full public view. Meanwhile, the younger boys continued to wind silk and to net silk and thread purses. During the middle years of the century when many fashionable people were visiting the Hospital, these purses, and also garters made by the small boys, sold well: from 1 July 1751 to 1 July 1752 such sales brought in £107 9s 9d. The quantity of purses needed to produce such a sum is revealed by an inventory made in 1759, which showed over 212 dozen purses on hand valued at £105 7s 3d. The making of purses and garters terminated in 1771, but the matron continued to sell those on hand down to 1786.[18]

In the period after the General Reception, the children at the Ackworth and Shrewsbury hospitals were taught to weave woollen cloth. We can gather some notion of the quantity of their work from the fact that on 17 December 1767, 562¼ yards of woollen cloth made by the children at Shrewsbury were sold at auction. By this time the children in London were spinning flax and weaving linen. In 1766 they wove 1622 yards valued at £55 11s. Some of the linen was

---

* This sum was part of an invalid legacy that had escheated to the Crown because the Court of Chancery had held that £1,200 bequeathed by Elias Paz, a Jew, to establish a yeshivah (school for Talmudic studies) constituted an improper use.

sold, some was used to make shirts and shifts for the children. But in all, the children's cash earnings from 1757 through 1771 amounted to £3184 1s 11d, or more than £200 a year.

In the 1770s the girls began to make shirts, shifts, handkerchiefs and household linens to order, while most of the boys were employed in knitting. By the 1790s, however, the boys were spinning worsted and yarn, although their earnings from this work proved small, while the girls, still sewing to order, earned just over £100 in 1796 and £107 in 1798. Over the years the income from the children's work formed only a small part of the Hospital's revenues, but the Governors did not on that account regard it as unimportant. For they believed that the work performed by the girls trained them to become good domestic servants and that bringing up the boys 'in habits of industry would tend to make them useful & profitable members of the Community'.[19]

Only one other item of income need be mentioned: rents. Until the development of the estate at the end of the century, the Hospital's rental income remained small, being derived chiefly from leasing a portion of its lands to a dairy farmer and from renting Powis Wells, a few small houses, and two alehouses on the estate. Several persons also paid small amounts to rent pieces of ground for gardens. And from time to time during the century small sums also came in from the New River Company for use of a strip of land through which its water pipe ran, and from Messrs Choice & Lover, butchers, for the privilege of grazing their sheep in the Hospital's courtyard.

In addition, from 1745 onward the Hospital received some rents from ten houses located at Garlick Hill and in the adjoining Sugar Loaf Court in the City of London. How the Hospital became the owner of these houses is something of a mystery. On 20 October 1744 John Milner and Taylor White purchased the property for £770, and they immediately executed deeds of it to the Hospital. But the Hospital's annual accounts do not show any expenditure to reimburse them, and the minutes do not record the vote of thanks to Milner and White that one would expect if they had made a gift of the property to the Hospital. Be that as it may, the property produced little income in proportion to the many problems involved in making repairs and collecting rents, so that in 1756 and again in 1758 the Governors contemplated selling it. But nothing came of the idea, and in 1791 we find the Governors executing a twenty-one-year lease of the houses at an annual rent of £69 clear of all taxes, which appears to be the most profitable arrangement made for the property in the course of the century, since in more than one year taxes and repairs had exceeded the rents.[20]

It is, of course, always easier to spend money than to get it. And sometimes the Governors spent more than they received, even though they frequently treated large benefactions and legacies as income rather than as additions to capital. Indeed, from 1772 to 1787 the Hospital's capital increased in only three years—by a total of £6118 3s 5d. During the other thirteen years expenses in excess of receipts nibbled away at its capital, reducing it by a total of £17,497 14s 11d, so that by 1788 the Hospital was more than £11,000 poorer than it had been when Parliament terminated all support at the end of 1771.[21] But operating in the red was not a new experience for the Governors who had had to borrow money more than once from the London Assurance Company to pay current bills while waiting for payment of the Parliamentary grants. And more than once they had appointed special committees to study ways and means of keeping down expenses or increasing revenues.[22]

Unfortunately, the annual accounts do not provide sufficient details to make possible a comparison of the items of expense from year to year. Obviously, some costs must have fluctuated widely depending on how many children were being cared for in London, how many at the branch hospitals, and how many by country nurses at any given time, to say nothing of the effect of rises and falls in the prices of food and other supplies. We can, however, learn something about the kinds of costs that the Governors had to meet from a very exact statement of expenses made for the year 1788. A summary of this statement follows:

Food (meat, flour, yeast, butter, milk, cheese, small beer, sugar, rice, salt, oatmeal):		£ 2414.11.10
Heat and Light (coal, firewood, candles):		475.18.7
Housekeeping supplies (soap, brooms, turnery-ware, tinware, and miscellaneous):		183. 8.1
Clothing, hats, shoes and stockings, mending, and household linens:		770. 1.9
Repairs:		213.13.2
Garden expense:		£ 52. 6.2
Wages:		
Preacher, Reader, organist, and two singers:	£ 205.0.0	
Secretary:	100.0.0	
Apothecary and 4 infirmary nurses:	70.0.0	
36 other employees:	341.9.6	
		716. 9.6

Taxes:	72.17.10
Printing, advertising, postage, stationery, and newspapers:	117.19.4
Apprentice fee and clothing for a handicapped boy:	22.13.6
Bibles and Prayerbooks:	9. 9.7
Medicines and extra nurses for inoculations:	93. 3.11
Coffins and burial fees:	5.10.0
Incidental expenses:	142.10.7

Total: £5290.13.10

In addition, the Hospital also incurred expenses of £1718 4s for the salaries of the country nurses and for transporting children to and from the country.[23]

In 1788, therefore, it cost just over £7000 to care for 192 children at nurse in the country and 317 children in London. At that time, the care of the children in the Hospital required a staff of forty-two (excluding the preacher, reader, organist and singers), which indicates a ratio of children to staff of eight to one. Apparently, such a ratio was not uncommon, for in the period from 1770 through 1772 the ratio ranged from five to one to eight to one.[24]

The Governors, of course, kept control of expenditures in their own hands, allowing the employees almost no authority to buy anything without prior approval. And the Committee never made purchases impulsively. Usually they obtained competitive bids from suppliers, and frequently they made comparisons of costs with officials of other institutions, most often Christ's Hospital. Invariably they aimed at neither the most expensive nor the cheapest but sought good, durable quality at a reasonable cost in any item purchased. They also attempted to check on deliveries to prevent short weight or the foisting of inferior merchandise upon the Hospital. They required that the steward and matron keep elaborate records to ensure control of the inventories of clothing, linens, food, furniture and other supplies. And they made use of the girls' labour in the house and that of the boys in the garden to keep down the number of employees. When clothing wore out, it was sold for rags. In short, the Governors tried to eliminate all waste and to minimize expenses.[25]

In some years their efforts succeeded better than in others, depending on the degree of co-operation obtained from the employees, on the amount of time that the Governors were willing to spend in personal supervision, and, in no small measure, on the personality of the resident treasurer. But, reviewing the financial situation of the Hospital over the entire period of sixty years, we may justifiably conclude that, for the most part, the Governors raised the Hospital's revenue with shrewdness and ingenuity and spent it with sound business judgment. The men who managed the Hospital combined good sense with good will and followed the principle enunciated by a special committee appointed in 1790 to investigate the Hospital's finances: 'that it is more consistent with the main Object of this Charity, and with the general Purpose both of Humanity and Policy, that a smaller number of Orphans should be kept well, than that a larger Number should be kept otherwise'.[26]

15

What They Wore and What They Ate

HOW TO CLOTHE THE infant foundlings engaged the Governors' attention long before they had to consider what to feed them. For in the beginning, the country nurses solved the latter problem, but the children arrived with no wardrobe beyond what they wore, and some of them wore very little. Anticipating the need several months before the first children were taken in, the Governors placed orders for sixty bundles of clothing, one to accompany each child to the home of its country nurse. Each outfit consisted of '4 Biggens, 4 long Stays, 4 caps, 4 neckcloths, 4 shirts and 12 clouts, and also the following woollen cloathing: a Grey Linsey mantle, a pair of Grey linsey sleeves, 2 white Bays Blanketts, 2 Rowlers, and 2 double Pilches'. A few months later each child, they decided, would need 'a Grey Linsey Coat and Petticoat, and a Grey Linsey Boddice Coat'.*

This description[1] of the first clothing of the foundling infants tells us four things: first, there would be no frills; second, the children would be warmly clad; third, there would be enough changes of linens and diapers to keep the children clean; and fourth, there would be no departure from the traditional practice of swathing an infant so tightly that it could move very little. A printed form of receipt for clothing signed by the country nurses in 1750 indicates few alterations: the Hospital no longer gave out rowlers; the infant's

---

* A biggen (biggin) was a close cap that bound the forehead tightly and was used to promote the hardening of the skull of newborn infants. Clouts were diapers. Bays (a variation of baize) was coarse woollen material with a long nap. Rowlers (rollers) were swaddling bands, i.e., narrow strips of cloth wrapped around a newborn infant's arms and legs to prevent free movement. A pilch was a triangular flannel cloth worn over the diaper. A boddice coat was an inner garment for the upper part of the body, reinforced with whalebone stays. Linsey was a material made of a mixture of wool and flax.

outfit now included two pairs of stockings, one pair of shoes, a comb and brush; and sleeves were now of linen instead of linsey.[2]

But up to the middle of the century the Governors appear to have made no other modifications in the clothing of the children at nurse, although one would have expected changes following publication in 1748 of Dr Cadogan's book on the care of infants and the Subcommittee's declaration in 1749 that the children were to be cared for by their country nurses 'conformable to the directions in Dr Cadogan's treatise'. That the Governors were not carrying out Cadogan's advice about infants' clothing was admitted by the Hospital's matron to the writer of an anonymous letter, received in 1750, which pointed out the disparity between recommendation and performance. For, said Dr Cadogan, nurses think

. . . a newborn Infant cannot be kept too warm; from this Prejudice they load and bind it with Flannels, Wrappers, Swathes, Stays, &c. commonly called Cloaths; which all together are almost equal to its own Weight; by which means a healthy Child in a Month's Time is made so tender and chilly, it cannot bear the external Air; . . . But besides the Mischief arising from the Weight and Heat of these Swaddling-cloaths, they are put on so tight, and the Child is so cramp'd by them, that its Bowels have not room, nor the Limbs any Liberty, to act and exert themselves in the free easy manner they ought. This is a very hurtful Circumstance; for Limbs that are not used will never be strong, and such tender Bodies cannot bear much Pressure . . . . To which doubtless are owing the many Distortions and Deformities we meet with every where; . . .

I would recommend the following Dress: A little Flannel Waistcoat without Sleeves; made to fit the Body, and tie loosely behind; to which there should be a Petticoat sew'd, and over this a kind of Gown of the same Material, or any other, that is light, thin, and flimsy. The Petticoat should not be quite so long as the Child, the Gown a few Inches longer; with one Cap only on the Head, which may be made double, if it be thought not warm enough . . . . the whole Coiffure should . . . neither bind nor press the Head at all . . . . laying aside all those Swathes, Bandages, Stays and Contrivances, that are most ridiculously used to close keep the Head in its Place, and support the Body . . . . Shoes and stockings are very needless Incumbrances, besides that they keep the Legs wet and nasty, if they are not changed every Hour, and often cramp and hurt the Feet: a Child would stand firmer, and learn to walk much sooner without them.[3]

Perhaps it was Dr Cadogan's influence that led the General Court to

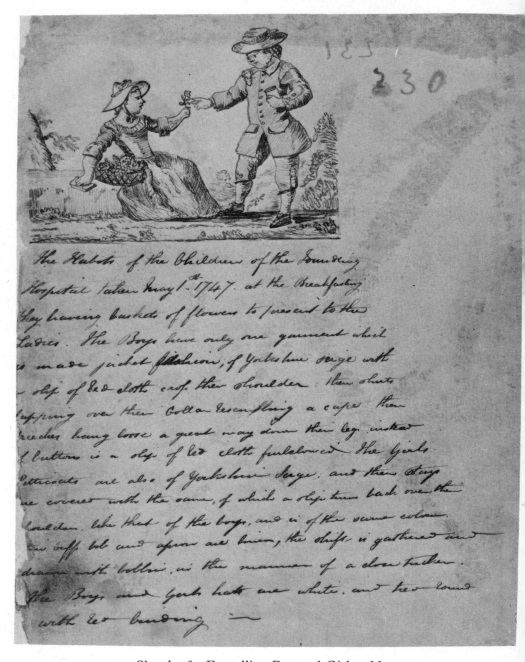

The Habits of the Children of the Foundling
Hospital taken May 1st 1747. at the Breakfasting
they having baskets of flowers to present to the
Ladies. The Boys have only one garment which
is made jacket fashion, of Yorkshire serge with
a slip of Red cloth cross their shoulder: their shirts
lapping over their collar resembling a cape. their
breeches hang loose a great way down their leg. instead
of buttons is a slip of Red cloth furbelowed The Girls
Petticoats are also of Yorkshire serge. and their stays
are covered with the same, of which a slip turn back over their
shoulder. like that of the boys, and is of the same colour.
their neff bib and apron are linen, the shift is gathered and
drawn with bobbin, in the manner of a close tucker.
The Boys and Girls hats are white. and turned round
with Red binding

11. Sketch of a Foundling Boy and Girl, 1 May 1747

decide in 1753 that the children should go barefoot during their years in the country in order to 'make them healthy & hardy',[4] but whether or not he succeeded in accomplishing further reforms in the dress of the infant foundlings after he became the Hospital's physician in 1754 is not clear.*

When the children returned to London from the country, they wore the Hospital's uniform. Hogarth had designed it in 1745 or 1746, and from a contemporary description we learn that:

> The Boys have only one garment which is made jacket fashion, of Yorkshire serge with a slip of red cloth cross their shoulder; their shirts lapping over their Collar resembling a cape; their breeches hang loose a great way down their legs, instead of buttons is a slip of red cloth furbelowed. The Girls Petticoats are also of Yorkshire Serge; and their stays are covered with the same, of which a slip turns back over their shoulders, like that of the boys, and is of the same colour. Their buff bib and apron are linen, the shift is gathered and drawn with bobbins, in the manner of a close tucker. The Boys and Girls hats are white, and tied round with red binding.[5]

From the beginning the colour scheme of the children's clothes was brown trimmed with red, and from the beginning the Governors ordered them made of good, sturdy woollen cloth: coats of brown drugget for all of the children, dresses of brown serge for the girls. For shifts and shirts the Hospital used Lancashire sheeting, and for the girls' caps, Irish linen. And the children had to wear shoes and stockings. In 1757 the Governors decided that both boys and girls should wear low-heeled shoes, and in 1760 the matron devised a new style of bodice for the girls, one made without any stiffening except buckram. But apart from this, the uniform apparently underwent very few changes in the course of the century.[6]

The children received their new clothes each year before the annual meeting in May. A list made on 24 January 1753 indicates that the Governors provided enough changes to ensure cleanliness: every year each girl received three bib-aprons, three shifts, two night and two day caps; and each boy received three shirts. Moreover, when a boy left to serve his apprenticeship, the Governors gave him a coat, waistcoat, breeches, three shirts, two pairs of stockings, two pairs of

---

* Cadogan's treatise, however, continued to be read. By 1782 it had gone through ten editions, had been reprinted in Philadelphia and Boston, and had been translated into both French and German. And it remained in print in Paris and London until at least 1805.

shoes, and a hat, a wardrobe that in 1761 cost £1 5s 11d. A girl about to be apprenticed received a coat, two petticoats, three shifts, three day caps, two night caps, two bibs and aprons, two pairs of stockings, two pairs of shoes, and a hat. The Governors also issued orders that the children's shoes 'be kept clean with strong brushes and soft with Neat's foot oil', and that their clothing be kept mended. And in 1790 the General Court, upon the recommendation of a special committee, directed that the children change their body linen twice a week.[7]

Clothing always represented one of the major items of expense. When made by seamstresses outside the Hospital, the cost of clothing a child for its first five years was calculated in 1751 to amount to £5 1s 10 1/2d, plus mending of linen at 4s a year and mending of shoes at 4s 4d a year. By 1759, the Hospital's employees and the older girls were making most of the children's clothes but, until the country hospitals could furnish large quantities of woollen fabric and the children in London could weave sufficient coarse linen, the cost of materials continued to make up a large item of expense. In the 1780s when the Governors once again had to buy materials, the cost of a boy's clothes for one year was estimated at £1 9s 3d, while clothes for a girl would amount to £1 7s 6d. By 1799 the cost of a boy's suit—coat, waistcoat, and breeches—had risen from its 1787 price of 12s 6d to 16s, and the cost of shoes and their repair had increased from 12s 3d to 14s for each child, a charge that covered four pairs of shoes a year.[8]

The wearing of uniforms by children in institutions did not, of course, originate with the Foundling Hospital. Christ's Hospital had long been called the Bluecoat Hospital from the fact that its boys wore long blue coats over yellow breeches and stockings. In the Amsterdam *Weeshuijs*, the children wore black wool outer garments, each displaying a small red, white, and black shield on the upper left sleeve. Children in the orphanage at Venice dressed in red uniforms. And in the Paris institution, the children were clad alike in brown.[9] There were practical reasons for such a custom: uniform clothing saved expense and eliminated the possibility of conflict among the children arising from envy.

But uniformity of clothing may have had unintended consequences. Although the Hospital's records offer no evidence, we may speculate that, on the positive side, uniformity of dress might have encouraged a sense of group solidarity, thereby fostering the individual child's sense of security through a feeling of belonging. On the other hand, uniforms would dispose people to see and think of the children not as individual human beings but as a faceless body. Moreover, the uniform set the children apart from all other children and labelled them as foundlings—bastards in the public mind. This would matter little while they were in the Hospital, but being marked as different by their clothes might have affected their ability to form close relationships with others or even made them targets for ridicule after they left the Hospital to serve their apprenticeships. Also, uniformity of dress might tend to discourage a child from thinking of himself as a unique personality possessing individual worth.

Uniformity, of course, prevailed as much in food as in clothing. All the children in the Hospital, except those in the infirmaries, shared the same menu. And because of the importance of food to the children's health and its high position in the scale of expenses, it became a matter for frequent discussion by the Governors, who never left the planning of menus to the matron, steward, or cook but throughout the century customarily sought the advice of a physician in constructing the weekly tables of diet.

During the first few years the Governors had to think only about food for the staff and for those infants who, for one reason or another, could not be wet nursed. Such children were fed pap, and tradition offered various methods of preparing it out of mixtures of flour or bread with water or milk. Some eighteenth-century recipes called for the use of rice flour or arrowroot with a flavouring of sugar, spice, or a drop of wine, a practice roundly condemned by Dr Cadogan. But we do not know exactly how the foundlings' pap was prepared until 1757, when the Governors decided to follow the recommendation of Mrs Elizabeth Sloane. Her advice was, first, to grate well-baked sea biscuit very fine; then, to moisten it with a little water, and add milk, making certain that it was not hot lest it make the pap glutinous, a method not unlike Dr Cadogan's direction to boil bread and water together until almost dry and then mix with fresh, unboiled milk. Two years later, however, the apothecary reported that the nurses were ignoring these directions and preparing the children's pap entirely without milk.[10]

The diet of the older children became a matter of concern when a substantial number of them began to return to London from the homes of their country nurses. In 1747 the Hospital's physician, Dr Conyers, drew up the first comprehensive table of diet, which is set forth in Appendix VI, together with similar tables for 1762 and 1790. The tables show that the Foundling Hospital conformed to the general meal pattern of both rich and poor in the eighteenth century: a light breakfast, a heavy midday meal, and a light supper.

We may also make several other observations from these tables. In the first place, the children ate meat three times a week in 1747, but by 1762 the number of meat meals had increased to five; in 1790 there were four. And this increase in meat consumption occurred in spite of

12. The Girls' Dining Room, 1773

the fact that meat rose in price after the middle of the century, a clear indication that the Governors did not sacrifice the children's health to expense. Further evidence of their willingness to place health before any other consideration can be found in the minutes of a meeting held in 1782 at which it was proposed to substitute suet puddings for meat twice a week. The Committee rejected the proposal because the Hospital's physician opposed it, 'as by Experience he has found that the Augmenting of Animal Food has greatly contributed to the better health of the children'.

The children did not, however, eat fish, eggs, or poultry. Probably the absence of fish can be attributed to its high cost, brought about by the tax on the salt used to preserve it, or, in the case of fresh fish, by the charges for transporting it from the coast. Then, too, the dubious quality of much of the fresh fish sold at Billingsgate would argue strongly against serving it. The omission of eggs and poultry, which seem, in any event, to have been regarded as luxuries, may have been a matter of custom: these foods did not form part of the diet of any London institution in the eighteenth century even though in the first half of the century such items were cheap.[11]

We can also see from the tables that bread constituted a staple of the children's diet: in 1747 and in 1790 it was the principal item of the evening meal, and in 1790 it served additionally as the children's breakfast three times a week. In 1762 the use of bread as the main part of the meal alternated between breakfast and supper. This was to be expected. In the eighteenth century bread formed the major item in the diets of the poor, of artisans and town labourers, and of workhouses and other institutions.[12] Less to be expected was the inclusion of potatoes in the children's diet as early as 1747, for they were by no means a customary component of institutional diets in the south of England during the eighteenth century.[13]

Another characteristic common to the three tables of diet is the omission of tea and beer. The vigorous opposition of Jonas Hanway while he served as a Governor undoubtedly accounts for the absence of tea, and a later generation of Governors apparently saw no reason to disagree with him. But the exclusion of beer is more surprising. Eighteenth-century men might debate the salubrity of tea drinking, but they generally thought of beer as a food rather than as an intoxicant, and it was certainly safer to drink than water from the Thames or from springs contaminated by the drainage of graveyards and sewers. Moreover, the girls, aged eight to sixteen, who resided in the Hospital of the Parish of St George Middlesex endowed by Henry Raine, received in 1754 'what beer they will drink' for both breakfast and supper every day, and also for dinner at least five times a week. In the same year the boys, aged ten to fourteen, at the Greenwich Hospital were given a quart of beer every day except Wednesday. And the children of Christ's Hospital also drank beer for breakfast.

The Foundling Hospital's records indicate, however, that from time to time the children, or at least some of them, did receive a ration of beer—for the staff, of course, the Governors always laid in an ample supply. In 1778 the Committee resolved to allow the children small beer* with their Sunday dinner, and a record made in 1787 shows that each child was given a half pint every Sunday and a similar quantity on Good Friday, May Feast Day, Charter Day, and Christmas. Some of the boys who performed exceptionally arduous work, such as those who assisted the gardener, also received a pint of beer every day, divided between dinner and supper.[14]

The children's diet may not have been quite as monotonous as the tables seem to indicate. We might conclude from examining them that the foundlings never ate any fruit, sweets, or vegetables before 1762 and only limited amounts thereafter. But this conclusion would not be entirely warranted, for other records indicate that from time to time the children ate foods not listed in the tables, such as an occasional apple or gooseberry pie, when apples were cheap or gooseberries in season. Plum puddings provided special treats for Christmas and Charter Day, and in the 1790s special buns were served on Good Friday. Raisins and currants frequently improved the rice puddings. And mention of the 'Fruit Walk' and 'melon ground' in 1755 suggests that the children may have enjoyed melons and other fruit in the summer.[15]

It seems probable, too, that the children ate vegetables, and perhaps a greater variety of them, than the tables of diet reveal. As early as 1749 the Governors were planning to enlarge the garden to supply the Hospital with vegetables, some of which were to alternate with meat in the children's diet. In 1761 the Hospital was raising at least part of its potato supply in a field adjoining the Hospital, and from time to time we find other vegetables mentioned in the minutes, such as beans, parsnips, Brussels sprouts and spinach. Long before century's end the garden encompassed four and a half acres, and we may form some idea of what it produced from a seed list made in 1791. That year the gardener planted peas, five varieties of beans, red and white radishes, spinach, potatoes, several kinds of cabbage, kale, cauliflower, broccoli, carrots, several varieties of lettuce, mustard, cress, celery, cucumbers, onions, leeks, parsnips, turnips, parsley,

* Small beer was weak beer with an alcohol content of 2 to 3 percent. A resolution of 1798 forbade serving porter to the children.

marjoram, summer and winter savory, and thyme. Probably some of these vegetables and herbs were planted in limited quantities to serve only the table of the staff. Nevertheless, everything suggests that the children's dinners included a few vegetables almost from the beginning, and that their variety and quantity increased over the course of the century. Obviously, however, any consumption of fruits or vegetables must have been largely seasonal because no means then existed for preserving such items except root-cellaring, for which the Hospital does not seem to have possessed extensive facilities.[16]

The tables of diet also hide another uncertainty: the nature of the bread, for it was not the same in all periods. In 1749 the Hospital purchased bread of the 'second sort', that is, made from stoneground wheat flour bolted through coarse cloths that permitted enough bran and germ to pass through so that the end product appeared 'dirty white' in contrast to the best quality of flour which, having been bolted through fine linen or woollen cloths, was a pale cream colour. By 1757 a servant, who functioned as both baker and brewer, was baking the Hospital's bread in its own ovens, and it seems likely that the Hospital may then have been using the best grade of flour since the Governors in 1758 pronounced the bread 'what this Committee could wish to have in their own Familys'. Moreover, during the wheat shortage of 1772–74, when Parliament authorized general use of 'standard' loaves made of darker flour containing more bran, the Governors tried a specimen and rejected its adoption for the Hospital. The wheat shortage of 1795, however, forced change upon them, and in midsummer they substituted rice for flour in the puddings and adopted the standard loaf, which was furnished by a baker in Guilford Street. By January 1796 the Governors had decided to use bread made of two-thirds wheat and one-third barley.[17]

A further hazard of accepting the tables of diet uncritically is that they tell us nothing about the size of the portions allotted to each child, although other sources do give some information on this point. From 1758 to 1790 the usual serving of meat weighed 8 ounces before cooking. In 1758 the bread allowance was 61 ounces a week; by 1784 it had risen to just under 74 ounces. In the same period, the cheese (probably Cheshire) allowance also increased from 3 3/4 ounces a week to almost 6 ounces a week. In 1758 a serving of milk was half a pint. Beyond this we know almost nothing. The size of the servings of broth, gruel, milk porridge, and vegetables appears nowhere; nor do the records show the precise recipes used for preparing the broth, which was sometimes made from shin beef and sometimes from ox heads, and which sometimes included rice, sometimes barley, and sometimes oatmeal, onions, herbs and root vegetables.[18]

An examination of the tables of diet of other institutions caring for children in the 1750s and 1760s offers no more detailed information but does make some degree of comparison possible. The children of Christ's Hospital breakfasted on bread and beer every day and ate bread with cheese or butter for supper six days out of seven. They were served meat (beef or mutton) five times a week. The boys at the Greenwich Hospital received only five ounces of bread a day (a little better than half the foundling children's allotment), a half pound of meat three times a week, six quarts of beer and four ounces of butter a week, and four dinners weekly of milk or pease porridge, water gruel, or the like. The girls at the Hospital of St George Middlesex lived largely on bread and beer. They ate three ounces of bread with beer for breakfast every morning; six ounces of bread, with an ounce of butter or two ounces of cheese, and beer for supper every evening; and for dinner four ounces of meat plus six ounces of bread and beer five days a week. On the other two days they ate rice milk or pease porridge accompanied by bread and butter. None of these institutions listed any vegetables at all in their tables of diet. The best of the lot would appear to have been the Asylum for Orphan Girls, which, in 1763, gave its children milk instead of beer and a considerable amount of vegetables. Breakfast consisted of rice milk, water gruel, or milk pottage. For supper the girls ate bread and cheese three times a week, barley broth twice a week, and twice a week potatoes, radishes and 'sallad'. Four dinners a week consisted of mutton and 'garden stuff', and the other three dinners were, respectively, hasty pudding, plum pudding, and rice pudding. These girls, in short, enjoyed vegetables at one meal or another every day except Wednesday.[19]

The children of the Paris hospital fared no better than those in English institutions, at least in 1740. Each day they received a pound and a half of bread and, on meat days, half a pound of meat with broth. Meat days alternated with 'les jours maigres' when they ate peas, beans, cheese and butter with their bread. But all of these diets pale beside the quantity and variety of the food consumed in the orphanage at Amsterdam. A list made in 1740 indicates that during the preceding year that institution had used enormous quantities of wheat, rye, white beans, maple peas, green peas, barley grits, oat grits, coarse oatmeal, wheat flour, rice, peeled barley, cheese, butter, syrup, vinegar, salad oil, beef, oxen, pigs, mutton, veal, beer, sweet milk and buttermilk. In addition, the children were given such extras as boiled eggs for Easter; radishes in May; gooseberries and lettuce in June; fresh peas, broad beans, and leeks in July; carrots in midsummer; currants, kale, apples, or white plums in August; cabbage, plums, and raisins in September; more cabbage and carrots in late autumn; and cakes in December.[20]

It seems certain, however, that the foundlings enjoyed a more ample diet, one of better quality and with more variety, than poor children who lived with their parents. The historians who have investigated the food consumption of the poor in eighteenth-century England agree that the diets of artisans and labourers living in towns were improving up to the middle of the century but declined from 1760 onward. This occurred because the cost of food, spurred by bad harvests, inflation, and the effects of war, rose by 40 percent while wages lagged far behind. By 1770 meat cost 4d to 5d a pound and butter sold for 8d a pound in London. As a result, wheat bread, potatoes and tea became the principal diet of the poor, with, perhaps, a little butter, an occasional herring, or a bowl of broth on Sundays. Sir Frederick Morton Eden tells us that in the south of England in the 1790s the poorest labourers ate dry bread and cheese, accompanied by tea, from week's end to week's end. Those whose earnings were slightly higher might afford meat once a week but never bought milk, for milk was too expensive—3 1/2d a quart in London. But even in the good years earlier in the century unskilled and casual labourers always lived close to the edge of existence. Indeed, the food provided for workhouse residents was probaly more adequate, and certainly more regular, than that of the labouring poor, for, Eden indicates, many of these establishments served meat dinners three or four times a week.[21]

It is equally unlikely that the food consumed by the poor of London could match in excellence that set before the foundling children, for the Governors took great pains to make certain that purchased items were of good quality. In an age when adulteration of foodstuffs was widely practised,* this demanded considerable vigilance. Fortunately, during much of the century the Governors could purchase milk from their cowkeeper tenant, a circumstance that guaranteed its freshness and freedom from the contamination that milk so often suffered by being carried through the streets of London in open containers exposed to filth of every kind. Later in the century when the Governors received a proposal to supply the Hospital with 'genuine scalded milk', they rejected it, 'not chusing to use any artificial milk', and in 1790 we find them recommending strict attention to make sure that the children's milk 'be unadulterated with

---

* The adulteration of foods and beverages was not stamped out until the enactment of the Sale of Food and Drugs Act in 1875.

stale milk or water'. Similarly, for many years the custom of baking bread in the Hospital's own ovens prevented its adulteration with alum, an all too common trick of London bakers. But the Governors still had to watch that suppliers did not deliver too coarse flour, rancid butter, sour beer, or musty meat, and did not cheat on weight.[22]

They also had to guard against excessive costs. One technique used by the Governors was to buy middle cuts of meat; another was to compare frequently the Hospital's costs for various items of food and the quantities consumed against similar data for other London institutions.[23] The importance of gathering comparative data becomes apparent when we reflect on the quantities of provisions that the Governors were dealing with. For example, a report made at midsummer 1784 shows that during the preceding year tradesmen had delivered to the Hospital 4228 pounds of butter, 9202 pounds of cheese, 9204 gallons of beer, and 92,400 pounds of flour.[24]

Not all of this food went to the children, of course, since most of the Hospital's staff received room and board as part of their compensation. And, eating apart from the children, they dined more copiously, although their breakfasts and suppers, for the most part, resembled those provided for the foundlings. The first table of diet ordered for the household in March 1741 allowed for a liberal use of meat:

> Upon Sundays Roast Beef, Mondays Stew'd Beef with Turneps and Carrots, Tuesdays Roast Mutton, Wednesdays Boiled Beef with Greens or Roots, or Pork with Pease Pudding in Winter, or Shoulders of Veal in Summer, Thursdays Stew'd Beef with Turneps and Carrotts, Fridays Roast Mutton, and Saturdays Boiled Beef with Greens or Roots, or Pork with Pease Pudding in Winter and Shoulders of Veal in Summer . . . . the Proportion of the said Diet [to] be at present Regulated at a Pound for each Head a Day one with another.[25]

Such a diet, which apparently the staff enjoyed for some years, originated, according to Thomas Bernard, in 'the over kindness and English feelings of the general committee', whereas, he said, in 1799 a weekly meat allowance to the staff of approximately a quarter of the amount allowed in 1741 was found to be sufficient. The servants' complaints about the quantity of it, however, do not entirely agree with Bernard's conclusions, although they still ate meat every day.[26]

Adding to all their other responsibilities, the Governors also took upon themselves at intervals the task of determining how well the kitchen staff prepared the food. They sampled specimens of the

Hospital's bread, they sipped the children's broth, and they tasted the puddings. What they found was not always to their liking. In 1790, for example, John Wilmot said on one occasion that the beef broth was 'as salt as brine', and Stephen White described a pudding served to the children in the infirmary as 'extremely bad, consisting of milk & flour & sugar boiled only to the consistency of thick paste'.[27]

From time to time the Governors also tried various experiments to improve the efficiency of the kitchen or the quality of the cooking. One of the most successful of such attempts was the renovation of the kitchen under the direction of Count Rumford during his long visit to London in 1795–96. The new equipment consisted of a built-in roaster large enough to hold 112 pounds of beef; a table mounted on castors to move the meat to and from the roaster; a built-in steam box capable of steaming 200 pounds of potatoes on a rack; a divided boiler, the larger side for boiling meat and the smaller for boiling greens; a similar divided boiler of lesser capacity; and a round iron boiler in which to cook milk porridge. All of the boilers were furnished with tightfitting covers that opened by balanced pulleys, so that each of them constituted, in effect, an early form of pressure cooker. The cost of this equipment and installing it amounted to approximately £150, but the design and arrangement of the various items, together with the system of flues, resulted in a 75 percent saving of fuel. Because the new methods lessened evaporation, the quality of the food was improved with less waste, and the compact arrangement of the equipment produced an early model of step-saving kitchen design that allowed the cook to perform her tasks more efficiently. It was, said a contemporary account, 'the first experiment of the kind, that has been made, on a large scale, in England'.[28]

But in spite of all the attention given by the Governors to the children's diet, it seems probable that they remained, in certain respects, malnourished. The absence of precise knowledge about the size of portions, composition of mixed dishes, and frequency with which seasonal fruits or vegetables were added to the diet makes comment on its nutritive value, of course, highly speculative. Nevertheless, it seems impossible that on meatless days the total calories that a child would have consumed could have exceeded fifteen hundred. Yet we now believe that a child between the ages of six and twelve needs two thousand to two thousand five hundred calories a day. On the other hand, because of the quantity and quality of the bread and the amount of milk allotted, the protein intake of the children would appear to have been adequate even on meatless days all through the century. These foods would also seem to assure the children of proper amounts of vitamins B_1 and B_2. Probably the amount of iron was also sufficient, except for the older girls, most of the time. But it seems almost certain that there must have been serious deficiencies in calcium and vitamins A, C, and D.

On days when the children ate milk porridge or gruel as well as bread and milk, their calcium intake was probably high enough, but on many days they received milk at only one meal. This pattern existed on six days a week in 1790 and on four or five days a week in the earlier periods. On such days eight ounces of milk could not possibly provide an adequate amount of calcium. The vitamin C deficiency would be present on any day that the children were served no fruit or vegetables. Therefore, if we take the tables of diet at face value, the children in 1747 would have received enough vitamin C only on Mondays when they dined on potatoes, assuming that each child ate at least two. As the frequency of serving vegetables increased, the probability of sufficient vitamin C in the children's diet would also have risen and may have reached an adequate level by 1762 when some form of vegetable was served at six dinners out of seven. The worst deficiency throughout the century, however, would seem to have occurred in the amounts of vitamins A and D. The only sources of vitamin A listed in the tables of diet are milk, cheese, butter, and 'greens', but on most days the menu would not include all of these foods, and, except when kale, spinach, broccoli or carrots were served, it would appear impossible that a child could have consumed more than half of the required amount of vitamin A each day. Also, we should not forget that the premise that the children did receive the necessary quantities of vitamins C and A from vegetables on any day rests on the assumption that the cook did not boil them too long, and that is indeed a doubtful assumption. Obviously, since the children ate no eggs or fish and little butter or cream, their diets fell far short of providing the minimum requirement of vitamin D.

Of course, the Governors did not think, as we do today, in terms of calories and vitamins. They wanted the children's diet to be ample and nutritious and considered it to be so because it had been prescribed by the Hospital's physicians. Certainly it was not a starvation diet, but it seems very likely that it lacked sufficient calories to encourage what we now consider normal growth and that its deficiencies in calcium and vitamins A, D, and sometimes C set the stage for many of the children's illnesses, as we shall see in the next chapter.

16

The Prevention and Cure
of Childhood's Ills

PROBABLY NO TOPIC engaged as much of the Committee's attention as the children's health: the variety and virulence of the diseases that so often plagued the foundlings disquieted the Governors greatly; how to prevent such illnesses worried them even more. And the means of prevention were not only few but frequently ineffective. For the most part, preventive measures consisted of separation of the sick from the well; destruction of contaminated clothing; fumigation; general cleanliness; outdoor exercise; immersion in cold baths, and similar activities designed to build up health and strength; inoculation against smallpox; and in the years before and after the General Reception, the examination of all infants brought to the Hospital in order to reject any who appeared diseased.

Such rejection was, in fact, the first preventive measure taken by the Governors, for on 4 March 1741 they inserted in the notice of the first admission the statement that 'no Child exceeding the Age of Two Months is to be taken in, Nor such as have the French Pox, Evil, Leprosy, or Disease of the like Nature, whereby the Health of other Children may be endangered. For the Discovery whereof, every Child is to be Inspected as soon as it is brought to the Hospital'.[1] But, of course, the unsophisticated examining techniques of 1741 did not screen out any but the most obvious ailments, and within a short time several children died. The most common cause of death was listed as convulsions.[2]

The death of the infant, Frances Hodges, on 8 April 1741 led to the Governors' second measure of prevention. Believing that the child was accidentally suffocated during the night, the Governors ordered 'That the Children in this Hospital do lye inside Beds or Cradles, and not in the Beds with the Nurses'.[3]

Separation of the sick from the well to prevent infection began soon afterwards. On 13 July the chief nurse noticed that one of the boys had broken out with what she thought to be smallpox, and she at once removed him to 'the room provided for the children that should happen to be taken with that distemper'. Fortunately, her diagnosis proved erroneous: the child had only a rash. But the prompt isolation of suspicious cases continued, with the Governors' approbation, all through the century. And in some periods children who appeared to be suffering from the most dreaded diseases—notably smallpox and venereal diseases—were removed from the Hospital for treatment elsewhere.[4]

During the General Reception the problems of caring for sick infants and of isolating them took on the aspects of nightmare. The Hospital's infirmary wards lacked the capacity to deal with the numbers involved, so that it became necessary to seek additional space outside the Hospital. With some anticipation of the need, the Governors in May 1756 had leased an old building, formerly a pottery, in an area known as the Brill, which was located near the present site of St Pancras Station. As soon as it had been converted into an infirmary, they arranged to transport sick children there by sedan chair. But within a year a second building had to be rented at Battle Bridge, in the same general area, chiefly for use as a place to inoculate the children against smallpox and to care for those afflicted with the itch. In the spring of 1759 the Governors appropriated from their tenant the Coach and Horses Alehouse just outside the Hospital's gates and transformed this building also into an infirmary. Later in the year they decided to make use of the Powis Wells buildings for the same purpose.

The acquisition of these additional buildings enabled the Governors to establish specialized infirmaries: until the early 1760s the children with infectious diseases were nursed at Battle Bridge or the Brill, while the Coach and Horses, used at first for children with the itch, continued to serve somewhat longer as a place for con-valescent children. From 1759 onward Powis Wells, because of the supposed beneficial effects of its waters, was used to treat children suffering from scrofula, scald heads, diseases of the eyes, and scorbutic eruptions. In the 1770s it was used chiefly to isolate children with the itch.[5]

The Governors achieved isolation, however, more easily than cleanliness. From time to time they waged combat against bedbugs (a 'Bugg Docter' performed the task at 4s a bed, 'no Cure no Money'); rats; lice and nits in the children's hair; and stinks and smells arising from tubs of wet diapers, poor ventilation in the wards, uncleaned privies, inadequate sewers, and drains without traps. Moreover, it required constant vigilance to see to it that lazy servants and nurses did not neglect the cleaning of the wards as well as the twice-a-day scrubbing of the children's hands and faces. The degree to which the Governors attained their goal of cleanliness rose and fell over the years, depending partly on the assiduousness with which they pried into the minutiae of daily routines, and partly on the supervisory ability of the matron.[6]

Above all, the Governors tried from the first to prevent the devastations of smallpox among the children, for in the eighteenth century smallpox was chiefly a disease of infants and children under three years of age, and in London, accounted for 10 percent of all deaths from 1721 to 1760. At the Governors' request, Dr Conyers performed the first inoculation of the children in March 1744, and while the procedure was under way the Committee met at the nearby Globe Tavern in order to escape the possibility of infection. This seemed a wise precaution for inoculation, unlike vaccination, produced in the recipient a case of smallpox, the severity of which, it was hoped, would be lessened by the elaborate course of preparation and the medicines, purges, and other treatment given after the inoculation. But while the induced disease lasted, it was just as infectious as smallpox contracted in the ordinary way and could be equally fatal.

When the procedure first came into use in England in the 1720s, the death rate was about one out of every fifty or sixty persons inoculated. So great a risk and the hazard of spreading the disease provoked debate about its desirability for some years, and the expense of the long periods of preparation and aftercare limited its use until mid-century largely to the wealthy. The Governors were indeed forward-looking in adopting inoculation so early, for even the smallpox hospitals for the poor, established in London between 1746 and 1768, did not inoculate children under seven years of age. Probably Dr Mead's strong approval and Sir Hans Sloane's advocacy of the procedure influenced the Governors' decision. In any event, the outcome of the first inoculation pleased them, and they decided to make it a rule to inoculate all children on their return from the country unless they had already had the disease or had been inoculated while at nurse. For, on occasions when epidemics threatened areas where the children were being cared for, the Hospital paid for the inoculations to be performed locally at a cost ranging from 10s each to three for a guinea.

In 1748 the Governors concluded that the procedure should be carried on outside the Hospital and, for some years, hired a house in Leather Lane for the purpose. By the end of April 1755, 211 children had been inoculated with only one loss of life and twenty failures to produce eruptive symptoms. In the 1750s, with the Governors' permission, Dr Cadogan experimented on several occasions with methods of inoculation other than the customary insertion of infectious matter into incisions in the children's arms, but the experiments involving external application of the inoculant proved unsuccessful. The Governors were not, however, as willing to embrace immediately the new technique of vaccination when Jenner published a report on his work in 1798, for the Hospital's physician was still inoculating the children in the usual way during the autumn of 1799.[7]

In spite of the Governors' efforts, some children died of smallpox contracted 'in the natural way', usually while at nurse in the country. But, apart from smallpox, the causes of death most often specified in the records were a great variety of fevers; measles; convulsions, often associated with teething; consumption; dysentery and diarrhea; mortifications; and in 1767–68, marasmus.[8] Although deaths from fevers outnumbered any other category, as we might expect since fevers caused eight out of ten deaths in the eighteenth century, I cannot describe them more specifically. The records mention eruptive fever, spotted fever, inward fever, putrid fever, purple fever, worm fever, nervous fever, and uncategorized fever. In 1763 an epidemic of 'eruptive fever' accompanied by 'ulcerous sore throats' swept the Hospital: 150 children lay in the infirmary at one time, and at least nine children died. Almost certainly this was scarlet fever, which at the same time was devastating southern England, for, the Secretary wrote, 'I heard from one of our seaports that of 1700 Inhabitants 1500 are Ill of this distemper at once'. In 1787 another epidemic of scarlet fever struck down over a hundred children, a number of whom died, and an epidemic of an unspecified fever brought death to several children in the winter of 1792. Probably some of the fevers were typhus or typhoid—the difference between them was not recognized until 1750. And from the fact that on several occasions the records list the cause of death as water on the brain, we might also suspect epidemic meningitis.[9]

After fevers, measles was the great killer. From time to time epidemics of measles ravaged the Hospital. In July 1746 forty-seven children contracted the disease, and four died. In 1766 there were seventy-four cases; in 1768 seven out of the 101 who were stricken by the disease died; in 1770 so many children were suffering from measles in the spring that the Governors suspended all apprenticing. And smaller epidemics also occurred in 1794, 1798, and 1800.[10]

We can only speculate about the deaths attributed to mortification and marasmus. A reference to a 'mortification in its bowels' or 'mortification in feet' would seem clearly to indicate gangrenous conditions. On the other hand, in the eighteenth century the word sometimes meant a state of torpor or unconsciousness preceding death. Therefore, the use of the word alone in the Hospital's records may well have described the child's dying condition rather than the actual cause of death. A marasmus is also an equivocal term. It always implied a wasting away of the body, which, of course, could lead to death, but it tells us nothing about the cause of the wasting away. Possibly it occurred in the aftermath of the epidemics of measles in 1766 and 1768, or it may have resulted from tuberculosis, since the records frequently mention cases of consumption. But because it appears as a cause of death only in a two-year period, we cannot discount the possibility of a diagnosis conforming to the doctor's current medical theories.

Less likely to cause death but more demanding of prolonged care on a day-to-day basis were those diseases designated as the itch, 'scrophulous' symptoms, scald head, inflammations or weakness of the eyes, and scorbutic eruptions. For readers unfamiliar with some of these disorders a brief description may be useful. The itch (scabies) unquestionably gave the most trouble. A highly contagious rash accompanied by violent itching but no fever, it could break out anywhere on the body except the face, although it was usually concentrated on the hands, wrists, feet and legs, and in the anal and genital regions. It was caused by a parasitic mite easily spread through clothing, bedding, or personal contact, and this, obviously, made control of the disease almost impossible in any institution. It was not, however, an affliction confined exclusively to institutions or to the poor, for Horace Walpole mentions several instances of the itch occurring in the upper levels of society.*

Scrofula, or the King's Evil, was a tuberculous condition of the lymphatic glands in the neck. Sometimes it also affected joints and bones, and its inflamed, ulcerated swellings, when healed, almost always left ugly scars. Scald head was a contagious ringworm of the scalp characterized by pustular patches that broke open and formed scabs. These would thicken and spread until the incrustations enveloped the whole head and face like a mask. Scorbutic eruptions were, of course, the blotches and scaly symptoms of scurvy, a disease that, as late as 1789, the Hospital's physician diagnosed among the children.[11]

Since scurvy is brought about by a deficiency in vitamin C, this fact

* Lord Edgcumbe, the 3rd Earl of Orford, and the Prince de Craon at one time or another suffered from the itch.

takes us back to our previous discussion of probable deficiencies in the children's diet. In addition to the evidence of vitamin C deficiency provided by the presence of scorbutic eruptions among the children, we also find records of many cases of lameness, crooked legs and other deformities, as well as purchases of supports for weak legs, all of which would strongly indicate the existence of the rickets that would result from the vitamin D deficiency in the children's diet. Rickets was, in fact, a very common disease among children in eighteenth-century London. In addition, the many cases of blindness and of weak or diseased eyes—'The Children in general seem to be extremely subject to distempered eyes', commented the Subcommittee's minutes on 15 September 1759—strongly support the premise that the children's diet did not contain sufficient vitamin A. Many of these children may have been suffering from xerophthalmia, although it is probable that smallpox caused some cases of blindness.[12] One final bit of evidence to support a theory of malnutrition among the children appears in a list of the children at the Ackworth Hospital who were suffering from various disabilities in 1771. The list described nine of them as 'dwarfs'. The significance of this data is that excessive shortness almost without fail indicates inadequate nutrition.[13]

The Governors themselves seem to have suspected a connection between diet and disease. In 1759 the Subcommittee noted that many children died or were constantly ill after returning to the Hospital from the country and, upon learning that 37 out of 158 children in the Hospital were afflicted with scald heads, recommended that an 'enquiry be made if the same children enjoyed health under their Nurses for 5 years because if they did it may be premised that the kinds of aliment given the children in the Hospital tho' good in itself is not so proper for them as that to which they used to have'.[14] Certainly, if the country nurses took Dr Cadogan as their guide, which the Governors intended them to do, they would have fed the children 'any kind of mellow Fruit, either raw, stewed, or baked; Roots of all sorts, and all the Produce of the Kitchen Garden'. But how nearly this ideal was achieved we do not know. Historians who have studied the diets of village and farm labourers in the eighteenth century generally indicate substantial differences between the diets of country folk in the north of England and those in the south and between the earlier and later parts of the century. Such differences, as well as those between one country family's local situation and another's, make any comparison of the quality of the children's diet while at nurse with their diet in the Hospital virtually impossible.[15] The Governors, too, did not pursue such a comparison, for even if the many other aspects of running the Hospital had not devoured their time, more urgent problems relating to the children's health constantly demanded their attention. The presence of venereal disease among the children taken in during the General Reception furnishes one example. Because of the potential threat to the nurses, the Governors felt compelled to deal with this problem as promptly as possible. In March 1759 they found so many children infected that they considered for a time the possibility of taking over a ward in the Lock Hospital for their treatment, and during the next seventeen months at least fourteen children were treated in that Hospital at a total cost of £48 15s. Many of the children did not survive the treatment, which was salivation produced by the administration of mercury. The cure, which lasted from a week or ten days to as long as ten weeks, was almost worse than the disease, bringing on fever, sleeplessness, swollen glands and tongue, sore mouth and throat, rashes and itching, followed by scaly incrustations, loss of hair and nails, and extreme pain.[16]

Whooping cough, often called 'chin cough', presented a continuing problem and sometimes proved fatal. The Governors frequently sent children so afflicted to the country for nursing. Consumptive children and those weakened by measles were also sent to the country to recuperate. In winter, chilblains required the staff's attention. More serious were cases of ruptures, for which trusses had to be secured; operations on children suffering from stones in the bladder; and amputations of limbs. All of these matters came to the Governors' attention, especially when the Hospital's surgeons deemed operations necessary. The decision to operate was far more serious in the eighteenth century than it is today, for surgery then was very crude, performed without anaesthesia, and accompanied by high mortality from loss of blood—transfusions were not given—or septic infection. Because of the uncertainty of the outcome and the intense fear induced in the patient, most people thought of operations as a last resort, and the foundlings did not differ from others in such feelings. For example, when Baron Wentzel offered to operate without charge on the eyes of a blind foundling, John Printer, to remove cataracts, the boy's 'irresolution prevented the Operation', and he remained blind for the rest of his life rather than submit to the procedure[17]

Accidents and the possibility of accidents burdened the Governors with still another source of worry. They tried to anticipate what might happen: they directed that iron guards be placed around the fireplaces to keep the children from falling into the fire, and they took precautions to secure the window sashes in such a way that the children could not fall out. But no one could foresee all the possibilities for accidents among so large a group of children. Only after a boy was killed as the consequence of sliding down a stair bannister did the Governors order an iron rail, with spikes affixed at intervals, to be mounted twelve inches above the bannister of every staircase in the Hospital.[18]

Fortunately, the Governors could call upon the best medical opinion of the time from among their own number to help them in their many difficult decisions affecting the children's health. There was, first of all, the eminent and wealthy Dr Richard Mead, who, like many other fashionable physicians, visited only his most socially prominent patients and prescribed for lesser folk, without seeing them, on the basis of the description of symptoms furnished him by their attending apothecaries. The foundlings, however, received his personal attention. Riding in a gilt carriage, drawn by six horses and accompanied by two running footmen, he came to Hatton Garden to examine the first children taken in and to advise what treatment should be given to those who were ill. Mead's ideas about the benefits of fresh air probably started the policy of sending ailing children to the country for their health. Another physician who devoted much of his time to the children in the early days of the Hospital was Dr Robert Nesbitt. Although less famous than Mead, he had studied under the great Dutch physician and chemist, Hermann Boerhaave, at Leyden and took a prominent part in the affairs of the Royal College of Physicians. Together, Mead and Nesbitt advised the Committee what medicines should be kept on hand, and the Royal College answered the Governors' queries about the advisability of wet nursing as against dry nursing and the propriety of allowing nurses to give restless children opiates to quiet them.

Another celebrated physician who gave advice in the early years was Sir Hans Sloane, who also served as physician to the children at Christ's Hospital. And we have already encountered Dr Cadogan's ideas about the care of the foundling infants. Apart from his association with the Hospital, Cadogan was a fashionable West End practitioner with a reputation for his treatment of the gout. Later in the century Sir William Watson, a botanist as well as a physician, advised the Governors for twenty-five years from 1762 to 1787. Dr John Mayo, who officiated as the Hospital's physician at the end of the century, also acted as physician to the Princess of Wales. Mayo probably created a greater stir than any other physician that ever attended the foundlings by bringing serious charges against the matron in 1790: he alleged that many of the diseases rampant among the children were directly attributable to her negligence of their diet, want of care for cleanliness, and inadequate supervision of the nurses.

From this recital one fact stands out: during the entire century the children enjoyed the advantage of medical supervision by some of the most eminent physicians of the time. And these men, who normally charged one or two guineas a visit, attended the children gratis. In addition, the Governors could always call on one or more surgeons, beginning with one of the original Governors, Peter Sainthill. Later in the century several men who practised dentistry also offered their services to the Hospital without charge.[19]

The key to day-to-day care, however, lay in the quality of the nursing, which varied from time to time because some nurses were lazy and some resisted any change in the traditional ways of doing things. It also depended on the degree of supervision exercised by the apothecary, who, in the beginning, visited the Hospital once a day. During this period the Governors permitted only the chief nurse to administer the medicines prepared by the apothecary—and no others—upon the prescription of one of the Hospital's physicians.

The General Reception, however, made necessary the employment of a resident apothecary, and as a result Robert McClellan was engaged in 1759 at a salary of £50 a year. As we have already noted, he remained at the Hospital until 1797. When he retired, the Governors decided that the Hospital no longer required an apothecary in residence and appointed as visiting apothecary Julian Mariner, who had grown up in the Hospital and had served as McClellan's apprentice.[20]

Until 1759 the visiting apothecary made up all medicines in his own shop or obtained them from the Apothecaries' Hall, but when McClellan came to live in the Hospital, an apothecary's shop was fitted up for his use. After his retirement, Julian Mariner continued to use it to prepare medicines for the children in the Hospital. By this time the shop contained 390 different drugs, 7 bottles of mountain wine, 6 bottles of vinegar, treacle, coarse sugar, lint, and such pieces of equipment as pewter syringes and a 'tobbaco clyster machine'. Among the drugs in the shop that a twentieth-century reader might recognize were: camphor, digitalis, jalap, opium, sal ammonia, ipecac, myrrh, alcohol, silver nitrate, calomel, magnesia, rhubarb, and cantharides (Spanish fly).[21]

Despite this repertory of drugs, the state of eighteenth-century knowledge about their true properties was such that few specifics existed: Peruvian bark (quinine) for malaria, mercury for syphilis, and sulphur for the itch. The apothecary used all of them in treating the children, especially since Sir Hans Sloane strongly advocated the use of the bark for fevers. Most of the drugs administered, however, had little effect on the course of the disease for which they were given but, unless they contained metallic substances such as antimony, probably did little harm. On the other hand, the common practices of purging, inducing vomiting, and bloodletting in the treatment of fevers, all of which were believed necessary to expel the cause, may have served only to weaken further children already critically ill.[22] Nevertheless, the Hospital's physicians authorized these forms of treatment: bloodletting by the use of leeches was practised as late as 1790. And from directions that the physicians prepared for the use of medicines in the country hospitals, we learn that they recommended for fever 'the fever powder of our own dispensatory, an Occasional Clyster, and Bark in Intermittents'; for worms, 'Wormseed—the best Medicine, Quicksilver, Rhubarb, & sometimes a little common Aloes, Crude Antimony,...and Magnesia, given discretionally 'till the Habit be corrected'; for diarrhea and dysentery, 'a vomit of Ipecacuana, especially in the beginning, Hartshorn drink, Nutmeg, Rhubarb at Intervals'.

The Hospital also supplied the country inspectors with rhubarb and magnesia to treat their infant charges for 'watery gripes', perhaps because Dr Cadogan thought so highly of *magnesia alba* as a 'lenient Purgative' effective against heartburn, 'green Stools, Gripes and Purgings'. Another item furnished to the country inspectors with instructions for its use was crab's claw powder or crab's-eyes, believed to be an antidote to diarrhea.* Modern ideas about the harmfulness of excessive use of laxatives did not exist. Quite the contrary opinion prevailed: a good purge was thought helpful in the treatment of almost any ailment and probably a general preventative of disease, a notion that accounts for Mr McClellan's practice of dosing all the children in a ward with a physic every three weeks, taking the wards by turns.[23]

If some of these methods seem ridiculous or harsh to us, we must remember not only the static state of pharmacology at the time but also the relatively few means of diagnosis available. The pulse watch came into use in 1707 but the fever thermometer, although employed in Holland, France, and Germany, was not widely utilized in England until the 1770s. For the most part, diagnosis depended upon observation of the patient's general appearance, respiration, tongue, region of pain, and signs of fever, and the appearance of extracted blood and urine. Moreover, few recognized that the treatment of

---

* Crab's-eyes were small stones found in the stomachs of crayfish and composed chiefly of carbonate of lime. In finely powdered form, it served as an antacid.

children required specialized knowledge. Only a handful of books devoted to the health and diseases of children appeared in England between 1689 and Cadogan's treatise in 1748. And, except among the wealthy, it was the apothecary upon whom fell the burden of making the first diagnosis and deciding whether to call in a physician or to treat the patient himself, a decision that he based not upon any course of formal training but upon what he had learned by apprenticeship to another apothecary and by experience.[24]

What diagnostic tools, if any, the Hospital's apothecary used I do not know. Nor have I found any indication that its apothecaries availed themselves of textbooks other than Cadogan's except for a handwritten copy of *Formula Medicamentorum* by Hugoni Smith, M. D., carefully transcribed into a book containing McClellan's notes on treatments from 1760 to 1762. Among other diseases, Smith's disquisition, which contained numerous prescriptions, discussed smallpox, measles, venereal diseases, and diseases listed as specific to children, i.e., teething, worms, scald head, whooping cough, and scrofula. That its recommendations did not depart from the customary practice of the time can readily be seen from the following extract relating to measles:

> The most degenerate symptom [of measles] is a peripneumony or inflammation of the lungs which frequently supervenes. Bloodletting becomes in the case a soverign remedy and may be boldly repeated according to the strength of the patient pulse and urgency of the symptoms. The antimoneal powder N. 1 is eminently serviseable and gentle Cathartics and Blisters after Bleeding may likewise be expedient, under some Circumstances an Emetic.[25]

For the most part, the Governors kept an open mind about new forms of health care except in their determination throughout the century that as many infants as possible should be placed with wet nurses in the country in spite of evidence that a child's chance of survival was approximately the same whether it was wet nursed or dry nursed.* Their conviction arose from the bad experience with dry nursing that they had had in the first year of the Hospital's existence. At that time Sir Hans Sloane had given his opinion, founded on fifty years' observation, 'that of three Infants bred without the Breast, two generally died, notwithstanding what he or others could do to help them'. The Committee had also observed

* From 2 June 1756 to 2 June 1757, 996 out of 2555 children wet nursed in the country died, a mortality rate of 39 percent, and 145 out of 375 dry nursed in the country also died, a mortality rate of 38.7 percent.

during the first year that the mortality rate for the children kept at Hatton Garden greatly exceeded that for those sent to the country to be nursed. This they attributed to the polluted air of London and the crowded conditions in the house. The consequence of these early events manifested itself in a firm resolution 'to send all Children which should be taken in, as soon as possible into the Country, to remain there until three Years of age; and that all such as would suck, should be nursed by wet Nurses only'.[26] Not everyone agreed with this view, and over and over again it came up for reconsideration, but, in the end, the policy remained unchanged.

On the other hand, the Governors willingly accepted the offer of Philip Jones in 1777 to apply his 'Spinal Machine for curing Distortions in Children on two of the Children of this Hospital', although 'the machines that must be made for each child' would cost three guineas apiece.[27] This brings to our attention one of the most insoluble problems to confront the Governors: what to do about deformed, blind, mentally retarded, epileptic, or otherwise handicapped children. Largely because of the policy of indiscriminate admission during the General Reception, the Governors found themselves burdened with many children afflicted with congenital defects, as well as those who had incurred permanent damage through malnourishment, neglect, or abuse at the hands of their parents. Some children, of course, suffered loss of limbs, blindness, or deforming scars as the result of disease or injury occurring after their reception into the Hospital. But however his handicap came into existence, such a child presented the Governors with a continuing problem.

Almost nothing in the way of treatment existed, but where any form of cure held out hope, the Governors tried it. They sent one paralytic girl to the hospital at Bath for treatment and another to be 'electrified'. They purchased trusses, leg braces, spectacles, and special shoes for children whom these devices might help. For the blind, the epileptic, and the mentally retarded, however, there was neither cure nor alleviation.

The care of such afflicted children, even in infancy, was attended with difficulties, and often the Governors had to pay the country nurses premiums to take them. Then, as the children grew older, the Governors discovered that many could not be apprenticed even though they offered larger fees with them. Tailors and shoemakers sometimes took lame boys, but no one wanted the deformed girls. One solution was to employ the handicapped children in the Hospital at whatever tasks they could perform and, as they grew older, to pay them servants' wages. For example, Joseph Stratford, whose speech defect rendered him almost unintelligible, was employed first as assistant to the baker and later as baker. And for a short period some of the handicapped children were kept busy making straw hats.[28]

The problem of dealing with these children became most acute when Parliament withdrew its support in 1771. On 6 June of that year the Ackworth Hospital held 120 children (38 boys and 82 girls) who were handicapped or 'weakly and very small', or who were afflicted with illnesses that made apprenticing virtually impossible. Of the 120, only 5 girls and 1 boy had been admitted before the General Reception. The Governors could hope, of course, that some of the small and weakly children or those who were suffering from sore heads, scrofula, worms, and the like would improve in health and later become eligible for apprenticing, but 18 were described as idiots, 32 were crippled or deformed, 4 were dumb, 7 were blind in one eye, 2 were epileptic, and one was ruptured. At the same time in the London Hospital 10 boys and 15 girls laboured under similar handicaps, while at Shrewsbury 2 children had diseased hips and one had a hernia.

By 1790 apprenticing and death had removed many of these children from the Governors' care, but twenty-seven of the girls (the oldest, admitted in 1749, being of 'weak understanding') still remained in the Hospital. Most of them could perform some work as teachers of the girls, assistants in the laundry, girls' nurses, or kitchen helpers, for which seventeen of them received £3 a year and their board, while six received no salary but were given board and clothing. Four, however, were incapable of any employment at all. Several boys, whose mental disorders made it impossible to keep them at the Hospital, were boarded out, usually in the country. Lievesly described one of these boys as a monster deformed in every limb, 'a perfect Ideot', and so extraordinary, in fact, that the Hospital's surgeon invited many other surgeons to look at him.[29]

Of the handicapped girls maintained in the Hospital in 1790, ten were either of 'weak understanding' or 'Ideotical', a situation that invited difficulties of several kinds, not the least of which one of the Governors set forth in the Visitors' Reports:

Monday 21st June 1790 Enquired into the behaviour of Cicely Sparks aged 33 years & upon her examination She acquainted me with the following particulars viz. That Hector Graham Apprentice to Mr. McClellan the Apothecary Aged 16 years first debauched her & had carnal knowledge of her Body that several times since he repeated it & likewise John Mott the Baker's Boy Aged 15 years did the same. Thomas Abingdon Col. Sharpe's Boy

Aged 17 years & several of the Apprentice Boys out of the House particularly William Vernon Aged 17 years apprentice to Mr. Besby Hair-dresser in Fetter Lane.[30]

As a consequence of her inability to refuse her seducers, this thirty-three-year-old idiot woman was believed to be pregnant—one more problem for the Committee to deal with.[31]

But the Governors never shirked such problems. Indeed, their attitude toward all of their handicapped charges was summed up in the disposition of the case of Ann Twigg, who, after being apprenticed twice, was returned to the Hospital in 1795 by her second mistress 'as being deficient in understanding'. The Committee, reflecting that 'it may be hurtful to the girl to be from under the immediate protection of this Charity', decided that 'she be permitted to remain in the Hospital and employed in such work as she may be found capable of'.[32] In short, the Governors accepted total responsibility for the handicapped foundlings, even for life.

17

A Christian and Useful Education

CARING FOR THE FOUNDLINGS' bodies took up far more of the Committee's time and thought than attending to their minds and souls, not because the Governors believed education and religious instruction unimportant but because they could plan and carry out this part of their work quite easily, and once set in motion, few problems arose. As we shall see, only one aspect of the children's education could be considered innovative. For the rest, the Governors adopted, apparently without much discussion, an educational programme typical of their time, one that required neither elaborate equipment nor a highly trained staff.

Victor Neuburg has pointed out that no real theory of popular education existed in the eighteenth century because the question of whether the children of the poor should be educated at all was still being debated. Those who opposed such education argued that the poor did not need education to do their work, and learning would make them too proud to perform servile tasks, dissatisfied with their lot, and, therefore, refractory and inclined to demand higher wages. This, they asserted, would undermine the whole structure of English society, for to be great, a nation must possess a vast pool of ignorant but contented people to do its drudgery.[1] As an anonymous commentator in the *London Magazine* put it in 1766, 'we have more occasion for having children bred up to labour than to any sort of learning'.[2]

The opponents of such views based their position on the necessity of teaching the children of the poor to read the Bible and also of indoctrinating them with proper precepts of subordination. Said George Chapman in 1773:

To reconcile the lowest class of mankind to the fatigues of constant labour, and the otherwise mortifying thoughts of a servile employment, pains should be taken to convince them, when young, that subordination is necessary in society; that they ought to submit to their masters or superiors in every thing that is lawful; that nature has formed us for action; that happiness does not consist in indolence, nor in the possession of riches, nor in the gratification of sense, nor in pomp and splendid equipage, but in habits of industry and contentment, in temperance and frugality, in the conscious-ness of doing our duty in the station in which we are placed.[3]

Beyond the objectives of religious instruction and social condition-ing, the proponents of education for poor children did not agree among themselves. Chapman and, earlier, James Nelson thought that in addition to reading boys should learn writing and simple arith-metic. Chapman also included instruction in psalmody—a natural suggestion from a Scotsman used to kirks without choirs—and thought that properly supervised, vigorous outdoor exercise would benefit the children by inuring them to fatigue and inclement weather.[4] But others, while agreeing upon the benefits of teaching poor children to read, did not approve of instruction in writing or arithmetic because such skills would qualify the children to become clerks and bookkeepers, thereby making them competitors of the sons of substantial tradesmen and lesser merchants. Dr Isaac Watts, a champion of the charity schools, spoke for many when he said: 'There are none of these Poor who . . . ought to be bred up to such an accomplished Skill in Writing and Accompts, as to be qualified for . . . [superior] Posts; except here and there a single Lad, whose bright Genius, and whose constant Application and Industry have out-run all his Fellows'.[5]

Undergirding both sides of the debate were Lockeian premises: that mental culture was not for mean men; that character was formed in early childhood; and that utility should constitute the guiding principle of education. All parties, in fact, wanted the same thing: to preserve the hierarchical structure of English society as they knew it, believing it to be the right and natural arrangement of human relationships. They differed over means, not ends.[6]

At first, the Governors aligned themselves with the proponents of education limited to reading. The plan for operating the Hospital formulated in 1740 stated that when the children returned from the country they were 'to be taught to read and instructed in the Principles of the Christian Religion, and brought up to Labour'.[7] And so the sewing and knitting mistresses taught both boys and girls to read by the traditional means of the hornbook,* the period of instruction lasting from the age of three to the age of six.[8]

In 1754 the Subcommittee raised the question whether the children should also learn to write, and they recommended the employment of a schoolmaster. But nothing came of these suggestions, and not until February 1757 did the Hospital engage a schoolmaster at £30 per annum plus lodging and a gown, a salary comparable to that usually paid to teachers in the charity schools. At the same time, the Governors decided 'that to every fifty of the Girls, who have attained their age of 6 years, a Mistress shall be appointed to teach them to work, read and write when required', such mistresses to receive £10 a year and board. But in May, when the Hospital finally advertised for schoolmistresses, no mention was made of writing. Instead, the mistresses were expected to instruct the girls in reading, spinning, knitting, and needlework, 'in such manner as may enable them to make useful Servants, and also in the Catechism of the Church of England'.

With the arrival of the schoolmaster, Joseph Redpath, came changes. Mr Redpath did away with hornbooks and, with the Governors' approval, ordered three thousand battledores;** two thousand half sheets containing the Hospital's prayers, the Creed, the Lord's Prayer, and the Ten Commandments; and three thousand sets of the first sixteen pages for a spelling book, each set sewed into a strong paper cover. In making use of battledores, the Governors anticipated a future trend, for this type of instructional material became very popular in the 1770s. At this time, too, the Governors divided the boys into two classes, so that each group attended school half a day and worked half a day.[9] By 1759 the schoolmaster was teaching some of the boys to write, and the schoolmistresses had to be able to give the girls similar instruction, if required, in addition to teaching them to read. Both the nurses and the schoolmistresses were expected to assist in teaching the children their prayers and the catechism.[10]

In schools for poor children, after they had learned the alphabet and how to spell, the Bible often served as their only reader, although suitable textbooks were in print.[11] The Hospital also used the Bible as a reader, but the Governors showed sufficient sensitivity to the

* A hornbook was a single sheet containing a printed alphabet, the nine digits, and the Lord's Prayer, with a protective covering of transparent horn, set in a frame with a handle. Such devices had been used in England at least as early as 1421 and from the end of the sixteenth century were the common means of instruction.

** Battledores were alphabets pasted on cardboard.

psychology of children to rescue the foundlings from the mindless rote learning then commonly employed in teaching children. In 1763 the Governors learned

> . . . that the Reading Mistress puts the Girls to reading Passages in the Scripture which it is absolutely impossible they can understand and consequently cannot read with any pleasure or improvement. [They thereupon] Ordered that she teach them to read in such passages as they can understand so that they may read with delight and that she explains to them in an easy familiar manner such parts as are most interesting that they may be improved in their understanding and at the same time learn to read with so much the greater ease. [And they] Ordered that the Boys Master observe the same rule.[12]

In addition to the Bible, the 'Instructions to Apprentices' was also used for pedagogical purposes, but apparently the Hospital's teachers took advantage of no other texts.[13]

Some of the children learned the first elements of reading at dame schools while still living with their country nurses—in the beginning, at the nurses' own expense. The Hospital's clerk, who made a visit of inspection in 1764 to several villages, reported that in Ewell twelve children were 'sent to School every day at the expence of their Nurses, and to Church three times a week'. A similar situation prevailed in Chertsey. At Epsom and Dorking, however, he found that none of the children attended school and 'but very few could tell their Letters; Tho' most of them could gabble over the Lords Prayer'. After receiving this report, the Governors decided to reimburse the nurses for the expense of sending the children to school, the cost of which usually amounted to 2d or 3d a week for each child. And this practice seems to have continued for at least the next twenty years.[14]

By the end of the century all of the boys were learning to read and write, and some of them were studying arithmetic. On 5 February 1800 the schoolmaster informed the Governors

> . . . that he had under his care 95 boys from the age of 5 to 14 years inclusive. Of this number 10 write legibly and read in the Bible, and of those, 8 are learning arithmetic, and in respect of education 5 of them are fully qualified to go out with credit as apprentices. That 10 are in the first rudiments of writing and in a state of improvement. That 25 are capable of reading in their spelling books, and the remaining 50 are learning their letters.

He also advised that 'with one exception all the boys who have been apprenticed during the last year were able to read and write their names'. At the same time the schoolmistresses assured the Governors that all of the girls who had gone out as apprentices could, with few exceptions, 'read in the Bible and work with their needles'.[15] A week later, the Committee decided that a class of not more than twelve older girls should be taught to write and cast accounts every Monday and Thursday afternoon. But, in fact, the Governors had been considering whether the girls should learn to write since the spring of 1796,[16] possibly because of Thomas Bernard's influence, for he would gladly have seen every poor person in the kingdom taught to read and cypher at public expense.[17]

Doubtless the Governors had not given the matter much thought in the earlier years of the century, for at that time no one could see any practical reason why girls destined to enter domestic service would need writing or arithmetic. But by 1773, Chapman was suggesting that poor girls learn to write and, if they had the inclination, study the common rules of arithmetic also. He justified his recommendation by the conviction that 'this early attention to their minds', which he considered quite as capable of learning as those of boys, 'would render them more diligent and more faithful servants' and, when they married, would 'render them more capable of instructing their children, and more attentive to their behaviour'.[18] Captain Coram had said the same thing almost forty years earlier in a letter to Dr Colman:

> . . . [it] is an Evil amongst us here in England to think Girls having learning given them is not so very Material as for boys to have it. I think and say it is more Material, for Girls when they come to be Mothers will have the forming of their Childrens lives and if their Mothers be good or Bad the Children Generally take after them so that Giving Girls a vertuous Education is a vast Advantage to their Posterity as well as to the Publick.[19]

The Governors, however, had not shared this view nor shown any inclination to lead the way in giving poor girls more education than they required to read the Bible. This state of educational backwardness the foundling girls shared with approximately 60 percent of their female contemporaries until the mid-1780s and with about 55 percent of them by 1800, a gradual improvement in the level of female literacy having taken place from the mid-1780s onward, possibly because of the Sunday School movement. Nevertheless, the foundling girls surpassed their French counterparts, for in 1790 only twenty-four out of eight hundred girls at the Paris institution could read.[20]

On the other hand, by 1800 the level of education achieved by the foundling boys exceeded substantially that of their contemporaries, for the number of men unable to sign their names in a marriage register hovered around 40 percent from 1754 to the end of the century, with a slight improvement in the final five years. But by this time the foundling boys were scoring close to 100 percent in the ability to write. The achievement of the boys appears even more remarkable when we consider the correlation of illiteracy with occupation. In all times and in all regions this correlation occurred because literacy possessed a varying functional value: in general, the only persons to acquire literary skills beyond elementary reading were those whose occupations or social status demanded them. In the retail trades, for example, only 5 to 10 percent of the men were unable to write; among craftsmen in textile, metal, and leather trades, 20 to 39 percent could not sign their names. But among husbandmen the number of nonwriters was 46 to 56 percent, and among labourers and servants, it was 59 to 65 percent.[21] Since, in theory, the foundlings were being trained to fill society's most laborious occupations and were, in fact, usually apprenticed to the sea service, to husbandry, or to tradesmen of the lower ranks, the paradox confronts us that from 1759 onward some of the boys, and by the end of the century virtually all of them, were receiving more education than they needed for the occupations to which they were apprenticed. Indeed, the boys were probably more literate in many instances than their masters and, therefore, more likely than they to become acquainted with the dangerous ideas appearing in the scandal sheets that dominated the public press in the last quarter of the century. Such a state of things may well explain the increase in the number of conflicts between masters and their foundling apprentices that we have already noted in Chapter 11.

Although the foundling children spent far more years in school than most poor children, for whom the average was about eighteen months,[22] years in school do not guarantee education, and we cannot judge how well the foundlings were taught because we know nothing about the qualifications of any of the schoolmistresses or of the schoolmasters who preceded Robert Atchison. But the qualifications set forth in Atchison's letter of application in 1780 would not seem to us impressive—yet he was hired—for he wrote:

Having been Inform'd that the Place of Schoolmaster to your Children will soon be vacant I beg Leave to offer myself for your approbation. I have no great Literary attainments, am by Profession a Mechanic, but my Eyes failing by Constant

Application Induced me to offer myself to your Service. My moral Character will (without the least Reserve) bear a Strickt Enquiry and can be well attested.[23]

His candidness about his eyesight may have been unusual, but his background was not. Teaching poor children was regarded as a humble position that required no special training. Anyone who could read, write, and do sums could fall back upon such an occupation in time of need or combine it with another trade, which many found necessary to do because teaching was generally ill paid. As Thomas Bernard put it, 'they who can do better quit teaching school for more profitable employment, while the lazy and inferior remain'.[24] Moreover, Atchison, like his predecessors, had so many other tasks assigned to him—investigating the characters of applicants for apprentices, collecting pew rents and keeping accounts for the chapel, reconciling differences between masters and apprentices— that he remarked in 1800 that 'from his being absent on the duties of the Hospital during the school hours and having no one to assist or officiate for him', he had not been able to give the children 'that regular course of instruction which otherwise he should feel himself enabled to do'.[25]

Whatever its deficiencies, the Governors wanted the children's education to serve useful purposes, and they held similar views about the foundlings' recreation. They always allotted time for play, not play for the fun of it but play for a purpose: to build strong, healthy bodies. As the Governors expressed it in 1749, they intended that the children's 'diversions be innocent, active, and requiring exercise'.[26] In fact, five years later the members of the Subcommittee conceived the idea that the Hospital should purchase 'some sort of Javelin or Dart', which the boys could learn to throw 'in order to inure them to a proper Sleight in throwing a Harpoon in the Greenland Fishery; whereby not only some dexterity will be acquired but their Chests opened and Strength increased; and this may also serve them for Pastime'.[27] The General Committee, however, took no action on this utilitarian proposal, although two years later they did accede to Mr Whatley's suggestion that the boys 'be learnt to exercise in a military manner'.

As for the girls, the Subcommittee ordered that they 'be exercised in walking upright and strong without wadling'. Indeed, walking about on the Hospital's property under the chaperonage of their nurses and schoolmistresses constituted the only provision made for their recreation all through the century, other than reserving a play space for them at the south end of the east colonnade. No one ever purchased special toys for the girls. If they played with dolls, then they must have been homemade—rag dolls dressed by the little seamstresses themselves.

The boys, on the other hand, from at least 1755 onward were given bats and balls, tops and whips; were taught how to use them; and were provided with outdoor play space adjacent to the Hospital.[28] The Governors also made similar provision for the children in the country hospitals. An account written by a visitor to the Shrewsbury hospital in 1771 notes that 'there is a large Piece of Ground allotted the Children to play in and what seems extraordinary there should be occasion for, a master is appointed to see that they do play'.[29]

For the foundlings, then, play formed a part of their overall training just as their religious instruction was inextricably interwoven with the lessons taught in the schoolroom, where, apart from the 'Instructions to Apprentices', the children's whole course of reading consisted of religious texts. In addition, efforts to teach the children the Catechism had begun in 1748 when the Governors directed the nurses to 'employ the Sunday Evenings in Instructing the Children in the Catechism, and hearing them Read the Scriptures'. And when the Committee appointed the Reverend John Waring Reader for the chapel at a salary of £40 a year, they charged him with the duty of catechizing the children publicly once a month.

In 1754 the Governors adopted a new schedule for catechizing the children. It provided for a public exercise every Sunday—in the chapel from Lady Day to Michaelmas and in the dining room after evening prayer during the rest of the year. The Reader was also expected to give an exposition of the Catechism over a period of twelve successive Sundays every year, beginning the first Sunday in May. Unfortunately, Mr Waring proved lax in these duties, and by January 1758 the Committee found it necessary to reprove him for failure to catechize the children from Michaelmas to Christmas. The same dereliction occurred again in the autumn and winter of 1758, and again in 1759.[30] But by this time the Governors had compensated in part for the Reader's neglect—he continued in his post until 1766—by engaging Mr Redpath, who added to his other duties that of teaching the boys the Catechism, while the schoolmistresses gave the girls similar instruction. During the next forty years arrangements for additional instruction by the clergy varied, but, in general, some provision was made for an exposition of parts of the Catechism by the Reader on one Sunday afternoon a month combined with an occasional public catechizing of the children in the chapel.[31]

The Governors also tried to ensure that the children would not forget their religious training during their apprenticeships. Not only

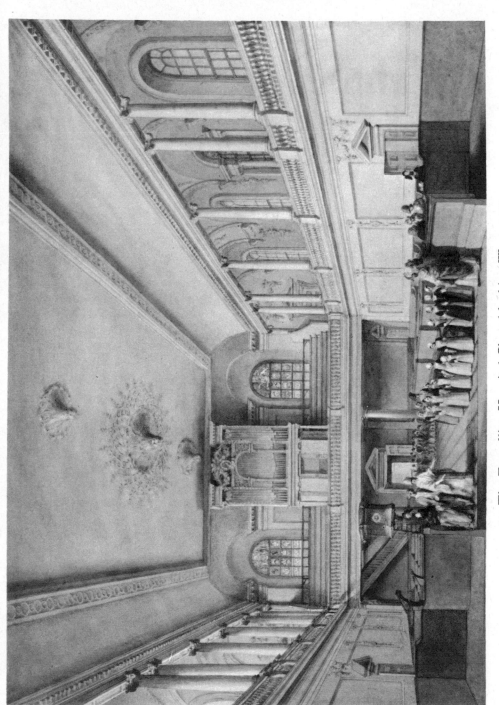

13. The Foundling Hospital Chapel looking West, 1773

did they give each child leaving the Hospital a Bible and Common Prayer Book, but they also delivered to each child's master instructions specifying what the Hospital regarded as his religious duty to his apprentice:

> As it is of the greatest moment to breed up Children in the Fear of God, as the best means of keeping them in Proper Subjection to their Masters, Mistresses, and Superiors, and as praying is the most effectual means to promote such Fear, and to inforce obedience to the Laws of God, you are hereby informed, that it is expected of You to take Care that this Child_____ Aged____says h__prayers constantly every Morning, as well as every evening, and you are to endeavour to give h__a due sence of what h__is about, and to this end, you must be careful that h__ repeats h__prayers in a Slow, serious & solemn Manner. And you are further to take Care that this Child do frequent the publick worship on the Sabbath day, in a sober, pious, orderly manner.[32]

Moreover, when the Governors visited the apprenticed foundlings, they were expected to examine the children to ascertain 'if they can read and say their prayers, and in such case to use their discretion in giving them a little Tract, The Abstract of the Bible, printed for the use of this Hospital'.[33]

Yet in spite of the Governors' concern for the children's religious instruction, no foundling was confirmed at the Hospital in the eighteenth century. The reason for this seeming neglect was that in the earlier part of the century most children left the Hospital to begin their apprenticeships while still too young to be confirmed. By the 1790s, however, the children were not, as a rule, apprenticed until they were thirteen to fifteen years old. Apparently the changed circumstances went unnoticed until, in May 1799, the Governors realized that thirty children of a proper age to be confirmed had been placed out during the preceding eighteen months and that another twelve who were fourteen years old remained in the Hospital. They at once concluded that if they could assemble the thirty apprentices on a Sunday, some forty-two children could be and should be confirmed at a private ceremony in the chapel. Whereupon the treasurer, Thomas Bernard, called upon the Lord Bishop of London for advice and assistance. The Bishop informed him that if the children could be properly prepared, he would 'under the peculiar circumstances of this Charity, vary in this Instance his general Rule, and Confirm every 4 years such Children as were fit, and not under the age of 13 years'. The Governors immediately ordered confirmation tracts to be printed and distributed so that 'the Charity may in the ensuing

Spring have the benefit of his Lordships benevolent Assistance'.[34]

The children's religious training during at least part of the century was further reinforced by their instruction in music. This was probably the most unusual feature of their entire education, for eighteenth-century opinion tended to regard teaching music to poor children as either unnecessary or likely to expose them to disreputable associations. For a short time early in the century the charity schools had taught singing in some of the schools, encouraged by parsons and congregations who enjoyed hearing the children's voices in the Sunday services, but in 1724 the Bishop of London had put an end to adding such frills to the education of children who should be learning only to become good Christians and good servants and beyond that needed nothing more.[35]

For the most part, until the 1770s, the Governors shared the views of their contemporaries. In fact, on 27 March 1765 the General Court informed Dr Lee at Ackworth that 'it is the opinion of this General Court that it is highly improper that the time of Charity Children should be employed in learning Musick or Singing'.[36] An exception had been made in 1753 when the Governors agreed that a seven-year-old blind boy, Tom Grenville, should be taught to play a harpsichord that had been given to the Hospital so that he might become 'a performer of Musick in the Chapel'. He learned so well that in 1758 the Governors authorized his teacher to instruct him in playing the organ at a cost of two guineas a quarter. The Governors also provided somewhat similar training for other blind children—John Printer in 1768, Blanch Thetford in 1771, and Mercy Draper in 1773. In the case of Mercy Draper, who possessed a very fine voice, the Governors remarked that such instruction 'may not only be advantageous to this Hospital but an Act of Justice to the Girl'.[37]

Meanwhile, sometime in the 1760s William Harrison, one of the most active Governors, began teaching 'such children as were capable of Instruction to sing Psalms, Hymns and Anthems in a Manner suitable to their capacities and situations'. The Governors took no official notice of his activities until 1771, probably in deference to public opinion while the Hospital was still receiving funds from Parliament. Then the Committee gave him its official thanks and asked him to continue his 'same kind Office' in collaboration with a newly appointed organist whose duties included teaching some of the children music.[38] The Governors evidently no longer thought such instruction a waste of time, and the reason for their change of mind appeared very plainly in the minutes of the Committee meeting of 19 May 1773 at which they concluded that those children who could become proficient in music might 'be of great use to this Charity by adding to the Fund for the support thereof'.[39] But the Governors still did not see fit to make such instruction general and resolved that no more than twenty children be taught music and singing. For about a month the Committee employed a signing master to teach these children. Then the General Court decided that the additional expense was unnecessary: the organist and Mr Harrison could do just as well 'in the usual manner'.[40]

In making its decisions, especially in respect to the instruction of Mercy Draper in singing, the Committee had the benefit of the advice of John Stanley, one of the Governors, who was a musician and composer of considerable ability and who was himself blind.* Stanley generously offered to teach the girl without charge if she could be sent to his home in Hatton Garden two or three times a week. In addition to promoting the career of Mercy Draper, which will be described in the next chapter, Stanley also played the organ in the chapel on special occasions, wrote three hymns or anthems especially for the Hospital's use, and directed the performances of the *Messiah* from 1769 to 1777.[41]

About a year after the Governors decided to dismiss the singing master, they were called upon to make a far weightier decision about training the children in music. In July 1774 Dr Charles Burney and Felice de Giardini, a famous violinist who had been a Governor of the Hospital since 1770 and had assisted with its musical programmes, approached the Governors with a proposal to establish a national music school at the Foundling Hospital. It was to be similar to the *conservatorios* in Venice and Naples that had so greatly impressed Dr Burney during his Italian tour in 1770. The plan envisioned two departments: one to teach girls singing, and the other to instruct boys in composition and instrumental performance. Children with no musical gifts at all could learn to transcribe music, or tune and mend instruments. Giardini and Dr Burney would act as supervising masters, for which each would expect a salary of £200 a year, but both would contribute musical compositions for the Hospital's use and would assist in any public performances. In addition, the school would need four assistant masters at £50 a year each, and in the first

---

* John Stanley (1713–86) served as organist at St Andrew Holborn for over fifty years and from 1734 onward also acted as organist at the Middle Temple. In 1779 he was appointed Master of the King's Band of Musicians, the highest professional honour obtainable. He composed both instrumental and vocal music, including oratorios and cantatas, and also invented a mechanical apparatus for teaching the theory of music to the blind, one of which devices was used by Tom Grenville.

year, instruments, books, and other supplies costing about £200.

If the Hospital itself could not provide sufficient good voices, it was proposed that children with the proper gifts be recruited from charity schools and workhouses, which could contribute toward the costs of their training. In time, it was hoped, the school might take in from all parts of the kingdom pupils who could pay for their instruction and thereby provide another source of income. Eventually, the proponents of the plan asserted, the school would pay its own way and bring in a profit to the Hospital, which could hire the boys out singly or in groups for musical performances in churches, oratorios, operas, plays and concerts. Their earnings, of course, would belong to the Hospital until they were twenty-one. Moreover, performances of sacred music, oratorios and anthems on Sunday evenings in the chapel would bring in substantial amounts, either from collections or from the sale of tickets. Above all, such a school would benefit the national economy by providing a pool of trained native musicians who could furnish the services for which foreigners were currently pocketing large sums of money.

Appealing both to the Hospital's urgent need for additional funds and the Governors' desire to prove the institution's usefulness to the nation, the scheme met with almost immediate approbation, at least on the part of Dr Burney's friends among the Governors. On 20 July the General Court resolved to accept the plan and to open a subscription roll to raise funds for beginning the project. According to Burney's biographer, Roger Lonsdale, this meeting was packed with Burney's supporters, and by the end of July they had plans for the school well mapped out. Then, something happened. Perhaps these men had second thoughts; perhaps they discussed the plan with the Hospital's solicitor; or perhaps Burney's opponents turned out in force. For on 3 August the General Court rescinded its previous action on the ground that the Act of Parliament of 1740 did not grant the Governors authority to employ the children in the manner proposed. Burney bitterly attributed the defeat of his plan to 'a small Junto, a Cabal . . . collected together from 2 or 3 neighbouring streets', which might well have been the truth, for it is likely that the Hospital's neighbours would not have welcomed the threat to their peace and quiet that a music school would offer.[42]

And so the musical training of the children continued 'in the usual manner', with Tom Grenville, now the Hospital's organist, instructing them. But by 1777 they were learning to chant the Te Deum at the morning service and the Magnificat at evening prayer, and by 1790 they were being taught singing on a regular schedule of one hour twice a week. That the Governors were moved to such an increase in the programme of musical training by practical rather than aesthetic considerations we may infer from the fact that in 1787 they were discussing 'what measures will be proper to be taken in order to preserve amongst the children a succession of Singers in the Chapel', and in 1796 they flatly refused to apprentice a boy because he was one of the chapel's singers. By then the Governors had recognized that the singing of the children was drawing many Londoners to the chapel services, which led to steadily mounting collections. In 1771 the collections totaled £101 1s 1d; in 1781, £216 13s; in 1787, £610 17s 9d; and in 1796, £1845 5s 3d.[43]

If the children paid heed to the words they sang, the texts of the anthems and hymns also served as a medium of instruction. They conveyed the message to the foundlings that God's goodness had provided for them, for which they owed him gratitude and praise. Many hymns of this type were simply metrical adaptations of the Psalms and expressed sentiments proper to any Christian. But some of the adaptations chosen for the children's use tactlessly reminded them of their origins. For example, the version of the Fifty-first Psalm included in the Hospital's hymnbook compelled the children to sing:

> Wash off my foul offence,
> And cleanse me from my Sin;
> For I confess my crime, and see
> How great my Guilt has been.
>
> In Guilt each part was form'd
> Of all this sinful frame;
> In Guilt I was conceiv'd and born
> The Heir of Sin and Shame.[44]

Other hymns were just as blunt. One, entitled 'A Hymn for the Children of the Foundling Hospital', written by Dr John Hawkesworth and set to music by Mr Stanley, contained these lines:

> Left on the worlds bleak waste forlorn,
> In sin conceiv'd, to sorrow born,
> By guilt and shame foredoom'd to share
> No mother's love, no father's care,
> No guide the devious maze to tread,
> Above no friendly shelter spread.[45]

We have no way of knowing how well the children understood the meaning of the words they sang. Perhaps such hymns gratified the listening congregation more than they humiliated the singers. Certainly, some of the hymns were addressed to the congregation, for they taught the children that they should be grateful to their human benefactors as well as to God. Handel's *Foundling Hospital Anthem*, composed in 1749, was aptly subtitled 'Blessed are They That Consider the Poor', and its words, adapted from the Psalms, must have warmed the heart of every listening benefactor with the assurance that the 'Charitable shall be had in everlasting remembrance', for 'The People will tell of their wisdom and the congregation will shew their praise', and 'Their reward also is with the Lord'.

Dr Paul Henry Lang has commented that the great difference between the Lutheran chorale and English church music is that the chorale gives expression to the mystical aspect of Christianity—the turning inward of the soul toward its own experience of God and away from the outward world—whereas English hymns and anthems function simply as accessories to a reasonable religion that gives proper attention to life on this earth.[46] Certainly the hymns used in the Hospital's chapel seem designed to serve as accessories to awaken impulses toward further generosity in the minds of the congregation and to remind the foundlings of the attitudes proper to children in their position.

Such reminders had, in fact, been enjoined upon the officers of the Hospital as early as 1749; they were to point out to the children often 'the lowness of their Condition, that they may early imbibe the Principles of Humility and Gratitude to their Benefactors, and to learn to undergo with Contentment the most Servile and laborious Offices'.[47] The Governors also urged persons visiting the Hospital 'that no familiar Notice may be taken of the Children, lest it should encourage them to forget the lowness of their Station'.[48] An attitude of this kind was by no means peculiar to the Governors of the Foundling Hospital. In 1789 the opening prayer of the Girls' Charity School in Sheffield was 'Make me dutiful and obedient to my benefactors, and charitable to my enemies. Make me temperate and chaste, meek and patient, true in all my dealings and content and industrious in my station'.[49] In short, the virtues emphasized to all poor children by every possible means were honesty, humility, gratitude, industry, and obedience to one's superiors, a combination that should have produced the perfect servant.

Gambling, swearing, indecent language or behaviour, drinking 'porter or spirituous Liquors', or any association of boys with girls were strictly forbidden, and these rules were fairly well enforced.[50]

But children are not angels, and some mischief was inevitable: breaking windows, playing with the clock pendulum, sliding on bannisters, begging from visitors, purloining a few coins out of the collection plate. Disciplinary measures had to be taken. From the beginning, however, the Governors determined that only a senior member of the staff should administer punishment. As early as 1743 they directed that 'no child of this Hospital shall be corrected, but by Order of the Matron and in her presence'. And in 1771 they dismissed the Hospital's baker for 'cruelly beating a boy of this Hospital'.[51]

As to the Governors' own disciplinary actions, the records present a strange pattern. From 1756 to 1775, punishments never appear in the minutes, but rewards are frequently mentioned. Children who excelled in some activity—gardening, darning, knitting, sewing, reading or writing—were presented with small rewards, such as a silver thimble, a pair of scissors, a silver threepence, a special hat, linen handkerchiefs, gingerbread, or even 'a Bible & Prayer Book, better bound than common, with initial Letters of the Boys & Girls Names in Gold Letters'. The point of such gifts was twofold: to incite the children 'thereby to Industry thro' the most powerful motive of self Interest' and 'to cause emulation in others'. Perhaps this policy was born of kindliness, but it probably owed something to current economic thought, which was beginning to argue that incentives to labour produced greater efficiency than deterrents to idleness.[52]

Be that as it may, the Governors ordered no special punishments during this entire twenty-year period except on one occasion. Immediately after the death of the boy who fell while sliding down a bannister, they posted a notice threatening any child who ever slid on a bannister again with confinement in a dark room, a diet of bread and water, and as many lashes as the Subcommittee might judge proper.[53] But apparently the Governors never had to carry out this threat, and the matron or schoolmaster dealt with all minor transgressions.

In 1777 an abrupt change in disciplinary procedures occurred. Soon after the publication in 1776 of Jonas Hanway's tract praising the benefits of solitary confinement,[54] the Governors, on 29 January 1777, ordered 'that a plan and estimate of the expence of fitting up a place for the solitary confinement of children who may misbehave be laid before the Committee'.[55] By 1779 this place of confinement, sometimes referred to as the Dark Room or the Lock-up Room but more often as the Prison, was in use. Between 1779 and the end of the century at least seven girls and four boys were incarcerated in this room on a diet of bread and water. Most of them were older children, already apprenticed, whose masters brought them back to the

Hospital to be punished for bad behaviour, but one was an eight-year-old boy who spent a week in solitary confinement before he became 'sensible of his faults and especially . . . owned to be a falsehood what he had before strenuously insisted on to be true'. Confinement for most children, however, lasted no more than three or four days, the object in all cases being to produce a change in the child's undesirable behaviour through a period of prolonged meditation upon his or her misdeeds.[56]

We should not, of course, lay the blame for this harsh punishment solely to Hanway's influence. For one thing, he did not attend any meetings of the Governors from 13 November 1776 to 14 May 1777, the period during which the plan for the 'Prison' took shape. Nor is there any reason to think that he intended his scheme for use by the Foundling Hospital. But neither is there any evidence that he subsequently opposed the Governors' action. Still a change in the Governors' thinking about modes of punishment certainly took place during the 1770s, and the pattern then established continued throughout the rest of the century. Whether the Hospital's 'Prison' may simply have represented an imitation of the manner in which the prisons at Clerkenwell and Tothill Fields dealt with refractory apprentices, or whether it may only have reflected an increasing tendency throughout English society to punish children by shutting them up in a dark closet in preference to beating them, I cannot say.[57]

Beyond discipline, beyond religious indoctrination, beyond practical skills, beyond reading and writing, however, another form of learning also took place in the Hospital on so subtle a level that probably no one realized it. This was the influence exerted upon the children by the total environment of the Hospital, with its cleanliness and order and a daily exposure to beauty such as most poor children never experienced. Day after day the foundlings saw specimens of the Hospital's great art collection hanging in their dining rooms, as well as those displayed in other rooms through which they passed from time to time. Week after week they heard and sang the music of the church, much of it of high quality. And in spring and summer, as they walked about the Hospital's grounds, they beheld colourful masses of flowers—scarlet, purple and white sweet peas, sweet alyssum, china asters, purple candytuft, yellow and rose lupines, petunias, wallflowers, double balsams, and purple stocks.[58] How could the children not add some sensitivity to beauty and the possibilities that life offers for it to their Christian and useful education?

18

Conclusion:
A Child of this Hospital

THE FINAL QUESTION—the one everyone always asks—is: what became of the foundlings when they had served their apprenticeships and severed their legal ties to the Hospital? We know that no one escapes the past, and so we wonder how the accident of acceptance into the Hospital instead of abandonment to a parish nurse or a workhouse determined the lives of the adult foundlings—their situation in the world and how they felt about and dealt with it.

Unfortunately, the records do not tell us what we would most like to know, except for some of the handicapped children who remained under the Hospital's protection all their lives. From the relatively few records relating to the other children's later lives we can surmise that, in the judgment of their betters, many turned out well: they became independent, decent, orderly, hard-working citizens, able to marry and support a family without further assistance from anyone. But how did their early history mark their personalities? Did they wonder forever who they really were? And how much did it matter to them? Did the conformity imposed by institutional life during childhood bring about internal rigidities combined with external docility and subservience? Or did it produce rebellious souls? Or inward tension and conflict between both extremes reflected outwardly in ambivalent behaviour? Were the adult foundlings ashamed of their origins and eager to escape and deny them? To what extent did the country nurses and their husbands, who served as the foundlings' surrogate parents in their most formative years, influence their lives by moulding the personalities with which they responded to all later experience? And the answer to all of these questions is that, for the most part, we do not know because most of the foundlings maintained no official contact with the Hospital after they left it, although a few must have maintained contact with each other, for the records

236

occasionally mention marriages between the Hospital's former wards.

We do know that some foundlings wondered for years who they really were and sometimes wrote to the secretary for information.* In 1785, for example, Sarah Billington, then twenty-eight, wrote 'desiring to be informed who are her parents; she having laboured for many years under the greatest anxiety of mind, wishing to know them'. But the most that the secretary could do was to send her a copy of the billet made upon her admission in 1757 and the token received with her.[1]

And we know, too, that some foundlings in later life still looked to the Hospital, as one looks homeward, for help in time of trouble. Usually the help was given. One young woman, unable to support her child when her soldier husband was sent abroad, brought the infant to the Hospital to be cared for much as a woman might leave her child with its grandmother, and the Governors took it in. Others appealed to be rescued from imprisonment for debt, for medical treatment, for aid in establishing a right to parish assistance. The secretary wrote to the parish officers of Farnham on behalf of one poor woman, 'who was one of the Children brought up in this Hospital' and whom parish officials had shunted from place to place without affording her relief. He reminded them of the woman's rights and their duties and ended his letter with a threat that the Committee would enforce her rights 'in a legal manner' if necessary. For a boy who had completed his apprenticeship with a silver caster but whose master died before the lad obtained his Freedom of the City, the Committee sought the help of the Hospital's solicitors.[2]

Several boys who became shoemakers solicited the Hospital for business. One of them, George Grafton, had overcome great difficulties before going into business for himself. Born with a bilateral club foot deformity so severe that his 'feet . . . turn inwards so that he is obliged to walk as on stumps', he underwent treatment—unsuccessfully—at the Hospital's expense when he was ten. As he grew older, the Hospital employed him to assist the schoolmaster. Finally, when he was eighteen, the Governors found a shoemaker willing to take the boy as an apprentice for a fee of £21. Six years later, in 1794, George went into business for himself and received a contract from the Hospital to furnish shoes for the children.[3]

We know most, of course, about the blind children who were brought up in the Hospital to careers in music. Tom Grenville, the first of these children to be so educated, has already been mentioned.

* The Coram Foundation still receives requests of this kind.

237

By 1766 Tom had learned all that the Hospital's assistant organist could teach him, and the following year, when he became twenty-one, he secured a position as organist for the parish of Ross in Herefordshire at £25 a year. In 1773 he came back to the Hospital as its organist at an annual salary of £40, and there he remained, with no advance in salary until 1796 when it was raised to £50. The Governors had, however, given him a piece of plate worth ten guineas in 1794 as a token of appreciation for his services. In 1797 he resigned his position to become organist of a parish church, and the Governors found it no easy task to replace him. According to Lievesley, Tom married and had one son and two daughters. In his later years when he fell upon hard times, the Governors granted him a pension of £10 per annum—later increased to £20—until his death in 1827.[4]

John Printer's story was somewhat similar. Born blind, he began to learn music at the age of twelve under the instruction of the Hospital's organist, and within four years he was himself serving as organist at St Katherine Coleman with a salary of £20 a year. Since he was only sixteen, the Hospital collected his salary and placed it out at interest for his benefit. In addition to his ability to play the organ, John possessed so fine a voice that when he reached twenty-one, the Governors decided to hire him as a singer in the chapel at £30 a year plus room and board and also arranged to invest his savings in a good mortgage. By 1787 John had also taken on the task of teaching the children of St Ann's parish to sing, and from time to time the Governors permitted him to sing in other parish churches for special occasions. In 1788 he gave up his residence at the Hospital to marry a 'careful wife', who took charge of his money much to his benefit and that of their two daughters. He, too, received a piece of plate from the Governors in 1794 and a raise in salary to £50 per annum in 1796. John's wife died in 1799, and at his request she was buried in the vault under the chapel. Shortly afterward he returned to live at the Hospital. A generous man—too generous, it was said, with friends and acquaintances who wanted to borrow money—he donated to the Hospital on 21 May 1800 'the valuable present of an Organ' at a cost of £60. In his later years he became crippled and unable to move about without assistance. He finally left the Hospital in 1815 to be nursed by a woman, who, according to Lievesley, 'made him her prey'. She married him and took all the assets he had acquired.[5]

All of the blind girl singers about whom we have any information met with unhappiness of one sort or another. The saddest story was that of Mercy Draper. Instructed by Mr Stanley, Mercy developed into an accomplished singer and for a number of years sang in the series of oratorios presented by Stanley each year during the Lenten season. She also sang on special occasions at various churches and chapels and sometimes at parties in private homes. Apparently, after reaching the age of twenty-one, she quit the Hospital and embarked on a singing career under Stanley's direction. But by 1783 she was refusing to sing any longer in Stanley's oratorios and wanted to return to the Hospital. Stanley, perplexed by her attitude, attributed it to her health, and the Governors allowed her to return as a singer in the chapel at £30 a year. But within a year it became obvious that she required constant attention, and by November 1784 her mind was completely 'disordered'. After much debate, the Governors decided to place her in a private asylum at Malling, Kent. The charges amounted to £40 per annum, but Stanley offered to contribute £15 a year toward the cost. And so she was taken away to Dr Perfect's madhouse on 1 February 1785. After Stanley's death and the exhaustion of her earlier earnings, which had been held in trust for her, the Governors seriously considered committing her to Bethlem Hospital as 'poor & mad'. Perhaps it was Jonas Hanway's legacy to her, together with the trust fund created for her benefit under the will of George Whatley, that rescued Mercy from this institution, or perhaps the Governors changed their minds. In any event, the records show that she continued to live in Dr Perfect's madhouse until her death in 1818.[6]

The unhappy aspect of the story of Blanch Thetford, who never left the Hospital, was an abruptly terminated love affair. Blanch lost her eyesight in infancy as the result of smallpox, but in spite of her total absence of vision, she learned to sew well and became a fine singer. In fact, she frequently sang with Mercy Draper at private parties and churches. When she reached twenty-one, the Hospital hired her, too, as a singer in the chapel at six guineas a year. In 1781 Blanch began to go out with a young man. When it came to the Governors' attention, they gave Blanch's suitor notice that they did not want him to come inside the Hospital's gates. Nevertheless, 'Mr Pew having since been seen going out of the Hospital arm and arm with Blanch Thetford', the Governors then ordered 'that the Porter at the Gate do not for the future suffer Mr Pew to come within the Hospital Gates'. Thus ended Blanch's short-lived romance. And so she lived out her life in the Hospital, sewing, knitting, singing in the chapel, and instructing a younger blind girl in music.[7]

The younger girl was Jane Freer, blind from birth, who had great musical talent. According to Lievesley, she could 'play upon every Instrument', and also sing well. She became an accomplished organist and also learned to play the guitar. But, says Lievesley, 'this

Child of Genius', whom a 'polished governess' might have trained to be 'the delight of Society', was so neglected by the matron that for some years she presented an increasing problem to the Governors and finally 'was obliged to be removed from the Hospital on account of her filthy habits and vulgar manners'.[8]

In contrast to the sad stories of these three girls, we can catch glimpses here and there in the records of some of the foundlings who succeeded in life in varying degrees. Ezekiel Hulse achieved the rank of a master tailor in Yorkshire, lived to a very old age in perfect health, and at the age of eighty-seven, Lievesley says, he could walk thirty miles in a day and was 'as upright as any man of 30'. Richard Stanton served his master so well that upon completion of the boy's apprenticeship, his master decided to retire and to give the boy his business, as well as allowing him to live gratis in his former master's house. In fact, a number of masters kept their foundling apprentices on as paid employees when they had served their time. One girl learned to be a shroud-maker and secured employment with an 'eminent Undertaker'. And Daniel Hay went into business for himself 'in the Glazing, Plumbing and Painting Branches'.[9]

The greatest success stories recorded, however, are those of Thomas Coram, the thirty-eighth child received, and Julian Mariner. Julian, as we already know, became the apprentice of the Hospital's apothecary, McClellan. In 1774 after his apprenticeship was completed, McClellan procured him a post as an assistant in the 'Chymical Warehouse at Apothecarys Hall', and he also attended lectures at hospitals in order to acquire greater proficiency. Julian saved his money and eventually purchased a partnership with a Mr Smith of Hatton Garden. When he died Smith left Julian a legacy of £1000, and he then married an heiress—a ward of Sir Samuel Romilly—who later went insane. By 1795 Julian had set up in business for himself in Kirby Street and substituted for McClellan during the latter's long illness in the summer of 1795. Thereafter he continued to assist his former master until McClellan's retirement, at which time Julian was elected the Hospital's apothecary. His patients, says Lievesley, were 'of the most respectable class', and 'he was much respected by them'. On 31 December 1828 Julian Mariner was elected a Governor of the Hospital, the first foundling to be so honoured, and when he died in 1831, he left the Hospital a legacy of £600.[10]

The foundling Thomas Coram was apprenticed when he was twelve to Henry Bird, Jr, a shipbuilder of Rotherhithe, to be employed in the sea service. If Lievesley's information was correct, this Thomas Coram followed so well in the footsteps of the Hospital's founder that in later years he was often seen riding up in his own carriage to attend services in the Hospital's chapel.[11]

From the fact that in later life only a few of the foundlings rose in the world, we should not, however, conclude that the Foundling Hospital was a failure. Few poor children anywhere in England rose in the world. Although social mobility—witness Captain Coram—existed within certain limits, the structure of British society did not encourage it. In this respect, therefore, the foundling children did not differ at all from their contemporaries, and in bringing up the children to become contented members of the labouring poor or of the lower levels of the crafts and trades, the Governors were, in fact, attempting to train the children realistically to fit into the kind of a world that willy-nilly they would have to live in. And so far as we can learn from the records that do exist, it would appear that until the last quarter of the century, when a certain amount of restlessness evidenced itself among the older apprentices, the Hospital's system of indoctrination worked fairly well for most of its wards—at least no evidence speaks to the contrary.

But we may legitimately wonder whether any of the foundlings ever became psychologically true counterparts of their contemporaries. In the first place, their personalities had been formed by two very different, and in some respects contradictory, influences: their years in the country and their years in the Hospital. Behaviourists would, I am sure, emphasize the conditioning by regimentation in the Hospital, whereas Freudians and those who practice transactional analysis would argue that the early years in the homes of the country nurses controlled. My own opinion, for whatever a non-psychologist's opinion may be worth, is that the early years in the country fixed the basic elements of the child's personality—provided the inward parental voices, as the transactional analysts would say—that thereafter determined how readily and how far the child would respond to the conditioning experience of life in the Hospital.

That the early years in the country had a powerful effect on the children cannot be doubted when we remember how often runaway apprentices went back to their nurses. Obviously, these children regarded their nurses' cottages as home and naturally so, for here they had known the mothering care that not only had kept them alive but also had fostered normal emotional development during the critical second half year of life;[12] here they had found their earliest adult models; here they had learned what family life was like, playing and working and sitting down to eat amid their foster brothers and sisters, from whom they acquired the habit of thinking of the cottage that sheltered them all as 'our house'.

When they were brought back to the Hospital between the ages of three and six (the age varied from time to time during the century), the foundlings were, in effect, transplanted country children. For many of them this separation from the only home they had ever known combined with introduction into a strange institutional environment must have been a traumatic experience, because the Hospital imposed upon the children an entirely different kind of life, replacing the comparative freedom of a small child in a country labourer's cottage with a strictly ordered existence. Now the child had to wear shoes and stockings, wash his face twice a day, use the necessary house instead of a corner of the garden or some other handy spot, eat at scheduled hours, play when told to play. And rarely did he escape the supervising eye of some adult.

But at the same time, the Hospital furnished the foundling with a larger substitute family: a group of many children whose situation corresponded to his own and a goodly number of adults who were kind even when firm. Moreover, it surrounded him with an environment that provided physical care and safety, consistent rules of behaviour consistently enforced, and the predictability of repetitious days and weeks, leaving little room for uncertainty. Thus, bit by bit the Hospital built up in many of the children a sense of security. The proof lies in the fact that so many of them returned to the Hospital, looking trustfully to the Governors to rescue them from harsh or unjust masters during their apprenticeships and from the vicissitudes of life in their later years. The foundling, in fact, could count on a more certain refuge in time of trouble than parish children or even the children of poor parents.

Some might argue that the Hospital programmed the foundlings to failure by its constant reminders of their shameful birth and lowly station. On the other hand, it admonished the foundling just as constantly that he had a purpose in the world: he had been saved to be useful. Moreover, he knew at first hand that he could be useful. Long before he went out to serve his apprenticeship, he realized that people would pay for the work of his hands: the purses, garters, fishnets, pieces of woollen and linen fabric, shirts and shifts that he and the other foundling children made earned money for the Hospital. He could, therefore, feel a sense of worth and self-respect, knowing that he was contributing toward his own support, which proved his usefulness.

In one respect, however, the Hospital failed the foundling: it did not prepare him with knowledge of what urban life outside the Hospital was really like, for the Governors had always made every effort to isolate the children from contact with anyone other than the

Hospital's personnel or fashionable Londoners who visited the Hospital with the Governors' approval. When the new apprentice accompanied his master through the gates of the Hospital, he encountered for the first time since his journey back from the country the sights, sounds, and smells of London's streets. To the foundling, whose only basis of expectation was the memory of a country village and whatever tales the Hospital's nurses or servants might have told him, much of what he saw, heard, and smelled in his first few weeks outside the Hospital must have come as a shock: filthy beggars with, perhaps, a nose half eaten away by disease, stinking sewage in open ditches, bloody offal flowing from the butchers' shambles, prostitutes inviting customers with obscene words and gestures, the stench of rotting bodies emanating from the open 'poor holes' in the church-yards, and until 1772 the skulls of rebels of the Forty-five stuck up at Temple Bar. All that London children of his own age and station in life took for granted presented to the foundling a new world, some aspects of which he was ill equipped to deal with. Innocent and gullible, the foundling was far more vulnerable to the crooked and the clever—unless his master shielded him—than the ragamuffins of the streets, because the sheltered life of the Hospital had prevented him from developing the quick-witted shrewdness of the street gamin, and the Hospital's regimentation and protectiveness had not taught him to think, act, or make judgments independently.

On the whole, however, there is a strong probability that the foundlings suffered no great psychological damage. They had known security from the day of their acceptance into the Hospital, which was more than most poor children knew, for even those with parents could never be certain of sufficient food from day to day. And the foundlings were not adrift emotionally: they knew their place in society and what was expected of them, and those expectations would not change because they were living in a time when change took place very slowly. The education and vocational training given them and the system of moral values instilled in their early years would serve most of the foundlings and serve them well for a lifetime. The evidence for this lies in the fact that throughout the century the Governors never found it necessary to change the Instructions to Apprentices.

The greatest emotional damage, therefore, that the foundlings were likely to have sustained was the feeling of rejection that might have accompanied the knowledge that their own parents had abandoned them. But, perhaps, for many the knowledge came too late to cause much harm. For most, the transitional experience had been to pass from one pair of loving arms to another, to move from a mother's breast to a nurse's, and usually this had taken place before the child was six months old. By the time the children were old enough to understand rejection intellectually, it would seem that a firm base of acceptance by their nurses may have already been sufficiently well established to counteract it.

Beyond these conclusions there is little more to be said about the children. In a sense they remained outside history: things were done to them and for them but not by them in any significant way. The protagonists were the Governors, and the Hospital was, at any one time, largely what the handful of active Governors made of it. Yet the Hospital never became Mr White's or Mr Hanway's or Mr Bernard's hospital, even though these men exerted strong influence in shaping its policies and practices. Instead, the Hospital gradually acquired a personality of its own based on the accretion of traditional ways of doing things and a continuity of administrative philosophy.

This philosophy, the product of the combined experience and thinking of all the active Governors over the years, guided the Hospital through the eighteenth century and largely determined its course in the years to follow. It embraced eight principles, although the Governors never set them forth in any formal statement. First, the Hospital's work must always expand to the utmost that its finances would permit. Its primary mission was to save lives and to educate and care for as many children as possible. Second, the rehabilitation of the mother was almost as important as saving the life of the child. Although this principle involved abandonment of the original plan of maintaining complete secrecy, it provided for such confidentiality concerning the woman and her circumstances as to permit her to find decent employment and keep the respect of friends and relatives, and it set the stage for the individual casework with unwed mothers still carried on by the Coram Foundation. Third, the Hospital accepted complete responsibility for all of the children that it received until they were twenty-one and even for life in the case of handicapped children. Fourth, the children and the Hospital's employees were to be kept isolated, as much as possible, from contamination by the outside world. Fifth, the Hospital, in order to ensure public support, must always show due respect for public opinion to the extent that even the appearance of evil, as well as evil itself, must be avoided.

Sixth, the standard of physical care, education, religious and moral instruction of the children was always to be kept high but suitable to the children's station in life. The application of this policy, however, produced discontinuities between theory and practice, for the Governors said and believed that they were training the children to become servants, seamen, farm labourers, and petty tradesmen. But, especially toward the end of the century, they were educating the children above the level required for such occupations and inculcating in them values and ways of behaviour more like their own than those of the labouring poor. The foundling's training, in short, reflected a gentleman's idea of how the labouring poor ought to live, but not, in fact, how they did live. Moreover, the standard of health care that the Governors provided for the foundlings not only exceeded that available to the offspring of the poor but, in many ways, exceeded that which their own children normally received, for no Governor maintained an apothecary in residence in his own home, nor would his children's health and diet have benefited from regular weekly supervision by the most eminent physicians of the time. Apparently the Governors, having rescued the children from almost certain death, felt an overwhelming compulsion to exert every means to preserve them. To do so, after all, justified the institution's existence.

The Governors' seventh principle was a willingness at all times to experiment with new ways of doing things but never to change merely for the sake of change. When they acted upon routine matters without much thought, they usually followed whatever customary pattern had been established. But when any special occurrence raised questions about old methods or suggested new ways of solving old problems, they never felt bound by tradition. Their criteria were that the new method not go against all that they had learned from past experience and that it promise to help more children or to care for the children in better ways. In short, the Governors—much like Captain Coram—welcomed constructive innovation while still holding fast to the principles, practices, and precedents that the years had demonstrated to be good.

And, finally, the Governors always regarded the children as individuals and not merely as numbered components of an undifferentiated group. True, each child received a number when it entered the Hospital, but without exception whenever the minutes, letters, or other records mentioned a child, its name appeared as well as its number. When the matron or steward filed accounts of their visits to children at nurse in areas near London, the Governors instructed them to make a report 'of each particular child by name'.[13] And, as we have seen, the Governors singled out the children's personal accomplishments for recognition with small rewards and gave individualized attention to the blind children so that they might develop their special talents. Moreover, beginning in the 1770s, efforts were made to try to prevent the children from being apprenticed to trades for which they seemed unsuited.[14] Indeed, the disposition of the Governors to see the children as individuals seems best summed up in a phrase that appears more often than any other in the Hospital's records: 'a child of this Hospital'. A typical entry respecting a child reads: 'Elizabeth Owen, No. 13518, a child of this Hospital'. She was not a number; she was a child with a name; more than that, she was the Hospital's child—the Governors' child, for whom they felt concern, interest, and responsibility.

At this point we might well ask what motivated these Governors who took such great interest in the children, struggled with so many difficulties and disappointments on their behalf, and spent endless hours in doing so. How typical were they of eighteenth-century men? I can answer neither question with certainty. Obviously, all of the active Governors shared humanitarian impulses, but to what extent religious convictions fuelled the energies of some, while a secular sense of responsibility for one's fellow creatures prompted the activities of others, it is impossible to know. The Governors performed their responsibilities and duties but did not talk about responsibility and duty in the abstract. Moreover, since few men ever do anything from single motives, we may speculate that for some of the childless men among the Governors their work at the Hospital served them—like Captain Coram—as a kind of vicarious fatherhood. And probably some who began their work purely out of a sense of duty, religious or secular, found in time that they had unconsciously turned duty into pleasure, because duty undiluted cannot be long endured.

Certainly, the active Governors were not typical. If they were, there would not have been so few of them. More likely, the great majority of the Governors, who paid their £50 and never attended a meeting, represented the average aristocrat or well-to-do gentleman of the time—men who possessed enough good will to give their money but not themselves to many worthy causes. For other charitable institutions in the eighteenth century experienced the same disproportion between the few who did the work and the many who contributed the money, a state of affairs that has changed little in two hundred years.

This book does not, of course, address itself, except indirectly, to the history of the family. Yet in view of the unsettled state of historical discussion about the relationship of parents and children in times past, which hinges on the extent of parents' affection for and attachment to their children,[15] it may be of some value to examine the evidence implicit in the history of the Foundling Hospital. To some extent it is open to two interpretations. If we gave full credence to the opinions expressed by the anti-Hospital pamphleteers of the General Reception period, we would have to conclude that large numbers of parents in the mid-eighteenth-century period readily surrendered their children to the Hospital's care, ridding themselves with no regrets of unwanted responsibility.

But we must look at this evidence with the scepticism appropriate to all polemics, the more so because there is factual evidence to the contrary. In the first place, we have the Governors' own description of the women who brought the first children to the Hospital on 25 March 1741: 'the Expressions of Grief of the Women whose Children could not be admitted were Scarcely more observable than those of some of the Women who parted with their Children'.[16] Secondly, there were among the tokens attached to the children many expressions of grief at parting with the child and of hope for being reunited with it in the future. Moreover, a substantial number of parents did claim their children, even unmarried mothers and unwed fathers of bastards. And parents often claimed their children long after relinquishing them to the Hospital. In 1764, for example, parents claimed a child admitted to the Hospital in 1750; in 1772 a parent sought a child admitted in 1751; and in 1780 a widow applied for the return of her two children received by the Hospital in 1759. One mother even sought employment in the Hospital in order to be near her child. Other parents, unable to remove their children from the Hospital, nevertheless came there to learn whether their children were dead or alive, one mother coming regularly every few months from 1798 to 1801.[17]

In the face of such evidence, it is difficult not to see strong proofs of a parental love that lasted for years. It seems obvious that these parents, most likely compelled by economic necessity, had placed their children in the Hospital to preserve them because they loved them, not merely to be rid of a nuisance. The evidence, too, of the great affection conceived by some of the country nurses for their nurslings and their desire and that of their husbands to adopt these children also argues strongly against adult indifference to or lack of affection for children. Moreover, the Governors' continuing watchfulness over the children after they left the Hospital to be apprenticed and their constant recognition of the children as individuals—children unrelated to them in any way but to whom they stood as surrogate fathers—provides still further evidence that there was no absence of love for children in eighteenth-century England.

On the contrary, it was the Governors' concern for the welfare of children that led to the General Reception, and although that experiment lasted only four years, it paved the way for the subsequent enactment of the Hanway Act, a step down the long road toward recognition of society's responsibility for providing adequate care for all of its children. After 1760, of course, the Foundling Hospital, because of its limited resources, could never again play a major role in providing that care: the need was too great. But even with unlimited funds it may be doubted whether the task could have been accomplished effectively by any associational charity given the dimensions of the larger problem of poverty, the small number of persons willing to volunteer their time to the enterprise, the state of medical and nutritional knowledge, and the absence of trained personnel. One can only marvel that during the General Reception the Governors did so much with so little.

The greatest accomplishment of the Foundling Hospital, however, was to set the pattern for incorporated associational charities that was first copied by the Marine Society, the Magdalen House, and the Female Orphan Asylum in 1756–58, and by innumerable institutions toward the end of the century when Evangelical influence encouraged the growth of many organized charities. Because the Hospital had already demonstrated successfully what an incorporated group of dedicated volunteers could do, no subsequent institution ever found its period of gestation so prolonged or its birth so difficult. The Hospital's organizational form and many of its fund-raising and other techniques were repeatedly imitated by its successors, both in England and in America, during the next two centuries. Thus, the patterns and the precedents that it established and the present-day work of the Coram Foundation remain as the continuing legacy of the Foundling Hospital—and of Captain Coram—to charitable organizations generally and to those helping children in particular. Every such institution is, in a sense, 'a child of this Hospital'.

Epilogue

THE HISTORY OF the Foundling Hospital does not, of course, end on 31 December 1799. The institution continued to care for children in London until 1926 when it moved, first to Redhill, and in 1935 to Berkhamsted. In 1954 the Governors, influenced by the trend toward noninstitutional forms of caring for children, disposed of the Berkhamsted property and placed the children in foster homes. The following year they changed the corporate title to the Thomas Coram Foundation for Children. This foundation still carries on work with unwed mothers and their infants by providing both adoption and foster care services. It also operates a day care centre for children, maintains a counselling service, and undertakes research in the field of child welfare. The institution's history in the twentieth century, as it was in the eighteenth, has been a record of experimentation and innovation.

But in the nineteenth century the Hospital saw only minor changes. The policy on restoring children to their parents remained the same; country nurses and their husbands still 'adopted' the infants they had cared for; parents still came to inquire about their children, and grown-up foundlings still came to inquire about their origins; supervision of apprenticed foundlings and investigation of the character of prospective masters continued; the isolation of the children from the outside world did not lessen. The children were still taught singing. And the Hospital's physician still fixed the foundlings' diet, which seems to have been just as lacking in nutritional adequacy as the Hospital's eighteenth-century diets, for the report of the Select Committee on Public Charities, published in 1840, remarked that 'few, if any, of the children brought up in this hospital attain an average height; . . . this fact is well known and admitted'.[1]

Continuity of personnel and royal patronage were as much features of the nineteenth century as of the eighteenth. Members of the Royal Family served as President during most of the century, beginning with the election of the Prince of Wales (later George IV) in 1809 and ending with George, Duke of Cambridge, who held the office from 1851 to 1904. And only three men acted as secretary throughout the century, one of them holding office for fifty years.[2] Continuity prevailed, too, among the country nurses: foundlings were often cared for by women of the same families for generations, many of them living in the same areas that had supplied nurses for the first foundlings in 1741.[3] Even the number of children on the institution's rolls at any one time remained relatively static, hovering between four hundred and five hundred, with a mortality rate in the early part of the century of 26 percent.[4] 'By the early part of the nineteenth century', say Nichols and Wray, 'the Foundling had reached a settled order of internal economy and administration from which it has had to depart only in accordance with modern progress'.[5]

Among the departures—and one that came soon after the close of the eighteenth century—was the decision, after experimental testing, to substitute vaccination for inoculation. Another change was the new policy of paying inspectors instead of depending on the voluntary services of charitably-minded men and women. The age for apprenticing gradually rose. In 1806 the Governors resolved that they would apprentice no child under fourteen years of age, and by mid-century it had become customary to delay the apprenticing of girls until the age of sixteen.[6] There were changes in educational practices, too. By 1836 a library had been created for the use of the older boys, and by mid-century the schoolmasters and mistresses were instructing the children not only in reading, writing, arithmetic, and the catechism, but also in English grammar and geography.[7] In 1862 the Governors appointed a drawing master, and in 1868 they sent several of the girls who had achieved academic distinction to training colleges.[8] On the other hand, troublesome girls now met with a new form of punishment: beginning in 1834, they were sent to Australia. Sea service, however, remained the solution for the problem of dealing with recalcitrant boys: from 1807 onward they were sent to the Marine Society for placement aboard ships. Caning at the discretion of the schoolmasters and mistresses also came into use.[9] But perhaps the greatest change in methods was the establishment of a band in 1847, an idea reminiscent of Dr Burney's plan of 1774. Usually about thirty boys aged nine to fourteen received instruction in instrumental music, and many of them later joined regimental bands or bands of the Royal Navy.[10]

The greatest change in policy, however, appears in a resolution, adopted in June 1801, stating that the principal object of the Hospital was the maintenance and support of illegitimate children. This policy continued in effect throughout the nineteenth century and into the twentieth. Although eighteenth-century Englishmen usually assumed that the foundlings were bastards, that, as we have seen, was by no means always the case. The Governors had never fixed any rules respecting legitimacy. But from 1801 onward the only children of legitimate birth admitted into the Hospital were the sons and daughters of soldiers and sailors killed in the line of duty. Between 1804 and 1814 only three legitimate children out of 349 were admitted, and in 1836 it was stated that no child of legitimate birth had been admitted in the last ten years.[11]

The Governors' decision to restrict admissions to illegitimate children was undoubtedly responsible for the most significant fact about the Hospital's history in the nineteenth century: it remained unique. No other foundling hospital or institution for the care of illegitimate children existed in London at least up to 1863. In that year Sampson Low, describing the charities of the metropolis, listed 640 institutions. These included medical hospitals; institutions for repentant prostitutes—of which there were twenty-two; societies for the benefit of poor clergy and dissenting ministers; homes for the aged; charities for the crippled, blind, deaf, and dumb; asylums for orphans of legitimate birth; Bible societies; home and foreign missionary societies; provident funds; parochial trusts; societies for the relief of prisoners; and societies for the improvement of public morals. But only one foundling hospital appears on the list.[12] In short, the Foundling Hospital, in contrast to the Magdalen House, had had no imitators.

This is a striking omission in an age that gave birth with the fecundity of rabbits to charitable enterprises of all kinds. Certainly the need had not disappeared nor even declined. For every child that the Foundling Hospital was able to receive, five were turned away.[13] For throughout England and Wales there continued to be a large number of illegitimate births. The average number per year from 1845 to 1848 in Middlesex County was 2200, or 40 per thousand births. The average for most counties was higher.[14]

Many of these children were born, lived out a short, neglected life, and died before they were a year old in workhouses. After 1834 there was, in fact, no other source of help for the unwed mother and her child because the New Poor Law provided for the illegitimate infant only through admission of its parent to the workhouse. Yet no appropriate facilities were made available there to care for babies. The Poor Law Commissioners ignored their existence, not even recognizing until 1842 that Anglican infants should receive baptism. And not until 1895 did the Boards of Guardians receive any instructions for dealing with their infant charges. Most often they left the care of such children to the feebleminded and aged female inmates of the workhouse, who performed their duties with scant supervision. The consequences appeared in the mortality rate of the infant population of workhouses: at the end of the century it was certain that one child in three would die. And as late as 1907 it was estimated that the death rate of such infants during their first year of life was between twice and three times that of children of the same age in the nation as a whole.[15]

Nineteenth-century London needed a dozen foundling hospitals, and one would have expected a response to that need at least comparable to the powerful pull on English purse strings exerted by repentant prostitutes or African missions. But a change had come over the spirit of English benevolence. It tended now to be more discriminating, more calculating, and less openhanded, less compassionate than the charitable giving of the past. It emphasized prevention and rehabilitation instead of simple relief of human misery. There were multiple causes for this change: Malthusian fears of overpopulation, and a population that was, in fact, expanding; rapid industrialization and urban growth that confronted Englishmen with new problems for which their previous experience had not prepared them; an increasing desire to incorporate a scientific approach into every activity; and the influence of Benthamite utilitarianism.[16] Most of these were reflected to some extent in the New Poor Law of 1834[17] with its principle of less eligibility and its objective of deterrence. All of them probably helped to create a climate of public opinion unfriendly to the establishment of additional foundling hospitals.

But undoubtedly the chief determinant of whether or not generous Londoners would pour out their largess for foundlings was the pervasiveness of Evangelical thought, which influenced social attitudes far beyond Clapham. It was not that Evangelicals were stonyhearted or indifferent to human need; they lavished time and money on many charitable endeavours. Indeed, their zeal for good works accounted for most of the eleemosynary institutions established in the early years of the century. But Evangelical values and priorities differed widely from those of the past: these men put the needs of the soul before those of the body, the relief of spiritual destitution before relief of physical distress. Henry Thornton saw quite clearly the difference between Christian and secular humanitarians: 'He [the Christian] is for mending the root; they are for lopping off the branches . . . . They are for improving the condition of men in this world, he is for securing to them heavenly felicity'.[18] 'The great business of life', said William Wilberforce, '[is] to secure our admission into heaven'.[19]

Such views, when translated into charitable action, inevitably resulted in institutions having as their first objective moral and religious ends: one might rescue a prostitute from the pangs of poverty and the miseries of disease, but this was only incidental to rescuing her soul from hellfire and starting her on the road to heaven. Moreover, Evangelicalism, which can be seen at its best in the generation of Wilberforce and Hannah More, tended in succeeding generations to lose its purity of purpose and to become narrower, distorted, and rigid, with adherents who were all too often canting bigots more intent on respectability than on religion. James Fitzjames Stephen sharply, and no doubt accurately, characterized the men of mid-nineteenth-century Britain who made virtually a career of philanthropy: 'No one expects that a person principally occupied in philanthropy will be very wise, very sympathetic, or very large-minded. We are rather apt to associate the name of a philanthropist with a certain narrowness of understanding, and not unfrequently with a good deal of coldness of temper'.[20]

Men of this ilk did not support the Foundling Hospital. Although most Evangelicals distributed their benevolence among numerous charitable organizations, many contributing to as many as twenty or thirty, few became Governors of the Foundling Hospital and even fewer participated in its governance. Of forty-seven vice-presidents and eight treasurers elected between 1770 and 1870, only seven appear in Ford K. Brown's list of ninety active Evangelical supporters of multiple charities. And among the Evangelicals who became Governors late in the eighteenth century or early in the nineteenth, a number were members of the Hoare and Thornton families, which had furnished Governors to the Foundling Hospital since 1739.[21]

The logic of most benevolent men of the nineteenth century prescribed that charity should relieve only the deserving, and the deserving, it is obvious, did not include bastards and foundlings. Why they and any institution caring for them were judged undeserving of help from respectable people was spelled out by John Brownlow, the Foundling Hospital's secretary, who wrote in 1847: 'But there are certain individuals who endeavour to smother their humanity under the plea, that the policy—*the good of society* as they term it—is against the existence of any institution which shall relieve distress arising out of an evil action'. His successor, W. S. Wintle, who revised Brownlow's history of the institution in 1881, did not find it necessary to change this statement.[22]

The 1840 report of the Select Committee on Public Charities made even clearer why there was no other foundling hospital in London. In the opinion of the writer of the report, even one was too many:

> Now if it be true, and few will controvert the assertion, that general and indiscriminate admission of all illegitimate children offered into an hospital of this description encourages prostitution, it is also certain that the grant of a charter for the foundation of an hospital for the reception, maintenance and education of *exposed and deserted* young children, tends to produce the same result, inasmuch as such a charter cannot be executed strictly without sanctioning and acting on the principle of general indiscriminate admission to the extent of the funds possessed, and it will follow that the charter of this hospital being of the nature just described, must, if so executed, be productive of evil results .... Now it would seem that not only does general indiscriminate admission encourage licentiousness, but that, for a like reason, any facilities afforded for disposing of the offspring of illicit connections, without compromising the reputation of the parents, have also a direct tendency to produce a similar result, and a tendency proportionable to the degree in which such facilities are afforded; and that the amount of mischief produced by any system, under which illegitimate children are provided for on such terms, can be always accurately estimated by observation of the number and class of the objects obtaining relief therefrom and the circumstances under which relief is given.
>
> If these principles be correct, it will follow that whilst all illegitimate children were admitted indiscriminately into this hospital, a general encouragement to vice was held out to the whole community, and that, under the system which now prevails, encouragement is in like manner afforded to a limited extent, that is, to those who are permitted to partake of the privileges conferred by it.[23]

This was the same argument against a foundling hospital that Captain Coram had encountered a hundred years earlier when he told Dr Colman that he had 'found Many weak persons ... [who] say such a foundation will be a promotion of Wickedness',[24] and the same disparagement that had prevented the merchants of Queen Anne's day from founding such an institution. Society's attitude toward foundlings had gone full circle from the beginning to the end of the eighteenth century, and by the nineteenth century it seemed as if nothing had changed. The plight of the foundling once more cried out for a Coram, yet no one stepped forward to take his place. But at least, despite all nineteenth-century criticism, the Hospital he founded still stood.

APPENDIX I

Chart I : The Lady Petitioners

Name	Date of Signing Petition	Age at Time of Signing	Father
Charlotte Finch, Duchess of Somerset	9 Mar. 1729	35	6th Earl of Winchilsea and 2nd Earl of Nottingham
Ann Vaughan, Duchess of Bolton	22 Apr. 1729	—	3rd Earl of Carbery
Henrietta Needham, Dowager Duchess of Bolton	25 Apr. 1729	46	Duke of Monmouth
Sarah Cadogan, Duchess of Richmond	22 Dec. 1729	23	1st Earl of Cadogan
Isabella Montagu, Duchess of Manchester	6 Jan. 1730	Not over 23	2nd Duke of Montagu
Anne Egerton, Duchess of Bedford	7 Jan. 1730	Not over 22	1st Duke of Bridgwater
Elizabeth Knight, Baroness Onslow	6 Apr. 1730	—	John Knight, merchant
Anne Pierrepont, Dowager Baroness Torrington	14 Apr. 1730	—	Robert Pierrepont, grandson of 1st Earl of Kingston-upon-Hull
Frances Berkeley, Baroness Byron	14 Apr. 1730	—	4th Baron Berkeley
Selina Shirley, Countess of Huntingdon	21 Apr. 1730	22	2nd Earl Ferrers
Juliana Hele, Duchess of Leeds	24 Apr. 1730	25	Roger Hele

Frances Feilding, Countess of Winchilsea and Nottingham	25 Apr. 1730	Not over 34	4th Earl of Denbigh
Frances Hales, Countess of Lichfield	27 Apr. 1730	32	Sir John Hales, 4th Bt and titular 2nd Earl of Tenterden
Dorothy Savile, Countess of Burlington	19 May 1730	30	2nd Marquess of Halifax
Elizabeth Bruce, Countess of Cardigan	19 May 1730	41	2nd Earl of Ailesbury and 3rd Earl of Elgin
Frances Thynne, Countess of Hertford	26 May 1730	31	Hon. Henry Thynne
Mary Tufton, Countess of Harold	5 July 1733	32	6th Earl of Thanet
Anne Lennox, Countess of Albemarle	6 Nov. 1734	31	1st Duke of Richmond
Anne Weldon Bernard, Baroness Trevor	2 Dec. 1734	64	Robert Weldon
Anne Seys, Dowager Baroness Ockham	21 Jan. 1735	45	Richard Seys
Margaret Cavendish Harley, Duchess of Portland	7 May 1735	20	2nd Earl of Oxford

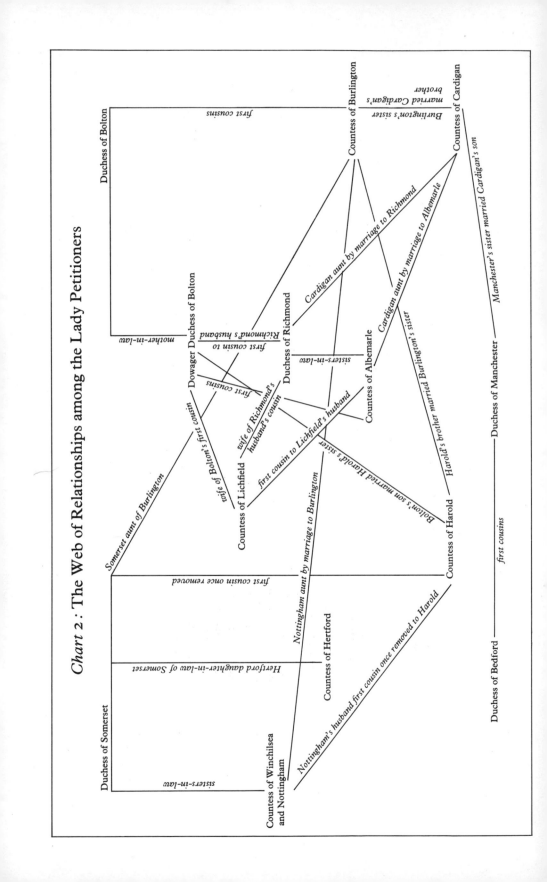

Chart 2: The Web of Relationships among the Lady Petitioners

APPENDIX II

Chart 1 : Analysis of Characteristics of the Men Proposed by
Thomas Coram to be Governors of the Foundling Hospital

Characteristics	Group I **	Group II *	Group III	Totals
Social Status:				
Nobility	20	9	60	89
Commoners	152	43	91	286
Totals:	172	52	151	375
Occupations of Commoners:				
Country Gentleman	6	4	25	35
Merchant	37	8	21	66
Banker	3	1	3	7
Lawyer	9	1	8	18
Physician or Surgeon	18	2	0	20
Army	3	1	1	5
Navy	8	1	1	10
Court or Government Service	11	6	9	26
Miscellaneous Commercial Occupations	7	0	2	9
Miscellaneous Noncommercial Occupations	4	1	0	5
	106	25	70	201
Unknown	46	18	21	85
Totals:	152	43	91	286
Members of Parliament in 1738:	22	10	40	72

259

Chart 1 (Contd.)

Characteristics	Group I **	Group II *	Group III	Totals
Very Wealthy Commoners:	13	3	15	31
Related to one or more of the Lady Petitioners:	13	7	11	31

Note: Group I, which Coram indicated on his list by**, consisted of those who had consented to act as Governors or who had subscribed one of his petitions. Group II, which Coram indicated by *, consisted of those who, he had been told, approved of his plan. Group III consisted of men considered by Coram to be suitable persons to promote his project.

Chart 2 : Age of Proposed Governors

	Mean	Median	Spread
Group I, 60 known:	46.5 Yrs	45.5 Yrs	21–79
Group II, 24 known:	46.4 Yrs	44.5 Yrs	21–78
Group III, 102 known:	48.3 Yrs	48.0 Yrs	23–80
Entire number for whom ages are known:	47.5 Yrs	47.0 Yrs	21–80

Note: Mode was not a significant measure in any group.

APPENDIX III

The Mortality of Children Admitted to the Foundling Hospital
25 March 1741–29 September 1760

Period	No. of Children Received	No. of Children Died	Mortality Rate	No. Nursed in the Country	No. Died in the Country	Country Mortality Rate
25 March 1741 to 2 Sept. 1742	136	74	54.41%	80	29	36.25%
2 Sept. 1742 to 29 Sept. 1752	864	379	43.87%	864	319	36.92%
Cumulative Totals:	1000	453	45.30%	944	348	36.86%
29 Sept. 1752 to 25 March 1756	344	249	72.38%	342	207	60.53%
Cumulative Totals:	1344	702	52.23%	1286	555	43.16%
25 March 1756 to 24 June 1758	7692	3334	43.34%	6843	2513	36.72%
Cumulative Totals:	9036	4036	44.67%	8129	3068	37.74%
24 June 1758 to 29 Sept. 1760	7290	5926	81.29%	5379	4129	76.76%
Cumulative Totals:	16326	9962	61.02%	13508	7197	53.28%

Compiled from data in Gen. Com. 1:237; Quarterly Account of the Children, vol. 1, 29 September 1752, 25 March 1756, 24 June 1758, and 29 September 1760, GLRO.

APPENDIX IV

Indenture of Apprenticeship for the first child apprenticed by the Foundling Hospital

This Indenture made the   day of   in the Twenty-fifth year of the Reign of our Sovereign Lord George the Second By the Grace of God of Great Britain, France & Ireland King, Defender of the Faith and so forth and in the Year of our Lord 1751, Between the Governors & Guardians of the Hospital for the Maintenance & Education of Exposed & deserted Young Children of the one part and Stephen Beckingham of the Parish of St George the Martyr in the County of Middlesex, Esq. of the other part, Witnesseth that the said Governors & Guardians have put & placed out and by these presents do put & place out John Bowles one of the Children of this Hospital Aged about   years apprentice to the said Stephen Beckingham with him to dwell & serve from the day of the date of these presents until the said Apprentice shall accomplish his full Age of Twenty four years according to the Statute in that case made & provided during all which Term the said Apprentice His said Master faithfully shall serve in all lawful Businesses according to his power wit & ability and honestly orderly & obediently in all things demean & behave himself towards his said Master and all his during the said Term, and the said Stephen Beckingham for himself, his Executors & Administrators doth covenant & grant to & with the said Governors & Guardians of the Hospital for the Maintenance & Education of exposed & deserted Young Children by these presents, That the said Stephen Beckingham, his Executors & Administrators, shall & will during all the Term aforesaid find provide & allow unto the said Apprentice meet competent & sufficient Meat, Drink and Apparel, Lodging, Washing and all other things necessary & fit for an Apprentice. And also shall & will provide for the said Apprentice that he be not any way a charge to the said Governors & Guardians during the said Term.—And at the End of the said Term the said Stephen Beckingham, his Executors & Administrators, shall & will make provide allow & deliver unto the said Apprentice double Apparel of all sorts good & new, That is to say, a good New Suit for the Holy Days and another for the working days and shall & will give Notice to the said Governors & Guardians of the place where such Apprentice shall go to reside or in case of the death of such Apprentice before he shall attain to the Age of Twenty four years shall & will give notice thereof to the said Governors & Guardians. In Witness whereof the said Governors & Guardians have to this present Indenture affixed their Seal and the said Stephen Beckingham hath put his hand & seal the day & year above written.

(Taken from General Committee Minutes 3:234–35)

Instructions to Apprentices

Hospital for the Maintenance & Education of Exposed & deserted Young Children, in Lamb's Conduit Fields.

INSTRUCTIONS to   upon being put Apprentice to   of   on the   Day of in the year 17   who on the   Day of was   years old.   is to serve h   till   years old.

YOU are placed out Apprentice by the Govrs. of this Hospital. You were taken into it very young, quite helpless, forsaken & deserted by Parents & Friends. Out of Charity have you been fed, clothed, and instructed; which many have wanted.

You have been taught to fear God, to love Him, to be honest, careful, laborious, and diligent. As you hope for Success in this World, and Happiness in the next, you are to be mindful of what has been taught you. You are to behave honestly, justly, soberly, and carefully in every thing, to everybody, and especially towards your   and Family; and to execute all lawful Commands with Industry, Chearfulness, and good Manners.

You may find many Temptations to do wickedly, when you are in the World; but by all means fly from them. Always speak the Truth. Tho' you may have done a wrong thing, you will, by a sincere Confession, more easily obtain Forgiveness than if by an Obstinate Lye you make the Fault the greater, and thereby deserve a far greater Punishment. Lying is looked upon to be the Beginning of every thing that is bad; and a Person used to it is never believed, esteemed, or trusted.

Be not ashamed that you were bred in this Hospital. Own it; and say that it was thro' the good Providence of Almighty God that you were taken care of. Bless Him for it; and be thankful to those worthy Benefactors who have contributed towards your Maintenance & Support. And if ever it be in your Power, make a grateful Acknowledgment to the Hospital for the Benefits you have received.

Be constant in your Prayers, and going to Chruch; & avoid Gaming, Swearing, and all evil Discourses: By this means the Blessing of God will follow your honest Labours, and you will also gain the Good-Will of all good Persons.

If you follow the Instructions which have all along been taught you, and which we now give you, you may be happy; otherwise you will bring upon your self Misery, Shame, and Want.

Note, Your Master will provide you Meat, Drink, Washing, Lodging, and Clothing: And he has agreed to pay you Five Pounds a year, for the Three last years of your Apprenticeship.

(Taken from General Committee Minutes 4:164–65, 17 April 1754)

Certificate of Good Conduct Given to an Apprentice

Foundling Hospital
London

This is to certify that George Farhill has honestly and faithfully served his Master Mr. Higgins for the Term of Seven Years and Six months ending the seventh day of May Eighteen Hundred to the Satisfaction of his Master and Mistress and the Credit of this Hospital where he had been preserved and Educated. In Testimony whereof and of the good Character of the said George Farhill a Donation of Five Guineas hath been this day presented to the said George Farhill and the Seal of this Corporation hath hereunto been affixed in the presence of the Governors and Guardians whose Names are hereunto Subscribed this fourth day of June in the Year of our Lord Eighteen Hundred.
Sealed with the Seal of the Corporation and attested by us.

Thos. Everett
Thos. King
Thos. Bernard
John Hunter
Wm. Harrison
Geo. Tennant

Signed and Sealed by order of the General Committee.

M. Lievesley, Secr'y.

(Taken from General Committee Minutes 23:297–98)

APPENDIX V

Summary of the Foundling Hospital's Income

1739–1756

Source	Total Received	Average per Year	Percentage of Total Income
General Benefactions	£ 37,419.10. 9	£ 2,201.0.0	34.79
Annual Subscriptions	8,388. 4. 0	493.0.0	7.80
Legacies	39,511.11. 0	2,324.0.0	36.73
Chapel (1746–56)	7,488. 5.11	681.0.0	6.96
Charity Boxes (1741–56)	2,746.16. 9	172.0.0	2.56
Rents and Interest	11,178. 6. 8	658.0.0	10.39
Children's Work (1747–56)	798.12. 1	80.0.0	.74
Miscellaneous Income	37. 5. 6	6.0.0	.03
Totals:	£ 107,568.12. 8	£ 6,615.0.0	100.00

(Data taken from annual accounts in *An Account of the Hospital*, 1759)

1757–1771

Source	Total Received	Average per Year	Percentage of Total Income
General Benefactions	£ 6,365.13. 1	£ 424.0.0	10.24
Annual Subscriptions	1,881. 9. 6	125.0.0	3.03
Legacies	32,096.15. 0	2,140.0.0	51.63
Chapel	1,684. 6. 7	112.0.0	2.71
Charity Boxes	574. 6. 6	38.0.0	.92
Rents and Interest	14,940.18. 7	996.0.0	24.03
Children's Work	3,184. 1.11	212.0.0	5.12
Miscellaneous Income	1,443.16. 2	96.0.0	2.32
Totals:	£ 62,171. 7. 4	£ 4,143.0.0	100.00

(Data taken from annual accounts in Foundling Hospital Library, vol. 16)

Summary of Certain Items of Foundling Hospital's Income
1772–1789

Source	Total Received	Average per Year
General Benefactions	£ 8,492. 9. 3	£ 472.0.0
Legacies	27,332.19. 3	1,518.0.0
Rents and Interest*	48,131. 8. 4	2,831.0.0

* Excluding missing data for 1782.

(Data taken from *The Report of the Committee appointed ... 12th May*, 1790, Appendix D; Record of Hospital's Income and Expenses, 1741–81, FHL 41, item 4; Annual account for 1772 in ibid, vol. 16; Annual accounts for 1783–89, GLRO, and loose copies at the Coram Foundation.)

In the following graphs the data on benefactions was taken from the Foundling Hospital's annual accounts; the data on economic fluctuations was taken from T. S. Ashton, *Economic Fluctuations in England*, 1700–1800, (Oxford, 1959), pp. 172–73

Total Legacies from 1739 to 1789

1739–1756:	£39,511.11.0
1757–1771:	32,096.15.0
1772–1789:	27,332.19.3
Total:	£98,941. 5.3

Average per year for 50 years: £1,979.0.0

Graph Showing Rise and Fall in General Benefactions to the
Foundling Hospital, 1739–1756

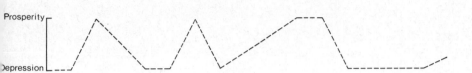

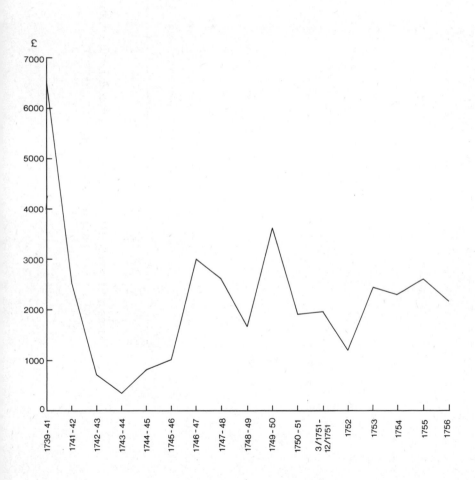

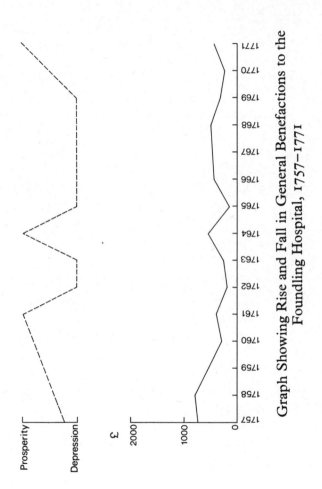

Graph Showing Rise and Fall in General Benefactions to the
Foundling Hospital, 1757–1771

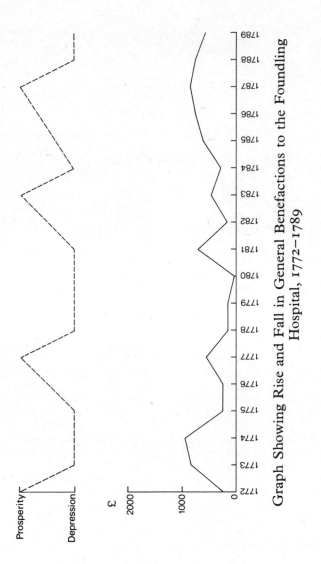

Graph Showing Rise and Fall in General Benefactions to the Foundling Hospital, 1772–1789

APPENDIX VI

Tables of Diet

1747

(Taken from General Committee Minutes 2:223–24)

In the Pork Season

	Breakfast	Dinner	Supper
Sunday	Broth	Roast Pork	Bread
Monday	Gruell	Potatoes	Milk & Bread
Tuesday	Milk Porridge	Boiled Mutton	Bread
Wednesday	Broth	Rice Milk	Bread & Cheese
Thursday	Gruel	Boiled Pork	Bread
Friday	Milk Porridge	Dumplins	Milk & Bread
Saturday	Gruell	Hasty Puddings	Bread & Cheese

In the Other Season

	Breakfast	Dinner	Supper
Sunday	Broth	Roast Beef	Bread
Monday	Gruell	Potatoes	Milk & Bread
Tuesday	Milk Porridge	Boiled Beef	Bread
Wednesday	Broth	Rice Puddings	Bread & Cheese
Thursday	Gruell	Boiled Mutton	Bread
Friday	Broth	Sewett Puddings	Milk & Bread
Saturday	Gruell	Hasty Puddings	Bread & Cheese

Gruell or milk porridge or pottage consisted of a thin mixture made by stirring oatmeal, rice, or another cereal into boiling water or milk. Gruell was sometimes made by stirring oatmeal into the liquid in which meat had been boiled.

A hasty pudding was a pudding made of flour and milk or water stirred into a thick batter. In the north of England and in Scotland, it was made with oatmeal and water and eaten with a little milk, beer, butter, or treacle topping it.

Dumplins was also a pudding made of dough, more or less globular in form. It might be plain or contain fruit and could be boiled or baked.

A sewett (suet) pudding was made of flour and suet, usually boiled in a cloth.

1762
(Taken from General Committee Minutes 8:186)

	Breakfast	Dinner	Supper
Sunday	Bread & Butter	Roast Beef & Greens	Milk Porridge
Monday	Gruel	Potatoes or Parsnips mash'd with Milk	Bread & Milk
Tuesday	Milk Porridge	Boiled Beef & Greens	Broth
Wednesday	Bread & Milk	Stewed Shins of Beef & Broth with Herbs & Roots	Milk Porridge
Thursday	Gruel	Mutton & Greens	Broth
Fryday	Milk Porridge	Stewed Shins of Beef & Broth with Herbs and Roots	Bread & Cheese
Saturday	Bread & Milk	Rice Pudding	Gruel

'Roots' referred to vegetables such as turnips, carrots, and the like. 'Greens' referred to green vegetables usually boiled, such as cabbage, kale, spinach, etc.

1790
(Taken from the General Committee Minutes 19:256)

	Breakfast	Dinner	Supper
Sunday	Bread & Butter	Roast Beef & Vegetables	Bread & Cheese
Monday	Milk Pottage	Boiled Mutton & Vegetables	Bread & Butter
Tuesday	Bread & Butter	The Boys, Rice Pudding; the Girls, Mutton Broth, thickened with Rice	Bread & Butter
Wednesday	Milk Pottage	Boiled Beef & Vegetables	Bread & Butter
Thursday	Milk Pottage	Broth thickened with Peas	Bread & Cheese
Friday	Milk Pottage	Boiled Mutton & Vegetables	Bread & Butter
Saturday	Bread & Butter	The Boys, Broth; the Girls, Rice Pudding	Bread & Cheese

LIST OF ABBREVIATIONS

AHR	*American Historical Review*
APC, Col.	Acts of the Privy Council, Colonial Series
CSP, A & WI	Calendar of State Papers, Colonial Series, America and West Indies
DNB	*Dictionary of National Biography*
FHL	Foundling Hospital Library
Gen. Com.	Minutes of the Foundling Hospital's General Committee
Gen. Ct.	Minutes of the Foundling Hospital's General Court
GLRO	Greater London Record Office
HMC	Historical Manuscripts Commission
Mass. Arch.	Massachusetts State Archives
MeHS	Maine Historical Society
MHS	Massachusetts Historical Society
PRO	Public Record Office
Sec. Cor. In	Correspondence of the Foundling Hospital's Secretary, In-Letters
Sec. Misc.	Reports and Miscellaneous items of the Foundling Hospital's Secretary
SLB	Letter Books of the Foundling Hospital's Secretary
Subcom.	Minutes of the Foundling Hospital's Subcommittee
WMQ	*William and Mary Quarterly*

NOTES

NOTES TO CHAPTER I

1. I am indebted to Miss E. M. Marshall, Children's Officer of the Thomas Coram Foundation for Children, for this legend.

2. *Private Virtue and publick Spirit display'd in a Succinct Essay on the Character of Capt. Thomas Coram* (London, 1751), p. 13. This anonymous pamphlet, published less than ten days after Coram's death, is usually attributed to Dr Richard Brocklesby.

3. No. 105 (11 July 1713).

4. Olwen H. Hufton, *The Poor of Eighteenth-Century France, 1750–1789* (Oxford, 1974), pp. 322–23.

5. Leon Lallemand, *Histoire des Enfants Abandonnés et Délaissés* (Paris, 1885), pp. 124–25.

6. Quoted in Lallemand, p. 111.

7. Ibid., pp. 131–35.

8. Saint Vincent de Paul, *Correspondance, Etretiens, Documents*, ed. Pierre Coste, 15 vols (Paris, 1920–60), 13:798.

9. Emily Green Balch, 'Public Assistance of the Poor in France', *Publications of the American Economic Association* 8, no. 4 (1893): 50–55; Mary Purcell, *The World of Monsieur Vincent* (New York, 1963), pp. 154–57; Shelby T. McCloy, *Government Assistance in Eighteenth-Century France* (Durham, N. C., 1946), pp. 212, 252; 'Translation of the King of France His Edict in June 1670', FHL 31:1–5; 'Memorial Relating to the Foundlings At Paris' (1728), ibid., pp. 14–15; *Abregé Historique de l'Etablissement de L'Hôpital des Enfans-Trouvés* (Paris, 1753), pp. 3–7, 9.

10. 'Regulation of the Hospital at Lisbon' (no date but undoubtedly from the eighteenth century), FHL 31:331; Jonas Hanway, *A Candid Historical Account of the Hospital for the Reception of Exposed and Deserted Young Children* (London, 1759), p. 31.

11. [Louis François] Benoiston de Chateauneuf, *Considérations sur les Enfans Trouvés dans les Principaux États de l'Europe* (Paris, 1824), p. 9; 'Epillogo de' Statuti del Pio Spedale della Pietà di Venezia' (no date but undoubtedly from the eighteenth century), FHL 31:339.

12. 'Berigt Wegens Het Aalmoeseniers Weeshuijs der Stadt Amsterdam', February 1740, FHL 31:65–66, 108–116; H. Brugmans, *Geschiedenis van Amsterdam*, 6 vols (Utrecht, 1972–73), 3:298–99.

13. David Owen, *English Philanthropy, 1660–1960* (Cambridge, Mass., 1964), p. 157.

14. William Maitland, *The History of London, from its Foundation by the Romans, to the Present Time* (London, 1739), p. 673.

15. Ernest Caulfield, *The Infant Welfare Movement in the Eighteenth Century* (New York, 1931), pp. 55–56; Jonas Hanway, *Letters on the Importance of the Rising Generation of the Laboring part of our fellow-subjects*, 2 vols. (London, 1767), 1:48–49, 68, 71; *An Account of the General Nursery or Colledg of Infants, set up by the Justices of Peace for the County of Middlesex with the Constitution and Ends thereof* (London, 1686), pp. 1–3, 7–10.

16. Ernest Harold Pearce, *Annals of Christ's Hospital*, 2d ed. (London, 1908), pp. 21, 26, 28, 31, 35.

17. Ibid., pp. 38, 247; Edmund Blunden, *Christ's Hospital: A Retrospect* (London, 1923), pp. 8, 12–13, 26–27, 54–55.

18. Elizabeth Cellier, 'A Scheme for the Foundation of a Royal Hospital . . . for the Maintenance of a Corporation of skilful Midwives, and such Foundlings, or exposed Children, as shall be admitted therein', in *The Harleian Miscellany*, 10 vols (London, 1808–13), 4:142–3, 145.

19. Hanway, *A Candid Historical Account*, p. 16.

20. [Thomas Bray], *A Memorial Concerning the Erection in the City of London or the Suburbs thereof, an Orphanotrophy or Hospital for the Reception of Poor Cast-off Children or Foundlings* (n.p., n.d.), pp. 21–22.

21. Robert Nelson, *An Address to Persons of Quality and Estate* (London, 1715), p. 212.

22. George Edward Cokayne, *The Complete Peerage of England, Scotland, Ireland, Great Britain, and the United Kingdom*, ed. Hon. Vicary Gibbs, 13 vols, 2d ed. (London, 1910–59), passim; G. E. Mingay, *English Landed Society in the Eighteenth Century* (London, 1963), p. 146; David Green, *Sarah Duchess of Marlborough* (New York, 1967), pp. 255–56; J. H. Plumb, *Sir Robert Walpole: The King's Minister* (London, 1960), pp. 79, n. 1, 113–14.

23. *The Crisis of the Aristocracy, 1558–1641* (Oxford, 1965), p. 9.

24. Henry Fielding, *The History of Tom Jones, a Foundling*, The Modern Library (New York, 1950), pp. 7–8.

25. J[oseph] Massie, *Farther Observations concerning the Foundling-Hospital* (London, 1759), p. 3.

26. Reprinted in *Gentleman's Magazine* 5 (September, 1735): 528.

27. Peter Laslett, *The World We Have Lost* (New York, 1965), p. 174.

28. Gordon W. Allport, *The Nature of Prejudice* (Cambridge, Mass., 1954), p. 31.

29. Ibid., pp. 380, 382.

30. 18 Eliz. I, c. 3, sec. 1.

31. Sidney and Beatrice Webb, *English Local Government*, vol. 7, *English Poor Law History, Part I: The Old Poor Law* (London, 1927), pp. 212–14; Caulfield, pp. 135–36; Hanway, *Letters on the Importance of the Rising Generation*, p. 104.

32. 9 Geo. I, c. 7.

33. Hanway, *Letters on the Importance of the Rising Generation*, pp. 12–13.

34. Jonas Hanway, *A Reply to C-----A-------, Author of the Candid Remarks on Mr. Hanway's Candid Historical Account of the Foundling Hospital* (London, 1760), p. 8.

35. *The Journals of the House of Commons*, 8 March 1715, vol. 18, p. 396.

36. Hanway, *Letters on the Importance of the Rising Generation*, pp. 12–13.

37. *Some Considerations on the Necessity and Usefulness of the Royal Charter Establishing an Hospital for the Maintenance and Education of Exposed and Deserted Young Children* (London, 1740), pp. 3–4.

38. 'Translation of the King of France His Edict in June, 1670', FHL 31:2.

NOTES TO CHAPTER 2

1. Thomas Coram, Memorial and Petition to the Archbishop of Canterbury, 1748, in William Stevens Perry, ed., *Historical Collections Relating to the American Colonial Church*, 5 vols (Hartford, 1870–73), 3:64–67; Thomas Coram, Affidavit, 7 January 1730, MeHS, *Collections*, 2d ser., *Documentary History of the State of Maine* 11:101–5; CSP, A & WI (1712–14): 20 August 1713, Thomas Coram to the Lord High Treasurer, p. 222; Thomas Coram, Memorial to Governor Joseph Dudley, 26 August 1703, quoted in Hamilton Andrews Hill, *Thomas Coram in Boston and Taunton* (Worcester, Mass., 1892), pp. 3–4; Thomas Coram, Petition to the King, 8 February 1727, PRO, PC 1/48.

2. Edgar Legare Pennington, *Anglican Beginnings In Massachusetts* (Boston, 1841), pp. 40–41, 47–48.

3. G. B. Warden, *Boston, 1689–1776* (Boston, 1970), pp. 34–36.

4. CSP, A & WI (1731): 12 March 1731, Capt. Coram to Mr Popple, p. 58; Thomas Coram, Complaint to the General Court at Boston, 5 March 1701, Mass. Arch. 40:649–50; Bernard and Lotte Bailyn, *Massachusetts Shipping, 1697–1714: A Statistical Study* (Cambridge, Mass., 1959), pp. 102–3.

5. The records relating to these lawsuits are to be found in the Records of the Court of Common Pleas, 1696–1702, for Bristol County, Mass., pp. 36–37, 39, 41–42, 52–53. See also Thomas Coram, Petition, 14 February 1701, Mass. Arch. 40:646.

6. James Pavior, Affidavit, 5 July 1701, MHS, Miscellaneous Bound Items, 1698–1702, vol. 6.

7. Thomas Coram, Complaint to the General Court in Boston, 5 March 1701, Mass. Arch. 40:649–50; Act to enable Thomas Coram to prosecute his appeal etc., 8 March 1701, Mass. Arch. 40:653–55. See also CSP, A & WI (1701): 14, 24, 26 February, and 5, 7, 12 March 1701, Minutes of Council in Assembly of the Massachusetts Bay, pp. 82, 98, 100, 107–8.

8. The records relating to these lawsuits are to be found in Records of the Court of Common Pleas, 1696–1702, for Bristol County, Mass., pp. 52–54. See also Records of the Court of General Sessions of the Peace for Bristol County, 1697–1701, pp. 69, 76.

9. Writ of Attachment against Thomas Coram, 24 December 1701, MHS, *Proceedings* 56:17–19.

10. Thomas Coram to the Secretary of the S.P.G., 18 September 1740, in Perry, ed., 3:342–3; Hill, pp. 11–12; Records of the Court of Common Pleas, 1696–1702, for Bristol County, Mass., p. 45; Thomas Coram, Complaint to the Justices of the Superior Court of Judicature for the County of Bristol, 11 September 1701, Boston Public Library, Department of Rare Books.

11. Records of Inferior Court of Common Pleas, 1702–1720, for Bristol County, Mass., pp. 22–23; Hill, pp. 3, 12; Thomas Coram to the Secretary of the S.P.G., 18 September 1740, in Perry, ed., 3:343–4.

12. Record Commissioners of the City of Boston, *Report Containing the Boston Marriages from 1700 to 1751* (Boston, 1898), p. 1; Thomas Coram to Dr Benjamin Colman, 24 August 1739, MHS, *Proceedings* 56:54; same to same, 13 September 1740, ibid., p. 55. Eunice Wayte was born 11 July 1677, the daughter of John and Eunice Roberts Wayte. Record Commissioners of the City of Boston, *Report Containing Boston Births, Baptisms, Marriages, and Deaths, 1630–1699* (Boston, 1883), p. 143.

13. CSP, A & WI (1712–14): 4 June 1713, Proposal of Disbanded Officers and Soldiers, p. 187; MeHS, *Collections*, 2d ser., *Documentary History of the State of Maine* 9: 16 October 1714, Thomas Coram to the Earl of Orford, pp. 342–44; H. B. Fant, 'Picturesque Thomas Coram, Projector of Two Georgias and Father of the London Foundling Hospital', *The Georgia Historical Quarterly* 32 (June, 1948): 83–87.

14. CSP, A & WI (1712–14): 17 June 1713, Reply of the Board of Trade to the Lord High Treasurer, p. 190.

15. Sheila Biddle, *Bolingbroke and Harley* (New York, 1974), pp. 253–56, 261–62, 268.

16. For a discussion of the claims to ownership, see Robert E. Moody, 'The Proposed Colony of Georgia in New England, 1713–1733', *Colonial Society of Massachusetts Publications* 34 (1943): 259–61.

17. Jeremiah Dummer to Mr Edward Hutchinson, 13 February 1717, MHS, Col. Edward Hutchinson Papers.

18. Jeremiah Dummer to the General Court of Massachusetts, 17 September 1720, Mass. Arch. 28:188–89 (also in Thomas Hutchinson, *The History of the Colony and Province of Massachusetts-Bay*, ed. Lawrence S. Mayo, 3 vols. [Cambridge, Mass., 1936] 2:184n).

19. Jeremiah Dummer to the General Court of Massachusetts, 8 April 1720, MHS, *Collections*, 3d ser. 1:142.

20. [Brocklesby], pp. 12–13. In a letter to the Countess of Huntingdon, 15 September 1739 (Hastings Collection, Henry E. Huntington Library, San Marino, California), Coram states that he has worked seventeen and a half years to establish a foundling hospital in London.

21. Coram to Colman, 22 September 1738, MHS, *Proceedings* 56:43.

22. John G. Sperling, *The South Sea Company* (Cambridge, Mass., 1962), p. 33.

23. I reached this conclusion from an analysis of data in Anthony Highmore, *Pietas Londinensis: The History, Design, and Present State of the various Public Charities in and near London* (London, 1810). Not only did distrust of the joint-stock company become traditional, but the so-called Bubble Act of 1720 (6 Geo. I, c. xviii, secs xviii–xxi) made joint-stock organization both costly and protracted.

24. Thomas Wentworth, Earl of Strafford, to Peter Wentworth, 28 September 1714, *The*

Wentworth Papers, 1705–1739, ed. James J. Cartwright (London, 1883), p. 423. Later, in 1718, Churchill was appointed to this post.

25. John M. Beattie, *The English Court in the Reign of George I* (Cambridge, 1967), pp. 41, n. 7; 275–76.

26. Coram to Colman, 30 April 1734, MHS, *Proceedings* 56:20. Bray received the living of St Botolph Without Aldgate in 1706 and resided there from 1708 to 1716 and from 1720 to 1730. H. P. Thompson, *Thomas Bray* (London, 1954), pp. 73–84. Coram probably became his parishioner after 1720.

27. [Bray], p. 12. Internal evidence indicates that this pamphlet (attributed to Dr Bray by Harvard College Library, to which a copy was given by Coram) must have been written after December 1727. Since Bray was ill in late 1729 and died on 15 February 1730, it was probably published in 1728 or early 1729.

28. Ibid., p. 26.

29. [Brocklesby], p. 16.

30. Thomas Coram, Pocket Book, FHL, vol. 98. In a pocket memorandum book, begun as a record of receipts and expenditures for the year 1729, Coram noted the date on which each of the lady petitioners signed. Significantly, he captioned the list: 'An Exact Account when each Lady of Charity Signed their Declaration', a clear indication that he had in mind the French model of Les Dames de la Charité.

31. Leonard W. Cowie, *Henry Newman, An American in London, 1708–1743* (London, 1956), pp. 16–18, 24, 102. On the other hand, the Duke's first wife, whom Newman would have known, died in 1722, and we cannot be sure that he knew the Duke's second wife, the signer of Coram's petition. According to the anonymous author (almost certainly John Holliday) of *An Appeal to the Governors of the Foundling Hospital on the Probable Consequences of Covering the Hospital Lands with Buildings* (London, 1787), p. 5, 'the recommendatory letters of Dr Mead gained . . . [Coram] admission into the mansions of the great'. Unfortunately, because of the tract's polemical nature and certain misstatements of fact, one does not know how much credence to give the quoted statement.

32. Cowie, pp. 165–66.

33. [Brocklesby], p. 14.

34. The genealogical information used to prepare Charts 1 and 2 was taken from Cokayne, the DNB, the general index (not yet published) of the *Yale Edition of Horace Walpole's Correspondence*, and many other sources.

35. [Samuel Smith], *Publick spirit illustrated in the life and designs of the Reverend Thomas Bray, D. D., late minister of St. Botolph Without Aldgate* (London, 1746), pp. 43–44; Coram to Colman, 30 April 1734, MHS, *Proceedings* 56:20; Thompson, pp. 97–99; John Wolfe Lydekker, *Thomas Bray, 1658–1730, Founder of Missionary Enterprise* (Philadelphia, 1943), pp. 30–32; Verner W. Crane, 'Dr. Thomas Bray and the Charitable Colony Project, 1730', *WMQ*, 3d ser. 19 (1962): 49–63; Verner W. Crane, 'The Philanthropists and the Genesis of Georgia', *AHR* 27 (October, 1921): 63–69. Crane's interpretation of Bray's role as the founder of Georgia has been challenged by Dr Albert B. Saye, but, to my mind, Crane's evidence is conclusive. Saye points out, however, that the idea of locating some sort of colony south of the Carolinas had been advocated at least as early as 1717 by various pamphleteers. Albert B. Saye, *A Constitutional History of Georgia, 1732–1945* (Athens, Ga., 1948), pp. 3–4. See also Fant, pp. 91–95.

36. Lydekker, p. 31; Saye, p. 10; CSP, A & WI (1730): 23 November 1730, Petition of Lord Viscount Percival and Others, p. 357; Crane, 'Dr. Thomas Bray', *WMQ*, pp. 55–56.

37. Geraldine Meroney, 'The London Entrepôt Merchants and the Georgia Colony', *WMQ*, 3d ser. 25 (1968): 230–44.

38. Thomas Coram to Henry Newman, 20 November 1732, *Notes and Queries*, 8th ser. 4 (1893): 266.

39. *Colonial Records of the State of Georgia*, ed. Allen D. Candler, 26 vols (Atlanta, Ga., 1904–16) 1:69, 71, 76–77, 85, 89, 97, 112; 2:25; *The Journal of the Earl of Egmont : Abstract of the Trustees' Proceedings for Establishing the Colony of Georgia, 1732–1738*, ed. Robert G. McPherson (Athens, Ga., 1962), p. 25.

40. Captain Coram to Henry Newman, 22 December 1733, *Henry Newman's Salzburger Letterbooks*, ed. George F. Jones (Athens, Ga., 1966), p. 407; see also pp. 74, 94, 395–96.

41. John Martin Bolzius to Capt. Coram, 28 July 1737, University of Georgia Library, Egmont Papers, vol. 14203, pt 1, p. 73.

42. Captain Coram to Henry Newman, 22 December 1733, *Henry Newman's Salzburger Letterbooks*, pp. 406–7.

43. Coram to Colman, 22 September 1738, MHS, *Proceedings* 56:47–48; Saye, pp. 29–30; Charles C. Jones, *History of Georgia*, 2 vols (Boston, 1883), 1:106–7, 114; *Journal of the Earl of Egmont*, pp. 6, 12, 48, 50–51.

44. *Journal of the Earl of Egmont*, p. 52.

45. Ibid., pp. 76, 86–87; CSP, A & WI (1738), p. 287.

46. CSP, A & WI (1734–35): 1 May 1735, Memorial of Thomas Coram and Petition of 102 Persons, pp. 413–15; copies of same with Coram's comments, FHL 28:203–6.

47. CSP, A & WI (1735–36): 11 July 1735, Coram's Reply to the Board of Trade with Estimate of Expenses, pp. 12–17 (copies of same, FHL 28:207–13); 6 April 1736, Proposals for Beginning a Civil Government in Nova Scotia, pp. 184–85; 14 April 1736, Coram's Comments thereon, p. 187; 2 June 1736, List of Proposed Trustees, p. 221 (copies of same, FHL 28: 214–16); (1737): 22 April 1737, Board of Trade to Committee of the Privy Council, pp. 120–21 (copy of same, FHL 28:218–19); APC, Col., vol. 3 (1720–45): 565; Memoranda of Thomas Coram, 6 February 1736 and 31 March 1738, FHL 28:221, 223; Coram to Colman, 2 March 1737, MHS, *Proceedings* 56:33; same to same, 9 July 1737, ibid., p. 37; Fant, pp. 95–97.

48. Coram to Colman, 21 September 1738, MHS, *Proceedings* 56:40–42.

49. Rev. Samuel Smith to Dr Colman, 29 January 1735, MHS, Colman Papers.

NOTES TO CHAPTER 3

1. Thomas Coram, Pocket Book, FHL, vol. 98.

2. Thomas Coram to the Countess of Huntingdon, 15 September 1739, Hastings Collection, Henry E. Huntington Library, San Marino, California; R. H. Nichols and F. A. Wray, *The History of the Foundling Hospital* (London, 1935), p. 15.

3. Copy of an Order of the Privy Council, 29 July 1737, with Petition of Thomas Coram attached, FHL 6:6–10.

4. Copy of Thomas Coram's List of Proposed Governors, 13 February 1739, FHL 42:53–59.

5. Coram to Colman, 22 September 1738, MHS, *Proceedings* 56:43.

6. The information used to construct the charts in Appendix II was taken from the DNB, Romney Sedgwick, *The History of Parliament: The House of Commons, 1715–1754*, 2 vols (New York, 1970); Cokayne; Meroney; and many other sources that produced only a single fact or date. I am well aware of the hazards here involved: inadequate or missing information about too many of these men makes statistical certainty impossible. To this must be added the possibility of erroneous identifications. Nevertheless, I believe the charts do provide a basis for tentative conclusions, which I may, perhaps, have stated somewhat more affirmatively than my evidence warrants.

7. Coram to Colman, 13 September 1740, MHS, *Proceedings* 56:55.

8. Coram to Colman, 24 August 1739, ibid., 56:54.

9. Thomas Coram to the Countess of Huntingdon, 15 September 1739, Hastings Collection, Henry E. Huntington Library.

10. Coram to Colman, 22 September 1738, MHS, *Proceedings* 56:43.

11. Petition of Thomas Coram to the Princess Amelia, with Coram's comments, 28 December 1737, FHL 6:3–5.

12. Petition of Thomas Coram to the Princess of Wales, FHL 6:11–13; copy in Houghton Library, Harvard University.

13. Coram to Colman, 22 September 1738, MHS, *Proceedings* 56:44; Vere Beauclerk to Thomas Coram, 17 June 1738, MHS, Colman Papers, vol. 2; Gen. Ct. 1:105; Gen. Com. 1:159.

14. Coram to Colman, 24 August 1739, MHS, *Proceedings* 56:53; H. F. B. Compston, *Thomas Coram: Churchman, Empire Builder and Philanthropist* (London, 1918), pp. 97–98.

15. [Brocklesby], pp. 16–19; Gen. Ct. 1:1–3; Governor Belcher to Jonathan Belcher, Jr,

8 May 1740, MHS, *Collections*, 6th ser. 7:221. Accounts of the first meeting of the Governors are also to be found in *London Magazine* 8 (1739): 627–28; *Read's Weekly Journal*, 24 November 1739; and *London Evening Post*, 20–22 November 1739. Although the Westminster Hospital was founded by voluntary subscriptions in 1719 and St George's Hospital in 1733, neither was incorporated during the eighteenth century. St George's Hospital was incorporated in 1834 (Local and Personal Acts, 4 and 5 William IV, c. xxxviii; J. Blomfield, *St George's, 1733–1933*, London, 1933, p. 54). The Westminster Hospital was incorporated in 1836 (Local and Personal Acts, 6 and 7 William IV, c. xx; Information kindly supplied by Mr E. S. Gower, Archivist, Kensington and Chelsea and Westminster Area Health Authority, South District).

16. [Brocklesby], pp. 15, 18; Coram to Colman, 22 September 1738, MHS, *Proceedings* 56:43; Governor Belcher to Thomas Coram, 31 August 1741, MHS, *Collections*, 6th ser. 7:411.

17. Coram to Colman, 22 September 1738, MHS, *Proceedings* 56:44–45.

18. Peter Laslett and Karla Oosterveen, 'Long-term Trends in Bastardy in England', *Population Studies* 27 (July, 1973): 260, 266–67, 282, n. 25.

19. Gen. Com. 3:16; 6:103–4.

20. [Bray], pp. 15–16.

21. Francis Bacon, 'Of Parents and Children', *Essays* (1612).

NOTES TO CHAPTER 4

1. Coram to Colman, 24 August 1739, MHS, *Proceedings* 56:53–54.

2. Cowie, p. 102.

3. Gen. Com. 1:7.

4. Gen. Ct. 1:4–7; Gen. Com. 1:1–5, 7–11, 13–16; *Daily Gazetteer*, 6 December 1739.

5. Gen. Ct. 1:10–12; Gen. Com. 1:16–18, 25; 'Reasons Why the Poor Children Educated in the Foundling Hospital should not Obtain a Settlement There', 1740, FHL, vol. 23. See Nichols and Wray, pp. 337–44, for provisions of the Act, which was 13 Geo. II, c. 29.

6. Gen. Com. 1:39.

7. Gen. Ct. 1:13–15; Gen. Com. 1:24, 27–31, 37–40, 65–66; *London Magazine* 9 (1740): 506.

8. Gen. Ct. 1:50; Gen. Com. 1:66–67, 73–74, 77–78, 80–82; *London Magazine* 9 (1740): 612.

9. Gen. Com. 1:42–53.

10. Gen. Ct. 1:20–22; Gen. Com. 1:37.

11. *An Account of the Hospital for the Maintenance and Education of Exposed and Deserted Young Children* (London, 1759), pp. viii–ix; Gen. Ct. 1:24–38.

12. *The Report of the General Committee For directing, managing, and transacting the Business, Affairs, Estate, and Effects of the Corporation of the Governors and Guardians of the Hospital for the Maintenance and Education of exposed and deserted Young Children; Relating to the General Plan for executing the Purposes of the Royal Charter, establishing this Hospital* (London, 1740), p. 4; *Abregé Historique*, p. 7; 'Berigt Wegens', FHL 31:81.

13. 'The Report of the Gentlemen appointed by the General Committee to peruse the Copys of the Establishments of Foundling Hospitals abroad, and to consider of a general Plan for executing this Charity', FHL 41: Item 1; *An Account of the Foundation and Government of the Hospital for Foundlings in Paris*, pp. 2, 7; 'Memoire concernant les Enfans Trouvés de la Ville de Paris', 1740, FHL 6: page 3 of document; 'The Hospitall at Paris', 1740, FHL 28:166–67; 'Berigt Wegens', FHL 31:74–76; 'Regulation of the Hospital at Lisbon', FHL 31:331. 'The Report of the Gentlemen, etc.' is essentially the same as *A Sketch of the General Plan For executing the Purposes of the Royal Charter Establishing an Hospital for the Maintenance and Education of exposed and deserted Young Children; As reported . . . on the 16th of July, 1740* (London, 1740).

14. 'Regulation of the Hospital at Lisbon', FHL 31:331–32; 'Memoire concernant les Enfans Trouvés', FHL 6: page 2 of document; 'The Hospitall at Paris', FHL 28:166; *An Account of the Foundation and Government of the Hospital for Foundlings in Paris*, pp. 13–14, 17–21, 25–26, 28–31; 'Berigt Wegens', FHL 31:65, 67, 94–95.

15. *An Account of the Foundation and Government of the Hospital for Foundlings in Paris,* pp. 13, 28.

16. Adriaan J. Barnouw, *The Pageant of Netherlands History* (New York, 1952), pp. 167–68, 172–73. Graphic evidence of Dutch women's participation in the government of eleemosynary institutions is to be found in Frans Hals's painting, *The Women Regents of the Old Men's Home at Haarlem* (1664).

17. Gen. Com. 1:34.

18. *Report of the General Committee,* p. 5; 'Report of the Gentlemen appointed . . . to consider of a General Plan', FHL 41: Item 1.

19. Lady Betty Germain to the Secretary, 20 July 1752; Lady Vere to a Governor (not named), 17 August 1752, Sec. Cor. In, 1752, GLRO.

20. 'Memoire concernant les Enfans Trouvés', FHL 6: p. 5 of document; 'The Hospitall at Paris', FHL 28:166–67; 'Regulation of the Hospital at Lisbon', FHL 31:332–33; 'Berigt Wegens', FHL 31:67; *Report of the General Committee,* p. 8.

21. 'Regulation of the Hospital at Lisbon', FHL 31:333; Hanway, *A Candid Historical Account,* p. 32; 'The Hospitall at Paris', FHL 28:166–67; *An Account of the Foundation and Government of the Hospital for Foundlings in Paris,* pp. 21–22; 'Berigt Wegens', FHL 31:67, 77–78, 80, 90, 92; 'Report of the Gentlemen appointed . . . to consider of a General Plan', FHL 41: Item 1.

22. Subcom. 1:29.

23. 'Berigt Wegens', FHL 31:71, 75; *An Account of the Foundation and Government of the Hospital for Foundlings in Paris,* pp. 2–6; 'Memoire concernant les Enfans Trouvés', FHL 6: p. 6 of document; 'Report of the Gentlemen appointed . . . to consider of a General Plan', FHL 41: Item 1.

24. Gen. Ct. 1:17; Gen. Com. 1:79, 93, 95–96, 99–101, 103–04, 106, 114, 116–17, 120–22, 124–27.

25. Daily Committee's Minutes, pp. 6–7, GLRO.

26. Ibid., p. 8.

27. Memorandum Book for the Admission and Disposal of Children, vol. 1, GLRO; Register of Baptisms, 1741–1838, GLRO.

28. Gen. Com. 1:129, 133–34, 145; Daily Committee's Minutes, pp. 9–10, 37, GLRO.

NOTES TO CHAPTER 5

1. Gen. Com. 1:176–77, 181–83, 190–91, 194.

2. Gen. Ct. 1:74, 76–81; Gen. Com. 1:199, 201–5, 209.

3. Coram to Colman, 13 September 1740, MHS, *Proceedings* 56:55.

4. Ibid.; Governor Belcher to Captain Coram, 25 October 1740, MHS, *Collections,* 6th ser. 7:332.

5. Coram to Colman, 13 September 1740, MHS, *Proceedings* 56:55. Eunice Coram was buried in All Hallows Church, London Wall, 21 July 1740; see *Index of Obituaries in Boston Newspapers 1704–1795* (Boston, 1968) 2:248.

6. Gen. Com. 1:258, 273, 277, 332.

7. Register of Baptisms, 1741–1838, GLRO.

8. Morris Lievesley, Notebook, FHL, vol. 24. Lievesley was secretary of the Foundling Hospital from 1799 to 1849 and had earlier served as clerk. According to his notes, he heard this story from Thomas Collingwood, secretary from 1758 to 1790, who said he remembered seeing Coram with the children.

9. [Brocklesby], p. 21; Thomas Bernard, *An Account of the Foundling Hospital in London, for the Maintenance and Education of Exposed and Deserted Young Children,* 2d ed., (London, 1799), p. 23.

10. FHL 42:61. This is a copy. Since Coram himself did not sign the petition, the principal evidence linking it to him is that this copy is in his handwriting. Although he often made copies of documents relating to matters in which he was himself involved—some are in the Foundling Hospital's archives—he never, to my knowledge, made copies of anything else. My own opinion

that the handwriting is Coram's has been reinforced by the concurring advisory opinion of Mr Roy P. Basler, Chief of the Manuscript Division of the Library of Congress, Washington, D. C.

11. *The Political Journal of George Bubb Dodington*, ed. John Carswell and Lewis Arnold Dralle (Oxford, 1965), p. 48.

12. Thomas Coram to Mr Austin, 31 January 1749, HMC, 9th Report, App. 2, p.478.

13. W. S. Macnutt, *The Atlantic Provinces: The Emergence of Colonial Society, 1712–1857* (Toronto, 1965), pp. 36–37; *Gentleman's Magazine* 19 (1749): 112–13, 185.

14. Charles C. Jones, 1:313, 428; James Ross McCain, *Georgia as a Proprietary Province: The Execution of a Trust* (Boston, 1917), pp. 235–39, 243; HMC, *Manuscripts of the Earl of Egmont: Diary of Viscount Percival Afterwards First Earl of Egmont* (London, 1920), vol. 63, pt 3, p. 78.

15. [Brocklesby], p. 26.

16. Gen. Com. 3:201–03; Letter of Joshua Paine to Sir William Pepperell (?), 9 April 1751, quoted at length in Samuel Jennison, Notes for a Biography of Thomas Coram, American Antiquarian Society, Worcester, Mass.; *London Advertiser*, 4 April 1751; *Read's Weekly Journal*, 6 April 1751; *London Evening Post*, 2–4 April 1751. Other newspapers and periodicals that carried accounts of Coram's death and funeral were the *Penny London Post, Whitehall Evening Post, Remembrancer*, and *Gentleman's Magazine* 21 (1751): 141, 183.

17. Albert Camus, *Le Mythe de Sisyphe* (Paris, 1942), p. 166.

NOTES TO CHAPTER 6

1. Gen. Ct. 1:81.

2. The description is Mme d'Arblay's, as quoted in Hugh Phillips, *Mid-Georgian London* (London, 1964), p. 208.

3. John Rocque's Map of London, 1746.

4. London County Council, *Survey of London*, vol. 19: *The Parish of St. Pancras, Part II* (London, 1938), p. 25; Register of Title Deeds, 1595–1803, GLRO.

5. Phillips, p. 207; Defoe, 1:328–29; Subcom. 1:174.

6. *Gazetteer and London Daily Advertiser*, 11 June 1756; Alfred Stanley Foord, *Springs, Streams and Spas of London: History and Associations* (London, 1910), pp. 168–69; Septimus Sunderland, *Old London's Spas, Baths, and Wells* (London, 1915), p. 81.

7. Gen. Com. 2:38–39.

8. Ibid. 3:177.

9. London County Council, *Survey of London*, vol. 24: *The Parish of St. Pancras, Part IV* (London, 1952), pp. 25–26, 30; Phillips, pp. 204, 206; Gen. Com. 1:340; Secretary of the Foundling Hospital to the Trustees of the Rugby School, 20 June 1744, Sec. Cor. In, 1744, GLRO.

10. Gen. Com. 1:218, 226–28; Building Plan, FHL, vol. 168; Benedict Nicolson, *The Treasures of the Foundling Hospital* (Oxford, 1972), plates 10 and 12.

11. Memorandum Book for Admission and Disposal of Children, vol. 1, GLRO; Gen. Com. 1:232–33, 238, 242, 304–05, 307–08, 326–27, 339, 342; 2:13, 42, 47, 53–54; *London Magazine* 11 (1742): 461; 12 (1743): 516.

12. Gen. Com. 2:98.

13. Gen. Ct. 1:134; Gen. Com. 2:174–77, 197, 199, 260, 268, 284, 338; Sketch and Description of the Children at the Breakfasting, 1 May 1747, FHL, vol. 39; *Gentleman's Magazine* 17 (1747): 245; *London Magazine* 6 (1747): 241.

14. Gen. Ct. 1:149.

15. Ibid. 1:150.

16. 'Vertue Note Books', Vol. III, *Walpole Society* 22 (1933–34): 135.

17. Ronald Paulson, *Hogarth: His Life, Art, and Times*, 2 vols (New Haven, 1971), 2:35, 37, 42–44, 56; Nicolson, chap. 3.

18. Quoted in Paulson, 2:93; see also Gen. Ct. 1:209.

19. Gen. Com. 2:179; 7:161.

20. Ibid. 3:110; Nicolson, p. 42.

21. Paulson, 2:50–51, 306–10; Nicolson, pp. 36–37.

22. Nicolson, p. 53.

23. Gen. Ct. 1:259; Gen. Com. 4:79–80; Subcom. 1:89.

24. Gen. Com. 3:7–9, 15–16.

25. Vol. 19 (1749): 235.

26. Paul Henry Lang, *George Frideric Handel* (New York, 1966), pp. 226, 484. I am indebted to Dr Lang's definitive biography and to chapter 5 of Nicolson for most of my account of Handel's association with the Foundling Hospital.

27. Lang, p. 21. For an account of the founding of Whitefield's Orphan House at Bethesda, see Eric McCoy North, *Early Methodist Philanthropy* (New York, 1914), pp. 22–23, and George Whitefield, 'An Account of Money Received and Disbursed for the Orphan-House in Georgia', in Grace Abbott, ed., *The Child and The State*, vol. 2 (Chicago, 1938), p. 26.

28. Gen. Com. 3:9.

29. Gen. Ct. 1:208.

30. Gen. Com. 3:109, 115–17, 328.

31. Lang, p. 333.

32. Ibid., pp. 355, 407.

33. Ibid., pp. 529, 534.

34. Gen. Com. 3:328; 4:86, 176; 5:70–71, 250; 6:137; 7:59.

35. Ibid. 4:145–46; Subcom. 1:211–12.

36. Quoted in Nicolson, p. 48. This copy may be seen today at the Coram Foundation.

37. Gen. Com. 7:59; Subcom. 3:140–41; *Sacred Musick, Composed by the late George Frederick Handel, Esq.; And Performed at the Chappel of the Hospital, for the Maintenance and Education of Exposed and Deserted Young Children; on Thursday, the 24th May, 1759. In Grateful Memory Of his many Noble Benefactions to that Charity* (London, 1759).

38. Gen. Com. 7:269, 430; 8:113, 259; 9:67, 212; 10:50, 204; 11:98; 13:164–66, 340; 14:147–49, 305; 15:164–66, 207, 325; 19:29.

39. Ibid. 3:324; 4:265–66; 5:3–4; 10:5; Subcom. 1:140; 2:51.

40. Gen. Ct. 1:212–13; Gen. Com. 2:160, 313, 316; 3:47, 96, 111, 150, 175, 275; 4:103, 115; *Gentleman's Magazine* 21 (1751): 330.

41. Gen. Ct. 1:267–71; Gen. Com. 2:332; *Gentleman's Magazine* 21 (1751): 426.

42. Gen. Com. 2:106–7.

43. Ibid. 3:282–83.

44. Ibid. 2:91, 163, 223–24, 322; 3:22, 96; 4:12, 37, 103, 115, 224, 281, 285, 310; Subcom. 1:27–29, 129–30, 170; 2:9.

Notes to Chapter 7

1. Gen. Com. 1:249.

2. Memorandum Book for Admission and Disposal of Children, vol. 1, GLRO; *Gentleman's Magazine* 19 (1749): 282.

3. Subcom. 2:75–76; *The Universal Museum* 2 (1763): 370. The Act of Parliament of 1740 provided that 'it shall be lawful for all and every person whatsoever to bring any Child or Children whatsoever to . . . such Hospital'. Nichols and Wray, p. 340.

4. Gen. Ct. 1:275.

5. Gen. Com. 5:33–34; *Gentleman's Magazine* 26 (1756): 147.

6. *Journals of the House of Commons* 27:567; Gen. Com. 5:54–55; *Gentleman's Magazine* 26 (1756): 201.

7. *Journals of the House of Commons* 27:592; Gen. Com. 5:60.

8. *A Candid Historical Account of the Hospital*, p. 24.

9. Ibid., pp. 11, 65.

10. *A Plan for the Establishment of Charity-houses for Exposed or Deserted Women and Girls and for Penitent Prostitutes* (London, 1758), p. 9.

11. Gen. Com. 5:60, 65–66, 68–69, 71, 75–76.

12. *Gazetteer and London Daily Advertiser*, 9 June 1756. *Read's Weekly Journal* and the *Public Advertiser* contained shorter versions of the quoted account, but other newspapers seem

to have ignored the event. It was mentioned, however, in the *Gentleman's Magazine* 26 (1756): 309.

13. Gen. Com. 5:83, 86, 92, 96; Sec. Cor. In, 1756, GLRO.

14. FHL 35:9–23; FHL, vol. 18.

15. Gen. Com. 5:161–62.

16. Matthew Prior, *Solomon on the Vanity of the World*, book 3. The written tokens quoted are from FHL, vol. 133. These and others are also to be found in Nichols and Wray, pp. 119–25.

17. List of the Parishes & Places whence 3300 Children came to the Foundling Hospital From 2 June 1756 to 2 June 1757, FHL 35:39–41. The other 1437 children came from counties outside the Bills of Mortality. Mr H. O. Wilson, Head Librarian of the Members' Library, London County Hall, very kindly supplied information about the economic status of the parishes included in this document.

18. Gen. Ct. 2:2.

19. Gen. Com. 5:151; A List of Children Received with £100 from 1756 to 1771, Sec. Misc., 1753/4–1795 bundle, GLRO.

20. Subcom. 2:100–101.

21. Gen. Com. 5:138, 312; 7:193, 196; Subcom. 2:96, 133; 3:92; FHL 10:73–74; FHL 11:212; FHL 35:47.

22. Gen. Com. 6:313; 7:193.

23. Quarterly Account of the Children, vol. 1, 24 June 1752, GLRO; Gen. Com. 3:272–73.

24. Places to Which 3300 Children were sent from the Foundling Hospital From 2 June 1756 to 2 June 1757, FHL 35:43–45.

25. Gen. Ct. 2:30; Gen. Com. 5:186.

26. Gen. Com. 5:230–31.

27. Ibid., 6:121, 124.

28. Ibid., 7:150–51.

29. Subcom. 3:34.

30. B. B. to the Governors, 20 February 1759. This letter was found, obviously misfiled, in the List of Sick at Battle Bridge and Brill Infirmaries, 1759, GLRO.

31. Gen. Com. 5:176; 6:21, 175.

32. Ibid., 5:138–39, 158, 236; Subcom. 3:8–9.

33. Gen. Com. 6:98; 7:27, 359; 8:217, 251; Subcom. 3:116, 153.

34. Subcom. 9:71.

35. Gen. Ct. 3:275.

36. Account of the Children, 31 December 1759, FHL 28:37.

37. Subcom. 2:153; 5:101, 131, 141.

38. Gen. Com. 10:274; Subcom. 3:8–9; Report of Secretary's Visit to Various Places, 4 April 1759, Sec. Misc., 1759 bundle, GLRO.

39. Letter of Thomas Fulljames, 30 September 1759, Sec. Misc., 1756–61 bundle, GLRO.

40. Anonymous letter to the Secretary, 29 May 1759, Sec. Cor. In, 1759, GLRO.

41. Gen. Com. 5:336; Subcom. 3:105.

42. Daily Committee's Minutes, pp. 19–20, GLRO.

43. Gen. Com. 2:248.

44. Ibid., 6:211, 229–30, 239; 7:326, 332, 345.

45. Ibid., 5:296; Subcom. 2:212.

46. Subcom. 2:149.

47. Ibid., 3:27–29.

48. Gen. Com. 5:129–30.

49. Ibid., 7:196.

50. Ibid., 7:172.

51. McCloy, p. 241, n. 21.

52. Hufton, pp. 342–43, 345.

53. Memoranda, Mainly Nurses' Certificates, GLRO; Sec. Misc., 1756–68 bundle, GLRO.

54. This brief sketch of village life is drawn largely from G. E. Fussell, *Village Life in the Eighteenth Century* (Worcester, 1948), and C. S. Orwin, 'Agriculture and Rural Life', in vol. 1 of A. S. Turberville, ed., *Johnson's England*, 2 vols (Oxford, 1933).

NOTES TO CHAPTER 8

1. 18 Eliz. I, c. 3, sec. 1.
2. 13 and 14 Charles II, c. 12.
3. 18 Eliz. I, c. 3, sec. 2.
4. 6 Geo. II, c. 31.
5. Dorothy Marshall, 'The Old Poor Law, 1662–1795', in E. M. Carus-Wilson, ed., *Essays in Economic History*, 3 vols (London, 1954–62) 1 : 299; E. M. Hampson, *The Treatment of Poverty in Cambridgeshire, 1597–1834* (Cambridge, 1934), pp. 165, 170–71; Webb, pp. 311–12; U. R. Q. Henriques, 'Bastardy and the New Poor Law', *Past and Present* 37 (1967): 103–8; Dorothy Marshall, *The English Poor in the Eighteenth Century* (London, 1926), pp. 207–21.
6. Gen. Com. 7:138, 183; Subcom. 3:212–14, 216–17; *Annual Register*, 5th ed. (London, 1769), 2(1759): 129.
7. Subcom. 3:38; The Several Informations of Sarah Gay, Widow, and others, 8 October 1758, Sec. Cor. In, 1758, GLRO; Affidavit of Elizabeth Brounsel, 11 August 1759, Petitions for Claiming Children, GLRO.
8. Mr R. Dingley's Acct. of a Child taken forcibly, 1758, FHL 11:149–50.
9. Gen. Com. 6:217–19.
10. Ibid., 7:19–20.
11. *Whitehall Evening Post*, No. 2074, 3–5 July 1759; Gen. Com. 7:88–89; Secretary's List of Prosecutions, 1760, Sec. Misc., GLRO.
12. Gen. Com. 6:296.
13. *The Tendencies of the Foundling Hospital in its Present Extent Considered In several Views . . . In several Letters to a Senator* (London, 1760), p. 10.
14. Taylor White to Mr Potter, February 1759, FHL 31:139.
15. Subcom. 3:143–44.
16. Ibid., 2:134.
17. Gen. Com. 6:296.
18. Hufton, pp. 345–46, 348.
19. Taylor White to Mr Potter, February 1759, FHL 31:142.
20. Subcom. 3:131; Sec. Misc., ca 1759–1776 bundle, GLRO.
21. Gen. Com. 6:212; Subcom. 3:227.
22. Subcom. 2:218.
23. Quarterly Account of the Children, vol. 1, 25 March 1756, 24 June 1758, 29 September 1760, GLRO. See also Hanway, *A Candid Historical Account of the Hospital*, p. 77.
24. Gen. Com. 6:127, 130–31.
25. Ibid., 6:247–48, 267–68.
26. Gen. Ct. 2:114, 119; Gen. Com. 7:55; Subcom. 3:103–4, 131; Hanway, *A Candid Historical Account of the Hospital*, p. 71.
27. Gen. Com. 6:193–94.
28. *An Humble and Free Address to the Most Noble President, The Right Honourable and Worthy Vice-Presidents, Governors, Trustees, and Guardians of the Foundling Hospital* (London, 1749), pp. 3–5.
29. Porcupinus Pelagius [pseud.], *The Scandalizade, A Panegyri-Satiri-Serio-Comi-Dramatic Poem* (London, 1750) p. 23.
30. Rev. Thomas Trant to Taylor White, 15 January 1757, Sec. Cor. In, 1757, GLRO.
31. Gen. Com. 5:273–74.
32. Sec. Misc., 16 April 1760, GLRO.
33. *Literary Magazine* 2 (1757): 166.
34. Gen. Com. 5:257–58, 263–64, 269. See Ruth K. McClure, 'Johnson's Criticism of the Foundling Hospital and its Consequences', *Review of English Studies*, n.s. 27 (1976): 17–26, for a full account of this affair.
35. Hanway, *A Candid Historical Account of the Hospital*, pp. 36–37.
36. Massie, *Farther Observations Concerning the Foundling Hospital*. Massie began the pamphlet in June 1758, added to it in October, and concluded it in 1759.

37. *The Rise and Progress of the Foundling Hospital Considered : and The Reasons for putting a Stop to the General Reception of All Children* (London, 1761), p. 38.

38. Jonas Hanway, *The Genuine Sentiments of an English Country Gentleman, upon the Present Plan of the Foundling Hospital* (London, 1759), p. 2.

39. Massie, p. 2.

40. *Candid Remarks on Mr. Hanway's Candid Historical Account of the Foundling Hospital and A more useful Plan humbly Recommended, in a Letter to a Member of Parliament* (London, 1760), p. 12.

41. Massie, pp. 1–2.

42. *The Tendencies of the Foundling Hospital*, pp. 13–15.

43. *Joyful News to Batchelors and Maids : Being a Song In Praise of the Fondling Hospital, and the London Hospital Aldersgate Street* (London, [ca 1760]).

44. *Rise and Progress of the Foundling Hospital*, pp. 33–34; *Gentleman's Magazine* 29 (1759): 622–23.

45. Massie, p. 2.

46. *Tendencies of the Foundling Hospital*, pt 2, p. 30.

47. *A Rejoinder to Mr. Hanway's Reply to C--A--'s Candid Remarks Comparing The New Plan of a Foundling Hospital . . . with the old one of our present Poor Laws* (London, 1760), pp. 33–34.

48. *Candid Remarks*, p. 17.

49. Ibid., pp. 8–10; *Tendencies of the Foundling Hospital*, pp. 35, 38; *Rise and Progress of the Foundling Hospital*, pp. 32, 39–43; Massie, p. 3; Hanway, *Genuine Sentiments of an English Country Gentleman*, pp. 4, 16–17.

50. *Rise and Progress of the Foundling Hospital*, pp. 6, 9–12; *Tendencies of the Foundling Hospital*, pp. 7–8.

51. Vol. 28: 240; same item in *Annual Register*, 5th ed. (London, 1768), 1 (1758): 93–94.

52. Dr Lee to the Hospital's treasurer, 18 February 1760, FHL 11:37.

53. Hanway, *A Candid Historical Account of the Hospital*, pp. 9–10, 41–45, 67, 75, 80–83, 86, 91–93, 95, 99–100, 110. See also Hanway, *A Reply to C-----A-------*.

54. *Some Objections to the Foundling-Hospital Considered By a Person in the Country to whom they were sent* (London, 1761). Although the British Library catalogue does not list an author for this pamphlet, I believe, from evidence in the Foundling Hospital's archives, that it was written by Dr Bolton. See Gen. Ct. 2:146; Secretary to Dean Bolton, 7 February 1760, SLB, vol. 3, GLRO; Draft of Treatise, FHL 31:145–56.

55. Vol. 29:54–55.

56. Hanway, *A Candid Historical Account of the Hospital*, pp. 36–37.

57. Ibid., pp. 38–39; Gen. Com. 7:26, 48.

58. *Journals of the House of Commons*, vol. 28, p. 571; Gen. Com. 7:57–58.

59. *The Parliamentary History of England from the Earliest Period to the Year* 1803 (London, 1813), 15 (1753–1765): 941–43.

60. Hanway, *A Candid Historical Account of the Hospital*, pp. 24–25.

61. Hufton, pp. 332, 344.

62. T. S. Ashton, 'Changes in Standards of Comfort in Eighteenth-Century England', *Proceedings of the British Academy* 41 (1955): 173, 176, 185.

63. Subcom. 3:149.

64. Gen. Ct. 2:126; Gen. Com. 7:177, 185, 187–88, 202–3, 212–13; Votes of the House of Commons, No. 26, 19 December 1759, FHL, vol. 16; *Journals of the House of Commons*, vol. 28, pp. 703, 707, 738, 747.

65. Gen. Ct. 2:127–28, 130–31; Gen. Com. 7:215, 217, 235; Register of Baptisms, 1741–1838, GLRO; *Journals of the House of Commons*, vol. 28, pp. 751, 753.

NOTES TO CHAPTER 9

1. Gen. Com. 7:247–49, 264, 284–86, 307, 408.

2. Taylor White to Dr Lee, 23 June 1761, SLB 3:90, GLRO.

3. Gen. Com. 8:137; 9:90, 238; 11:249–51; Subcom. 6:69–70.

4. 'A Particular Account of Moneys received of His Majestys Echequer [*sic*] by the Governours and Guardians for the Maintenance and Education of exposed and deserted Young Children in Virtue of Parliamentary Grants to His Majesty from the Year 1756 to 31st December 1764', FHL, vol. 23.

5. *Journals of the House of Commons*, vol. 30, pp. 310–11.

6. Gen. Ct. 2:255–57.

7. Nichols and Wray, pp. 157–81.

8. Taylor White to Sir Rowland Winn, 27 April 1765, SLB 3:309, GLRO.

9. Ibid.

10. Ibid.; same to same, 2 May 1765, SLB 3:310, GLRO.

11. Jonas Hanway to Mr Collingwood, secretary of the Foundling Hospital, 29 February 1764, FHL 31:185–97. The pamphlet was *A Proposal for saving £70,000 to £150,000 to the Public; at the same time rendering 5,000 young persons of both sexes more happy in themselves and more useful to their country, than if so much money were expended on their account* (London, 1764).

12. (London, 1758), pp. 5–6.

13. Gen. Com. 9:228–33; same item in FHL 43:7–9.

14. 'The Case of the Governors and Guardians of the Hospital for the Maintenance and Education of Exposed and Deserted Young Children', FHL vol. 1; Gen. Ct. 2:161.

15. Gen. Ct. 2:277–78; Gen. Com. 9:236.

16. Gen. Ct. 2:278–79; Taylor White to Sir Roland Winn, 27 April 1765, SLB 3:310, GLRO.

17. Gen. Com. 9:238, 261, 288, 325–6.

18. Ibid., 10:46, 65; *London Magazine* 35 (July 1766): 342–43.

19. Taylor White to Dr Lee, 11 May 1767, SLB 3:381; Gen. Ct. 2:328; 3:1; Gen. Com. 10:187, 211–12.

20. Gen. Com. 11:182–83.

21. T. S. Ashton, *Economic Fluctuations in England, 1700–1800* (Oxford, 1959), pp. 152–55.

22. Gen. Com. 12:254–58, 268–69; Registers of Apprentices and of Children Claimed, 1751–1896, vol. 1, GLRO.

23. *Journals of the House of Commons*, vol. 33, p. 326; Gen. Com. 13:120–21, 160–61.

24. Hanway, *A Candid Historical Account of the Hospital*, pp. 81–82.

25. Daniel Defoe, *A Tour Thro' the whole Island of Great Britain* (1734–37; 2 vols, reprint ed., London, 1927), 2:602.

26. Arthur Young, *A Six Weeks Tour through the Southern Counties of England and Wales* (Dublin, 1768), pp. 52, 88, 151.

27. Letter from Taylor White, 29 August 1758, Sec. Cor. In, 1758, GLRO.

28. Gen. Ct. 3:10–11, 258, 294–95; Gen. Com. 10:317; 12:161–62, 206; 14:31, 40, 157; 15:187; 16:149, 203, 205, 208–09; Nichols and Wray, pp. 157–81.

Notes to Chapter 10

1. Gen. Ct. 2:7, 230; Gen. Com. 1:255; 5:125; 8:130; 9:50; Register of Apprentices and of Children Claimed, 1751–1896, vol. 1, GLRO.

2. 5 Eliz. I, c. 4.

3. 43 Eliz. I, c. 2. The pertinent provisions of both acts can be found in Abbott, 1:91–98.

4. Nichols and Wray, p. 341.

5. 7 Geo. III, c. 39; Gen. Com. 7:250–51.

6. Gen. Com. 3:66–68.

7. Ibid., 3:236, 268; Subcom. 1:106.

8. Gen. Com. 3:238–39.

9. Ibid., 4:250–51, 275; Contract Book, 1742–1756, GLRO.

10. Gen. Com. 4:9, 5:44.

11. Gen. Ct. 1:244, 250, 341; Gen. Com. 3:296; 4:23–24, 221; 5:40, 47, 116.

12. Gen. Com. 4:160, 164–5; Subcom. 2:52–53.

13. George Kearsley, *Kearsley's Tables of Trades, For the Assistance of Parents and Guardians, and for the Benefit of those Young Men, Who wish to prosper in the World, and become respectable Members of Society* (London, 1786), passim.

14. Gen. Com. 7:367, 395, 397; 14:76, 105.

15. Ibid., 14:114, 157; 16:95–96; Subcom. 9:195.

16. Gen. Com. 9:252, 267–69, 284–85; 10:171; 11:73–74, 86–88, 154.

17. Clerk's Report of his Journey to Chertsey, etc., 18 July 1759, FHL 28:58.

18. J. Richards to Mr Collingwood, 23 February 1770, Sec. Cor. In, 1770, GLRO.

19. Antoine de Saint-Exupéry, *Le Petit Prince* (Paris, 1946), pp. 72–74.

20. Taylor White to Dr Lee, 16 June 1761, SLB 3:87, GLRO.

21. 16 and 17 Geo. V, c. 29.

22. Gen. Com. 8:154–55.

23. Gen. Com. 9:241, 343; Certificates of Good Character and Settlement of Masters, 1769, GLRO.

24. SLB, vol. 5, passim, GLRO.

25. Gen. Com. 13:130–31.

26. Rev. J. Richards to Mr Collingwood, 3 January 1771, Sec. Cor. In, 1770, GLRO; Subcom. 9:69.

27. Subcom. 9:154, 203.

28. Letter of Thomas Stanton, 2 February 1771; Mary Sheppard to Mr Collingwood, 3 March 1771; same to same, 21 April 1771, Sec. Misc., 1752–92 bundle, GLRO; Subcom. 9:154–55.

29. Subcom. 9:83–84.

30. Registers of Apprentices and of Children Claimed, 1751–1896, vols 1 and 2, GLRO.

31. Gen. Ct. 3:46; Gen. Com. 12:31; 13:13; 14:187; Subcom. 5:27.

32. Gen. Com. 5:153; 9:182; 11:144; 15:258; Secretary to Rev. Mr Gardnor, 14 February 1771, SLB 5:52.

33. Gen. Com. 8:22, 43–44, 46; 15:6, 8; Subcom. 9:152; William Dutton to Mr Collingwood, 15 May 1770, Sec. Cor. In, 1770, GLRO; Baron Dimsdale to Mr Collingwood, 19 December 1770, ibid.

34. Information of Elizabeth Owen and other witnesses before Francis Wood, Justice of the Peace, and Recognizance binding over Joshua Fox, John and Hannah Walker, 12–13 April 1771, Sec. Cor. In, 1771–72, GLRO.

35. Copy of Subcommittee Minute, 29 October 1774, Sec. Misc., GLRO.

36. Gen. Com. 15:22, 125–26.

37. Inquisition before the Coroner at Manchester and Evidence of Witnesses, 12 April 1771, Sec. Cor. In, 1771–72, GLRO.

38. Gen. Com. 13:162–63, 243.

39. Ibid., 9:263; *Annual Register*, 2d ed. (London, 1772), 10 (1767): 190–97.

40. Gen. Com. 8:297–98; 10:269–70, 292, 299, 304; 11:290–91, 306; 12:301, 309; 13:236–37; 14:8, 134, 152, 168–69, 178.

NOTES TO CHAPTER 11

1. Gen. Com. 7:118; Paper of Dr Brocklesby, 31 July 1759, FHL 28:168. This was the same Dr Brocklesby who wrote the first biography of Captain Coram.

2. Gen. Ct. 2:142–43, 185; Gen. Com. 7:265–66; Soldiers' Children Received, FHL 34:5.

3. Gen. Ct. 4:95–96.

4. Gen. Com. 20:137, 151, 154, 160–61; 21:156–60, 163, 175; John Heriot to the Secretary of the Foundling Hospital, 29 January 1794, FHL 34, Item 16-A; John Charles Beckingham to the Secretary of the Foundling Hospital, September 1794, FHL 23, Item 29.

5. Gen. Ct. 2:2; 4:277; Gen. Com. 22:287; A List of Children Received with £100 from 1756 to 1771, Sec. Misc., 1753/54–1795 bundle, GLRO; Account of Children Received with £100 each from 25 March 1760 to the 31 Dec. 1780, FHL 30, Item 41; Gen. Com. 1781–99, passim.

6. Gen. Ct. 2:224; Gen. Com. 10:58; 12:29; and vols. 8–12, passim; Sir Clifton

Wintringham to the Governors of the Foundling Hospital, 17 August 1768, FHL 10:103; Billets for Admission, GLRO.

7. Petitions for Admission of Children, 1768–69, GLRO.

8. Hufton, pp. 320, 324–5.

9. Petitions for Admission of Children, 1780–99, GLRO.

10. Gen. Ct. 2:304, 314–15; 3:30, 54, 162, 170, 180, 278–79, 309, 324; 4:28–29, 252; Gen. Com. 9:141–42; 11:109; 12:208–10; 13:156, 187, 335–36; 20:66; Subcom. 9:7; Account of Children Received from 25 March 1760 to the 31 Dec. 1781, FHL 35:155–56.

11. Gen. Com. 9:91–92; 16:86; 20:37, 71, 100, 187, 209–10; 21:251, 279; Subcom. 9:155.

12. Gen. Com. 7:250, 254; 21:290–93.

13. McCloy, pp. 248, 254.

14. Account and State of the Children, vol. 2, GLRO.

15. Gen. Com. 20:331.

16. Ibid., 21:234–39.

17. Gen. Ct. 4:236–37.

18. Account of Children Received from 25 March 1760 to the 31 Dec. 1781, FHL 35:155–56; Thomas Bernard, *An Account of the Foundling Hospital*, p. 64.

19. 7 Geo. III, c. 39.

20. John Pugh, *Remarkable Occurrences in the Life of Jonas Hanway, Esq.*, 3d ed. abridged (London, 1978), pp. 142–3.

21. Ibid., pp. 142–47. The act of 1762 was 2 Geo. III, c. 22. In support of his proposals Hanway wrote *Serious Considerations on the Salutory Design of the Act of Parliament for a regular, uniform Register of the Parish-Poor in all the Parishes within the Bills of Mortality* (London, 1762); *An Earnest Appeal for Mercy to the Children of the Poor, etc.* (London, 1766); and *Letters on the Importance of the Rising Generation* (London, 1767).

22. Gen. Ct. 2:304–5, 307, 316–17, 321, 323; Gen. Com. 10:173–74; Subcom. 6:161–63, 169, 175. For a detailed account of the Hanway Acts, see James Stephen Taylor, 'Philanthropy and Empire: Jonas Hanway and the Infant Poor of London', *Eighteenth-Century Studies* 12 (Spring, 1979): 298–304.

23. Gen. Com. 10:244–45, 250, 252–54, 259–60.

24. Taylor White to Dr Adams, 31 August 1769, SLB 4:253, GLRO; Gen. Com. 11:30, 348.

25. Gen. Com. 12:123–24, 132, 147, 151, 258, 282, 307, 316, 342; 13:12, 17, 50, 77, 97, 109.

26. E. N. Williams, *Life in Georgian England* (London, 1962), p. 109.

27. Gen. Com. 14:56–57, 65, 68, 70; 15:30–32, 34, 37, 111–12, 160; 18:234; 20:115–16, 118.

28. Subcom. 9:94; *The Report of the Special Committee appointed by the General Court of the Governors and Guardians of the Hospital for the Maintenance and Education of Exposed and Deserted Young Children* (London, 1771), p. 5.

29. Ibid., pp. 25–28.

30. Ibid., pp. 9–10, 13–14; Jonas Hanway, 'General Remarks on the Report of the Special Committee appointed to consider the State & Expences of the Foundling Hospital', October 1771, FHL 31:209–222; 'Examination of Printed Report by Mr. Hanway', FHL 35:110–22; Gen. Ct. 3:97–98, 100, 102–6.

31. An Account of the Receipts & Payments for Parish Children in Ten Years, 1777–86, FHL 30, Item 50; An Account of the Expences of the Foundling Hospital Detailed under their respective Heads, Specifying likewise what Increase of Expence the Parish Children cause to the Hospital From 31st Decr. 1787 to 31st Decr. 1788, Extracted from the Hospital Books, Sec. Misc., 1788, GLRO; Weekly Reports and State of the Hospital, 1786–88, GLRO.

32. Gen. Ct. 4:158; Gen. Com. 21:123.

33. Bernard, *An Account of the Foundling Hospital*, pp. 65–66.

34. Gen. Ct. 4:17–21; Gen. Com. 18:26; 19:240–41; 22:200–201; 23:202–3, 211–12; Visiting Committee's Reports, 21 May 1790, 26 May 1790, 7 June 1790, GLRO; Bernard, *An Account of the Foundling Hospital*, pp. 65–68.

35. Gen. Com. 18:281, 343–44; O. Jocelyn Dunlop, *English Apprenticeship & Child Labour* (London, 1912), p. 259.

36. Gen. Ct. 4:54–55.

37. Register of Apprentices and of Children Claimed 1751–1896, vol. 2, GLRO; List of Children Apprenticed Visited by the Schoolmaster from January 1791 to January 1792, Sec. Misc., 1758–92 bundle, GLRO.

38. Petitions/Applications to Take Apprentices 27 September 1785, GLRO.

39. Gen. Com. 16:243. Other instances may be found in Gen. Com. 18:187, 251–52.

40. Ibid., 22:66, 124–26.

41. Ibid., 20:279–80, 286; 21:241, 252–53; 23:172–73.

42. Ibid., 19:106, 254; 20:319; 21:129, 162; 22:220–21, 236; 23:118, 152.

43. Ibid., 22:255, 260, 271, 300, 304, 318–19; 23:81–82; George Unwin, *Samuel Oldknow and the Arkwrights* (Manchester, 1924), pp. 172–74.

44. Bernard, *An Account of the Foundling Hospital*, p. 71.

45. Report of R. Atchison, 10 December 1805, FHL 11:153.

46. Gen. Com. 23:225–27.

47. Bernard, *An Account of the Foundling Hospital*, p. 67.

48. Gen. Com. 20:217; 21:213–14.

49. Ibid., 23:280–81. For the form of certificate given, see Appendix IV.

50. Gen. Ct. 4:6; Gen. Com. 15:309; 18:11, 54, 295, 339–40.

51. Gen. Com. 20:50–52.

52. 'Report of the Situation of the Children, Apprenticed by the Churchwardens etc. of the United Parishes of St. Margaret and St. John in the City of Westminster, to the Cotton Manufactory of Messrs. H---, at M----, in the County of York; and to the Manufactory for Spinning Woollen Yarn, belonging to Messrs. J---- and T----, at Cuckney Mills, near Mansfield, Nottinghamshire: Addressed to the Workhouse Board of the said Parishes, April 10, 1797', *European Magazine and London Review* 34 (October, 1798): 265–68.

53. Gen. Com. 22:127–28, 132–33, 151–52; Dunlop, pp. 257–58.

54. Bernard, *An Account of the Foundling Hospital*, p. 65; Gen. Com. 21:311, 323; 22:265, 269–70; Matron's Reports on Children in the Country, 1798–1843, GLRO.

55. Account and State of the Children, vol. 2, 31 December 1780 and 31 December 1794, GLRO.

56. Gen. Com. 18:98; 20:333.

NOTES TO CHAPTER 12

1. Gen. Com. 12:296–97; Subcom. 3:228.

2. Gen. Ct. 3:187.

3. Ibid., 3:223–25; Gen. Com. 15:193–94; 16:71.

4. Gen. Ct. 3:243, 247–48; 'The Memorial of the Several Persons . . . being Owners or Occupiers of Houses in Queen Square', 30 June 1779, FHL 30, Item 42.

5. Gen. Com. 3:295, 298, 315; 10:197; 11:31, 161; 17:173–74, 301; Subcom. 12:144.

6. *An Appeal to the Governors of the Foundling Hospital*, pp. 8, 14–19, 32–33; Gen. Com. 18:293.

7. Gen. Ct. 3:333–34.

8. Ibid., 3:335–37; Rev. Dr Stephen White, *A Vindication of the Governors of the Foundling Hospital, for having determined to let the Land adjoining to the Hospital on Building Leases* (London, ca 1787–88); John Holliday, *A Further Appeal to the Governors of the Foundling Hospital, etc.* (London, 1788), pp. 1–17.

9. Gen. Ct. 3:340–41; Gen. Com. 19:35–36; Petition to Lord North, President, to call a Special Meeting, April 1788, Sec. Misc., 1753/54–1795 bundle, GLRO.

10. *The Proceedings of the Select Committee for Letting the Lands Adjoining to the Foundling Hospital, on Building Leases* (London, 1790), pp. 1–5; Gen. Ct. 4:2, 51.

11. Gen. Ct. 4:58–59; Donald J. Olsen, *Town Planning in London* (New Haven, 1964), fig. 64.

12. Gen. Ct. 4:78.

13. Ibid., 4:152–54; Olsen, pp. 78–80.

14. Gen. Ct. 4:198–99; Olsen, p. 82. I have curtailed my discussion of the details of developing the estate because Dr Olsen has already covered the same material so thoroughly in

chapter 5 of his book that I can add very little to it. Less complete but accurate treatments of the development of the Foundling Hospital estate are also to be found in Sir John Summerson, *Georgian London*, rev. ed. (New York, 1970), pp. 167–70, and London County Council, *Survey of London*, vol. 24, chap. 3. See also Nichols and Wray, chap. 33.

15. Gen. Com. 19:109–11; Case and Questions presented to the Hospital's Solicitor, 24 January 1789, FHL 41, Item 5.

16. Gen. Ct. 4:57; Gen. Com. 19:205–06; 20:234–37.

17. Information, Defendant's Answer, and Affidavits in the Action between Sir Archibald Macdonald, Knt, his Majesty's Attorney General, at the Relation of Edward George Lind, Esq., Informant, and The Governors and Guardians of the Hospital for the Maintenance and Education of exposed and deserted young Children and Stephen White, L.L.D., Defendants, December 1792-January 1793, FHL, vol. 43.

18. Petition of Henry James Layton, 27 September 1797, Sec. Misc., 1741–97 bundle, GLRO; Gen. Com. 21:217, 299; 22:6.

19. Gen. Com. 21:59; Olsen, pp. 81–82.

20. Gen. Com. 20:201–2; 21:123, 125–26.

21. Newspaper clipping, marked 1792 but not otherwise identified, in file of Foundling Hospital Prints, Maps and Prints Room, GLRO.

22. Gen. Com. 22:49–51, 54, 59, 63, 67, 148, 234–35.

23. Nichols and Wray, pp. 283–84; Olsen, p. 223.

24. Gen. Com. 20:48, 126; 21:77; 22:6; Olsen, pp. 82–84; *Survey of London* 24:29, 41–42; R. Horwood, 'Map of London', 24 May 1799, Section C, Maps and Prints Room, GLRO.

25. Gen. Com. 23:174.

NOTES TO CHAPTER 13

1. Nichols and Wray, p. 343.

2. Morris Lievesley, Notes, FHL, vol. 24.

3. Hanway, *Genuine Sentiments*, p. 26.

4. Gen. Ct. 2:290, 292, 310; 3:281–83, 287; 4:37–39, 42, 56–57, 60, 112, 130–31, 191–92, 196–97, 205–7; Gen. Com. 21:96–98.

5. Gen. Com. 1:68, 103, 110–11, 117; 16:122; 20:162; 21:74; 23:110; Daily Committee's Minutes, 1741–42, GLRO; Visiting Committee's Reports, 1790–91, GLRO.

6. Nichols and Wray, pp. 345–90, 412–13.

7. Rev. James Baker, *The Life of Sir Thomas Bernard, Baronet* (London, 1819), passim. Bernard did not become a baronet until 1810, which was subsequent to his resignation as treasurer of the Foundling Hospital.

8. Gen. Ct. 1:39.

9. Ibid., 4:62–63.

10. Gen. Com. 2:77. It appeared in the *Daily Advertiser* on 19 December 1745.

11. Gen. Com. 4:321–22; 14:244–45; 15:215–16; 23:133; Taylor White to Dr Lee, 26 May 1761, SLB 3:75–76; same to same, 16 June 1761, SLB 3:86, GLRO; Anonymous letter to Taylor White, 14 October 1763, Sec. Misc., 1763 bundle, GLRO; *Morning Chronicle and London Advertiser*, 26 November 1773 and 13 May 1776.

12. Gen. Com. 2:93; 3:11, 267; 4:270, 312; 21:324.

13. Gen. Ct. 2:182; Gen. Com. 2:280; 3:28, 38; 4:97, 103; 8:282; 13:334; 17:53, 59, 312; 21:14; Subcom. 5:126–27; Secretary to Mr Magee, 29 June 1765, SLB 3:317, GLRO.

14. Nichols and Wray, pp. 312–14.

15. Gen. Ct. 2:103–04, 161.

16. Gen. Com. 2:285; 4:158–59; 5:194, 211–12, 225–26, 229, 243–44; Subcom. 2:109–10; Daily Committee's Minutes, p. 16, GLRO.

17. List of Nurses and Servants in the Service of the Hospital on 8 April 1760, FHL 10:73–74; Weekly Reports on the State of the Hospital, 1771–73, GLRO; An Account of the Expenses of the Foundling Hospital . . . from 31st Decr. 1787 to 31st Decr. 1788 Extracted from the Hospital Books, Sec. Misc., 1788 bundle, GLRO; Minutes of the Committee of Accounts, 1795–1843, vol. 1: 31 May 1795, GLRO.

18. Gen. Ct. 2:117; Gen. Com. 15:66; Letters of Recommendation for Mrs Elizabeth Leicester, 13 July 1759, Sec. Misc., ca 1759–1776 bundle, GLRO; Report of John Wilmot, 19–26 May 1790, Visiting Committee's Reports, GLRO; Lievesley.

19. Gen. Com. 19:307; 20:7, 37, 45; 22:68–69; Nichols and Wray, p. 216; Lievesley.

20. Gen. Com. 2:7; 5:18; 6:66; 8:195, 309–10, 316, 332; 12:269, 275; 19:293; 22:209, 308–9.

21. Gen. Ct. 1:148; Gen. Com. 2:149, 153–54, 220; 5:215, 218; 6:9–10, 280; 7:97–99; 17:312; 19:258; 21:289–90; 22:28, 42–43; Subcom. 3:114; Letter of thanks from the Boys' Nurses, 27 September 1760, Sec. Misc., 1760 bundle, GLRO; *An Account of the Hospital*, pp. 20–30.

22. Gen. Com. 8:41; Register of Servants, 1758–71, GLRO.

23. Gen. Com. 5:215–16; 16:167–68; 17:333; Subcom. 15:66; Application of Robert Atchison, 21 March 1780, FHL 28: 125–26; Nichols and Wray, pp. 272–73.

Notes to Chapter 14

1. Gen. Ct. 1:18, 46, 71; Gen. Com. 1:1–2, 29, 31, 40, 62–64, 70–72, 76–83, 114–15, 139–40, 145, 147, 158–59, 167–68, 211, 215.

2. Gen. Ct. 1:67, 115; Gen. Com. 4:217–18, 232–33; 9:14–15; 18:61–62; *Gentleman's Magazine* 20 (October, 1750): 473; Huzzoramall, Executor of the Estate of Omychund, to the Governors, 13 February 1765, FHL 45:88; Cash Received on Account of Omychund's Bequest, 7 February 1781, FHL 35:295.

3. Gen. Com. 16:110–11.

4. Ibid., 23:109, 126.

5. Ibid., 1:147.

6. FHL 41, Item 14.

7. Gen. Com. 17:289.

8. Legacy Book, 1727–1799, GLRO.

9. See Appendix V.

10. Legacy Book, 1727–1799, GLRO.

11. Ruth K. McClure, 'New Channels of Beneficence: A Portrait of Pre-Evangelical Associational Charity, 1739–1758' (Master's essay, Columbia University, 1968), pp. 54–56.

12. Gen. Ct. 1:137–38; Gen. Com. 1:19, 133, 139–40; 2:31, 147, 233; 4:143.

13. Gen. Ct. 1:137–38; Gen. Com. 1:89; 2:241; 8:212; 9:12, 337; 10:154; 11:41; 12:244; 13:92.

14. Appendix V; T. S. Ashton, *Economic Fluctuations in England*, pp. 172–73.

15. Gen. Com. 4:250–51, 275; 5:15; 7:95; 9:180, 320; 10:35–36; 11:306; 12:240–41, 334; Daily Committee's Minutes, p. 42, GLRO; *Annual Register*, 2d ed. (London, 1772) 9 (1766): 85; *London Evening Post*, 2–4 January 1755; *Gentleman's Magazine* 25 (January 1755): 40.

16. Gen. Ct. 1:65, 93–94, 127–28, 130; 3:16; 4:133–34, 137, 142, 175, 193; 7:428, 430; 8:119, 204; 13:85; 21:69, 285; 22:160; 23:50; *Preachers of Sermons in aid of the Funds of the Foundling Hospital from 1760* (London, 1905), pp. 3–4.

17. Gen. Ct. 1:14; 4:58–59; Gen. Com. 17:99; 20:77, 222; 21:50; 22:64; Subcom. 1:89; 2:18, 51.

18. Gen. Ct. 1:212–13, 248; Gen. Com. 2:160, 205, 322; 3:47, 146, 173, 175, 186; 18:166; Subcom. 1:11, 24, 241; 3:164–65; 9:258.

19. Gen. Ct. 4:17–21; Gen. Com. 7:305, 405; 8:39, 314; 12:2; 14:16–17, 41, 161; 15:77, 100, 126–27; 20:60, 198, 257; 21:195; 22:200–201; Subcom. 5:220; 9:123; Secretary to Dr Lee, 26 March 1761, SLB 3:62, GLRO; Cloth made by the Children from 1 January 1766 to 31 December 1766 inclusive, FHL 28:35; Handbill giving particulars of an auction of woollen cloth manufactured by the children at Shrewsbury, 17 December 1767, FHL 35:97; Report of Mr Filmer, 2 March 1791, Visting Committee's Reports, GLRO; Appendix VI.

20. Gen. Ct. 4:48; Gen. Com. 1:203–5, 291–92; 2:37–38, 189–90; 4:83; 5:42; 6:302; 7:75; 12:269; 20:3, 190–91, 297; Subcom. 3:81, 244.

21. A Statement of the Increase or Decrease of the Estate of the Foundling-Hospital From the Year 1771 to the Year 1788, FHL 30, item 51.

22. Gen. Ct. 3:312–13, 330–31; 4:119–24; Gen. Com. 6:247; 7:199.

23. An Account of the Expences of the Foundling Hospital Detailed under their respective Heads . . . From 31st Decr. 1787 to 31st Decr. 1788 Extracted from the Hospital Books, Sec. Misc., 1788 bundle, GLRO.

24. *The Report of the Committee Appointed by the Annual General Court of the Foundling Hospital, Of 12th May 1790* (London, 1790), Appendix C; Gen. Ct. 3:143–45.

25. Gen. Ct. 3:289; 4:119–24; Gen. Com. 7:103–6; Subcom. 1:224; 2:51, 55–56; Report of Contracts for Meat Delivered to Christ's Hospital, 6 January 1762, FHL 35:73; Thomas Nugent to George Whatley, 18 March 1765, FHL 10:107–9; J. Perry, Steward of Christ's Hospital, to Thomas Collingwood, 26 May 1770, FHL 10:162; *An Account of the Hospital*, pp. 22–23, 26–27.

26. *The Report of the Committee Appointed . . . 12 May 1790*, p. 6.

NOTES TO CHAPTER 15

1. Gen. Com. 1:103–4, 106–7.

2. Sec. Cor. In, 1751, GLRO.

3. William Cadogan, *An Essay upon Nursing, and the Management of Children From their Birth to Three Years of Age*, 6th ed. (London, 1753), pp. 9–12; Anonymous Letter, 24 January 1749 O. S., Sec. Cor. In, 1749, GLRO; Subcom. 1:28.

4. Gen. Ct. 1:275.

5. Sketch and Description of the Children at the Breakfasting, 1 May 1747, FHL, vol. 39; Gen. Com. 2:91; *Gentleman's Magazine* 17 (June, 1747): 284.

6. Gen. Com. 2:91–92; 7:252; Subcom. 1:167–70; 2:102; Secretary to Mr Hargreaves, 30 December 1769, SLB 4:309.

7. Gen. Ct. 4:17–21; Gen. Com. 8:65; 9:43; Subcom. 1:167–69; 2:102; 6:35; 15:45; Expence of the Clothes delivered with a Boy when Apprenticed at age ten, 31 December 1761, Sec. Misc., ca 1752–1775 bundle, GLRO.

8. Gen. Com. 7:110; Subcom. 1:102–3; Secretary to Mr Alexander Fleming, 10 June 1767, SLB 3:384; Expense of Diet, Clothing, etc. for One Year, 1787, FHL 28:144–46; Contracts, 1767–1851, bundle for 1796–1800, GLRO.

9. 'Berigt Wegens', FHL 31:81; 'Memoire concernant les Enfans Trouvés', FHL 6: page 6 of document; 'Epillogo de' Statuti del Pio Spedale della Pietà di Venezia', FHL 31:342.

10. Gen. Com. 2:223–24; 4:242; 7:91, 156; 16:34; 17:159–60; Subcom. 2:109–10; 3:207; Cadogan, pp. 21, 23; Report of Mr McClellan, 19 December 1759, FHL 28:106; J. C. Drummond and Anne Wilbraham, *The Englishman's Food: A History of Five Centuries of English Diet* (London, 1939), p. 291.

11. Gen. Com. 17:160; T. C. Barker, J. C. McKenzie, and John Yudkin, *Our Changing Fare: Two Hundred Years of British Food Habits* (London, 1966), pp. 95–97, 101–2; John Burnett, *A History of the Cost of Living* (London: Penguin Books, Ltd., Pelican Books, 1969), p. 136; C. Anne Wilson, *Food and Drink in Britain* (New York, 1974), pp. 47–48, 52; Drummond, pp. 227–28.

12. Drummond, pp. 263–65, 268–69; Elizabeth W. Gilboy, *Wages in Eighteenth-Century England* (Cambridge, Mass., 1934), pp. 27–28; Sir Frederic Morton Eden, *The State of the Poor*, 3 vols (London, 1797), 1:496.

13. Drummond, pp. 259, 265, 268.

14. Gen. Ct. 3:143–45; Gen. Com. 16:109; 22:191; Subcom. 1:246–48; Account of Servants etc. to whom Beer is allowed, 29 November 1787, Sec. Misc., 1741–97 bundle, GLRO; Blunden, pp. 59–60, 85.

15. Gen. Com. 5:326; 21:60, 105–6, 126; Subcom. 2:33; 3:233; 12;97; Memorandum about the children's diet, ca. 1756–68, Sec. Misc., 1756–68 bundle, GLRO; Calculation of Rice Pudding for the Children, 6 February 1773, ibid., ca. 1752–1775 bundle.

16. Gen. Ct. 3:290; Gen. Com. 7:377; 17:64–65; 21:187; Subcom. 1:27–29; List of seeds for the Kitchen Garden, 11 April 1791, Sec. Misc., 1753/54–1795 bundle, GLRO.

17. Gen. Com. 3:99–100; 6:25, 278; 14:252; 20:293, 310; 21:17; Drummond, pp. 41, 222.

18. Gen. Com. 15:38, 224; 19:250; Subcom. 3:69–71, 203–4; 15:41; The Present

Allowance to the Servants and Children of the Hospital, 24 September 1784, Sec. Misc., 1784, GLRO.

19. Subcom. 1:246–48; Blunden, pp. 59–60, 85; *An Account of the Institution and Proceedings of the Guardians of the Asylum or House of Refuge, situated on the Surry Side of Westminster-Bridge, for the Reception of Orphan Girls residing within the Bills of Mortality, whose Settlements cannot be found* (London, 1763), p. 18.

20. 'Memoire concernant les Enfans Trouvés', FHL 6: pp. 10–11 of document; 'Berigt Wegens', FHL 31:82–89.

21. Eden, 1:286, 496–97, 532; Burnett, pp. 133, 136, 168, 184–86; Drummond, pp. 231, 258–59, 261; Gilboy, pp. 27–28.

22. Gen. Ct. 4:17–21; Gen. Com. 1:294, 298–99; 2:307; 10:78; 18:111–12, 114–15; Subcom. 15:77; Drummond, pp. 222, 230–32; Wilson, p. 262.

23. Gen. Com. 4:175; 8:241; Steward of St Bartholomew's Hospital to George Whatley, 28 May 1770, FHL 10:166; same to same, 31 May 1770, FHL 10:170; Report on costs of Meat used at St Thomas's Hospital, Guy's Hospital, London Hospital, and Christ's Hospital, 5 February 1774, FHL 35:139–40; T. S. Ashton, 'Changes in Standards of Comfort in Eighteenth-Century England', p. 175.

24. Provisions delivered into the Hospital from Midsummer 1783 to Midsummer 1784, Sec. Misc., 1741–97 bundle, GLRO.

25. Gen. Com. 1:20.

26. Bernard, pp. 17–18; Gen. Com. 20:217.

27. Report of John Wilmot, 24 May 1790, and Report of Stephen White, 16 June 1790, Visiting Committee's Reports, GLRO; Gen. Ct. 4:17–21.

28. *Account of the kitchen fitted up at the Foundling Hospital, under the direction of His Excellency Count Rumford* (London, 1796), pp. 1–3; Society for Bettering the Condition and Increasing the Comforts of the Poor, *Reports* 1:89–97; Charles Maechling, Jr, 'Count Rumford: Scientific Adventurer', *History Today* 22 (April 1972): 251; Sir Benjamin Thompson, Count Rumford, *Essays, Political, Economical, and Philosophical*, 3 vols (London, 1800–1802), 3:100–101, 103, 115, 225.

NOTES TO CHAPTER 16

1. Gen. Com. 1:116–17.

2. Memorandum Book for Admission and Disposal of Children, vol. 1, GLRO.

3. Gen. Com. 1:132; Daily Committee's Minutes, p. 21, GLRO.

4. Memorandum Book for Admission and Disposal of Children, vol. 1, GLRO; Gen. Com. 4:18, 144; 5:263; 6:35; 13:169.

5. Gen. Com. 5:73–74, 78, 188, 204; 7:35, 67; 11:18; 13:280–81, 283–84; Subcom. 2:91, 114, 134; 3:91–92, 197, 232–33, 238; 15:31; Memorandum of a lease with John Cocks, Esq., 31 May 1756, Sec. Misc., 1756–61 bundle, GLRO; Infirmary Weekly Reports on the Sick, 1761–1923, vols 1 and 2, GLRO; Apothecary's Notes on treatment, ca. 1760, GLRO; *Survey of London* 24:102–3, 114.

6. Gen. Com. 4:68–69, 73, 166; 17:333, 342; 19:65–67; Subcom. 3:103–4; 5:17, 31, 126, 129; 12:151; Letter from Lady Vere, 13 January 1753, Sec. Cor. In, 1753, GLRO; Report of W. L. Kingsman, 27 May 1790, and Report of J. Holliday, 21 July 1790, Visiting Committee's Reports, GLRO.

7. Gen. Ct. 1:108; Gen. Com. 1:288, 327; 2:280; 3:42–43, 255, 267; 4:270; 5:48; 10:132, 220–21, 231–32; 23:140; Subcom. 2:91–92; 3:228, 238; *An Account of the Hospital*, p. xiii; Lester S. King, *The Medical World of the Eighteenth Century* (1958; reprint ed., Huntington, N.Y., 1971), pp. 321–22; Sir D'Arcy Power, 'Medicine', in *Johnson's England*, ed. A. S. Turberville, 2:282; C. D. O'Malley, 'The English Physician in the Earlier Eighteenth Century', in *England in the Restoration and Early Eighteenth Century*, ed. H. T. Swedenberg, Jr (Berkeley, 1972), p. 152; William R. LeFanu, 'The Lost Half-Century in English Medicine, 1700–1750', *Bulletin of the History of Medicine* 46 (July–August 1972): 339; Charles Creighton, *A History of Epidemics in Britain*, 2 vols (2nd ed. with additional material by D. E. C. Eversley, E. A. Underwood, and L. Ovenall, London, 1965), 2:504, 506, 511, 531; E. St John Brooks,

Sir Hans Sloane, The Great Collector and his Circle (London, 1954), pp. 88–92.

8. Memorandum Books for Admission and Disposal of the Children, vols 1 and 6, GLRO; Register of Grown Up Children, GLRO; Register and Situation of Children, vol. 1, GLRO.

9. Gen. Com. 5:90; 18:300; 20:22–23, 28; Secretary to Dr Lee, 10 June 1763, SLB 3:238; King, p. 123; O'Malley, p. 153; *The Information and Complaint made to the Last General Court . . . By Dr. Mayo . . . with the Proceedings of the Committee of Enquity thereon* (London, 1790), p. 6.

10. Gen. Com. 12:280; Memorandum Book for Admission and Disposal of Children, vol. 1, GLRO; Treatment and Prescription Book for Measles, 1766–1800, Medical Miscellaneous, GLRO.

11. Gen. Com. 3:218; 4:296, 299; Present State of Children in the Infirmaries, 29 March 1760, Sec. Misc., 1760 bundle, GLRO; Robert Hooper, *Lexicon Medicum, or Medical Dictionary* (London, 1831); William A. R. Thomson, *Black's Medical Dictionary*, 22d ed. (London, 1955); Sir Arthur Salusbury MacNalty, *The British Medical Dictionary* (London, 1961); W. A. Newman Dorland, *The American Illustrated Medical Dictionary*, 22d ed. (Philadelphia and London, 1951); *Information and Complaint . . . by Dr. Mayo*, p. 34; W. S. Lewis et al., eds, *The Yale Edition of Horace Walpole's Correspondence* (New Haven, 1937–), 9:37, 17:95; 32:97, n. 12.

12. Gen. Com. 6:213; 16:6; Subcom. 9:59–60, 174, 212–13; List of the Children in Ackworth Hospital mentioning how each child is employed and also the Infirmities those labour under which render them unfit to be placed out Apprentice, 6 June 1771, Sec. Cor. In, 1771–72, GLRO; Drummond, pp. 322–23, 325; James Nelson, *An Essay on the Government of Children Under Three General Heads: Viz. Health, Manners and Education*, 2d ed. (London, 1756), p. 96; Miriam E. Lowenberg et al., *Food & Man* (New York, 1968), pp. 19, 188, 191, 193; G. Melvyn Howe, *Man, Environment and Disease in Britain* (New York, 1972), p. 144.

13. Subcom. 9:174; Lowenberg, p. 195.

14. Subcom. 3:216, 224.

15. Ibid., 1:27–29; Cadogan, p. 35. For discussions of the diets of village folk and farm labourers, see Drummond, p. 245; T. S. Ashton, 'Changes in Standards of Comfort', p. 177; Eric Kerridge, *The Farmers of Old England* (London, 1973), p. 160; Burnett, pp. 167–68.

16. Gen. Com. 5:129–30; 7:22, 58, 201, 234, 281, 308, 394; Statement of Account with the Lock Hospital, Sec. Misc., 1758–92 bundle, GLRO; Hooper.

17. Gen. Com. 1:237; 7:190, 369–70, 377, 394–95, 400; 9:96, 177; 14:335; 15:181, 221; 18:121; Subcom. 5:32; O'Malley, p. 148; Power, pp. 268–69; LeFanu, p. 334.

18. Gen. Com. 2:107; 14:193; 16:15.

19. Gen. Com. 1:54–55, 112–13, 129–30, 165; 16:38; *Information and Complaint . . . by Dr. Mayo*, pp. 9–11; LeFanu, pp. 328, 335, 338–39; O'Malley, p. 155; King, p. 23; Blunden, p. 62; G. F. McCleary, *The Early History of the Infant Welfare Movement* (London, 1933), p. 16; DNB, s.v. 'Mayo, John' and 'Watson, Sir William'.

20. Gen. Com. 1:155–57; 6:318; 14:306; 22:67–69, 84.

21. Subcom. 3:111; Inventory of Medicines in the Apothecary's Shop, 1798, Medical Miscellaneous, GLRO.

22. O'Malley, p. 154; Hooper; Thompson; Brooks, pp. 87–88; King, pp. 128–29.

23. Gen. Com. 5:206, 298; 19:210; Subcom. 2:146–48; 3:18–19; Cadogan, pp. 37–38; Lievesley.

24. LeFanu, pp. 328–29, 337, 339; O'Malley, p. 153; Power, pp. 272–73; John Rendle-Short, 'Infant Management in the 18th Century with Special Reference to the Work of William Cadogan', *Bulletin of the History of Medicine* 34 (March-April, 1960): 98.

25. Apothecary's Notes on Treatment, ca 1760, p. 55, GLRO.

26. *An Account of the Hospital*, pp. x–xii; Places to Which 3300 Children were sent from the Foundling Hospital From 2 June 1756 to 2 June 1757, FHL 35:43–45.

27. Gen. Com. 16:6.

28. Gen. Com. 6:97–98, 175, 213; 7:408–9; 10:38; 13:213; 14:208, 257; 15:52, 231; 16:100, 178; 18:345; 22:62, 113, 148; 23:90, 97; Subcom. 2:236; Bill of G. Grafton, 29 October 1796, and Bill of William and James Lauries, 1 April 1797, Minutes of Committee of Accounts, 1795–1843, vol. 1, GLRO.

29. Subcom. 9:174, 212–13; List of the Children in Ackworth Hospital . . . and also the

Infirmities . . . which render them unfit to be placed out Apprentice, 1771, Sec. Cor. In, 1771–72, GLRO; List of Handicapped Children 8 December 1794, Sec. Misc., ca 1770–92 bundle, GLRO; A List of such Foundling Children who from various Causes could never be placed out of the Hospital to provide for themselves, Visiting Committee's Reports, GLRO; Lievesly.

30. Report of B. Filmer, 21 June 1790, Visiting Committee's Reports, GLRO.

31. Report of John Wilmot, 20 May 1790, ibid.

32. Gen. Com. 20:252–53.

NOTES TO CHAPTER 17

1. Victor E. Neuburg, *Popular Education in Eighteenth Century England* (London, 1971), pp. 1–4.

2. *London Magazine* 35 (July 1766): 343.

3. George Chapman, *A Treatise on Education with A Sketch of the Author's Method* (Edinburgh, 1773); pp. 73–74.

4. Ibid., pp. 71–72; Nelson, p. 367.

5. Isaac Watts, *An Essay Towards the Encouragement of Charity Schools* (London, 1728), p. 37. Jonas Hanway expressed the same view in 1759 in his *Genuine Sentiments of an English Country Gentleman*, p. 33.

6. John Lawson and Harold Silver, *A Social History of Education in England* (London, 1973), pp. 174–76; Neuburg, p. 1.

7. *The Report of the General Committee . . . relating to the General Plan*, p. 8.

8. Gen. Com. 2:198; Subcom. 1:24, 28.

9. Gen. Com. 4:196; 5:193–94, 197, 252–53, 335–36; 6:6; Subcom. 1:231; 2:127; Neuburg, pp. 23, 59.

10. *Regulations For Managing the Hospital for the Maintenance and Education of exposed and deserted Young Children* (London, 1759), pp. 22, 30–31; Subcom. 3:123.

11. Neuburg, pp. 65, 71, 89.

12. Subcom. 5:184.

13. Gen. Com. 15:125.

14. Ibid., 9:71–72, 76, 236; 10:38; 17:334; Clerk's Report of his Journey to Epsom, etc., 2 May 1764, FHL 30, item 25.

15. Gen. Com. 23:202–3.

16. Ibid., 21:83; 23:211–12.

17. Thomas Bernard, *Of the Education of the Poor, Being the first part of A Digest of the Reports of the Society for Bettering the Condition of the Poor : and Containing a Selection of those Articles which have a Reference to Education* (1809; reprint ed., London, 1970), p. 32n.

18. Chapman, pp. 96–98.

19. Coram to Colman, 2 March 1737, MHS, *Proceedings* 56:33.

20. McCloy, p. 245.

21. R. S. Schofield, 'Dimensions of Illiteracy, 1750–1850', *Explorations in Economic History* 10 (Summer, 1973): 445–46, 449–50.

22. Ibid., p. 452.

23. Application of Robert Atchison for Position of Schoolmaster, 21 March 1780, FHL 28:125–26.

24. Bernard, *Education of the Poor*, p. 27; Neuburg, pp. 17–18, 23; Lawson and Silver, pp. 189–90.

25. Gen. Com. 16:225, 280; 23:202–3.

26. Subcom. 1:29.

27. Ibid., 1:215–16.

28. Gen. Com. 4:115; 5:45, 51; 7:42; 20:305, 310; Subcom. 2:9, 102; 3:205; 12:120.

29. 'From Liverpool to Worcester a Century and a Half Ago', *Notes and Queries*, 12th ser. 3, no. 57 (1917); 64; no. 58 (1917): 89.

30. Gen. Com. 1:254; 2:286; 4:37, 39, 44–45, 205; 6:64, 304; 7:183.

31. Gen. Ct. 3:66–67; Gen. Com. 13:20; 18:267, 269; 22:7; Subcom. 2:159.

32. Gen. Com. 5:9; 11:186.

33. Ibid., 13:187–88.

34. Ibid., 23:69–71, 83.

35. Blunden, p. 19; M. Gwladys Jones, *The Charity School Movement* (Cambridge, 1938), pp. 80–81.

36. Gen. Ct. 2:252.

37. Gen. Com. 4:115; 6:114; 11:45; 13:245; 14:110, 157; Subcom. 1:199.

38. Gen. Ct. 3:84–86; Gen. Com. 13:89–90.

39. Gen. Com. 14:163.

40. Gen. Ct. 3:156–57; Gen. Com. 14:167–68.

41. Gen. Ct. 3:156–57; Gen. Com. 14:312, 315; 15:97, 224, Gerald Finzi, 'John Stanley (1713–1786)', *Proceedings of the Royal Musical Association* 77 (1952): 65–69, 71–72; Tony Frost, 'The Cantatas of John Stanley (1713–86)', *Music & Letters* 53 (July 1972): 285.

42. Gen. Ct. 3:172–74, 177–78; Roger Lonsdale, *Dr. Charles Burney: A Literary Biography* (Oxford, 1965), pp. 149–53; Jamie Croy Kassler, 'Burney's Sketch of a Plan for a Public Music School', *Musical Quarterly* 58 (April 1972): 227–34; Nichols and Wray, pp. 211, 247–48.

43. Gen. Com. 15:220, 332; 18:325; 19:240–42; 21:120; Appendix V.

44. *Psalms, Hymns & Anthems Used in the Chapel of the Hospital for the Maintenance & Education of Exposed & Deserted Young Children* (London, 1774), p. 66.

45. Ibid., p. 51.

46. Lang, p. 208.

47. Subcom. 1:29.

48. Gen. Com. 3:30.

49. *The Poor Girls' Primer: for use in the Sheffield Girls' Charity School* (1789), as quoted in M. Gwladys Jones, p. 75.

50. Gen. Com. 3:29–30; 22:191; Subcom. 1:29, 107; 12:112.

51. Gen. Com. 1:288; 13:240; 22:191; Subcom. 1:88–89; 12:142; 15:68.

52. Gen. Com. 7:393; 9:19; Subcom. 2:95; 5:45; 6:33, 70, 73; 9:77, 244; A. W. Coats, 'Economic Thought and Poor Law Policy in the Eighteenth Century', *Economic History Review*, 2d ser. 13 (1943): 44–45.

53. Gen. Com. 14:194.

54. *Solitude in Imprisonment, With proper profitable Labour And a Spare Diet, The most humane and effectual Means of bringing Malefactors, who have forfeited their Lives or are subject to Transportation, to a right Sense of their Condition; with Proposals for Salutory Prevention* (London, 1776).

55. Gen. Com. 15:284.

56. Ibid., 16:176, 182; 17:144, 177–78; 21:253; 22:15, 31, 180, 198, 203, 310.

57. Hanway, *Solitude in Imprisonment*, pp. 74–76; Lloyd deMause, 'The Evolution of Childhood', in Lloyd deMause, ed., *The History of Childhood* (New York, 1974), pp. 42–43.

58. Gardener's seed list, 11 April 1791, Sec. Misc. 1753/54–1795 bundle, GLRO.

NOTES TO CHAPTER 18

1. Gen. Com. 18:102.

2. Ibid., 12:72; 13:216, 218; 20:342–43; Subcom. 9:137–38; 15:33; Edward Russell to the Committee, 3 September 1770, Sec. Cor. In, 1770, GLRO; Secretary to the Parish Officers of Farnham, 10 February 1796, SLB: 1795–1810, GLRO.

3. Gen. Com. 16:259–60, 279; 18:277; 19:30, 46; 20:167, 267.

4. Gen. Ct. 3:137; 4:174–75; Gen. Com. 10:106; 11:4; 20:166; 22:47, 61–62, 74–75; Lievesley; Nichols and Wray, p. 244.

5. Gen. Ct. 4:174–75; Gen. Com. 11:45; 14:62; 16:27, 57; 18:258; 19:79–80; 20:166; 23:171, 183, 283; Subcom. 12:56, 61; Lievesley; Nichols and Wray, pp. 235–37.

6. Gen. Com. 15:79, 85, 156–57, 192–93, 201, 218, 280, 288, 299–300; 17:201, 209, 342; 18:2, 36, 40–41, 53, 214, 276–77; 22:31–32; Pugh, p. 194; Nichols and Wray, p. 239.

7. Gen. Com. 13:245; 15:192–93, 218, 288, 299–300; 16:240; 17:11, 13; 20:166; 21:87, 175; Lievesley.

8. Gen. Ct. 4:220; Bill of Preston, 1 February 1800, Minutes of Committee of Accounts, 1795–1843, vol. 2, GLRO; Lievesley; Nichols and Wray, pp. 240–44.

9. Gen. Com. 23:38; Certificate of William Hughes, 5 May 1801, Petitions of Apprentices for Gratuities, 1800–1859, GLRO; Application of Susannah Bannister, 13 April 1785, Petitions to Take Apprentices, 1785, GLRO; Lievesley.

10. Gen. Com. 14:306; 20:273, 299; 22:84; Lievesley; Nichols and Wray, pp. 274, 397.

11. Contract Book, 1742–1756, GLRO; Lievesley.

12. L. Joseph Stone and Joseph Church in *Childhood and Adolescence: A Psychology of the Growing Person* (New York, 1957), p. 62, cite studies showing that a child deprived of consistent mothering by the same person, such as babies kept in institutions throughout infancy, become apathetic, intellectually and physically retarded, and eventually may show behaviour similar to that of adult psychotics, especially when separation from consistent mothering occurs in the second half of the baby's first year.

13. Bernard, *An Account of the Foundling Hospital*, p. 65.

14. Gen. Com. 14:145.

15. Ivy Pinchbeck and Margaret Hewitt, *Children in English Society*, 2 vols (London, 1969–) 1:301–3, 305; David Hunt, *Parents and Children In History: The Psychology of Family Life In Early Modern France* (New York, 1970), p. 195; Philippe Ariès, *Centuries of Childhood: A Social History of Family Life* (New York, 1962), pp. 38–39, 368–69, 400–404; John R. Gillis, *Youth and History: Tradition and Change in European Age Relations, 1770–Present* (New York, 1974), pp. 7–12, 16–17, 20–21; deMause, pp. 25, 33–34.

16. Daily Committee's Minutes, pp. 6–7, GLRO.

17. Gen. Com. 4:41; 7:228–29; 8:113, 118; 9:73; 15:87; 16:283; Subcom. 3:145; Receipts for Children, 1797, GLRO; Petitions for Claiming Children, 1772, GLRO; Sec. Misc., 1759–1770–1792 bundle, GLRO.

Notes to Epilogue

1. Parliamentary Papers, *Reports from Commissioners*, Vol. 4, pt 1, *32d Report of the Commissioners for Inquiring Concerning Charities*, Part VI (London, 1840), pp. 786–87, 790, 792, 794; Nichols and Wray, pp. 154, 246.

2. Nichols and Wray, p. 412.

3. Ibid., p. 100.

4. Brownlow, *History and Objects of the Foundling Hospital*, p. 70; *32d Report of the Commissioners*, pp. 783, 793.

5. P. 317.

6. Nichols and Wray, pp. 116, 150–51, 196; Brownlow, *History and Objects of the Foundling Hospital*, pp. 78–79.

7. Annotated copy of the *32d Report of the Commissioners for Inquiring Concerning Charities*, Part VI, pp. 780, 790, in the FHL, vol. 136. The annotations are dated 1856–57.

8. Nichols and Wray, p. 319.

9. Ibid., pp. 154, 196, 319; *32d Report of the Commissioners*, p. 790.

10. Nichols and Wray, pp. 278, 320–21; Brownlow, *History and Objects of the Foundling Hospital*, pp. 124–26.

11. Nichols and Wray, pp. 92, 96, 100; Brownlow, *History and Objects of the Foundling Hospital*, pp. 55–57; *32d Report of the Commissioners*, p. 780.

12. Sampson Low, Jr, *The Charities of London* (London, 1863), pp. vii–xi. An earlier list, with no mention of a foundling hospital, is to be found in J. C. Platt and J. Saunders, 'Charities of London', in *London*, ed. Charles Knight (London, 1844) 6:337–52. Similarly, Anthony Highmore's *Pietas Londinensis* (London, 1810) lists only the foundling hospital established by Captain Coram. And Ford K. Brown's *Fathers of the Victorians* (Cambridge, 1961), which lists dozens of charitable institutions founded from 1552 to 1844 (pp. 332–40), mentions no other foundling hospital.

13. Brownlow, *History and Objects of the Foundling Hospital*, pp. 70–71.

14. Henry Mayhew, *London Labour and the London Poor* (London, 1861–62; reprint ed., New York, 1968) 4:468.

15. Sidney and Beatrice Webb, *English Poor Law History, Part II, The Last Hundred Years*, Vol. 8 of *English Local Government* (London, 1929), pp. 300, 302, 304–6, 310.

16. Owen, pp. 97, 183, 498–9; G. D. H. Cole, 'A Retrospect of the History of Voluntary Social Service', in *Voluntary Social Services: Their Place in the Modern State*, ed. A. F. C. Bourdillon (London, 1945), pp. 13–14.

17. 4 and 5 William IV, c. 76.

18. Quoted in Standish Meacham, *Henry Thornton of Clapham, 1760–1815* (Cambridge, Mass., 1964), p. 143.

19. William Wilberforce, *A Practical View of the Prevailing Religious System of Professed Christians in the Higher and Middle Classes in this Country, Contrasted with Real Christianity* (London, 1797), p. 221.

20. *Essays By a Barrister* (London, 1862), p. 43. See also Owen, p. 98.

21. Brown, pp. 354–58; Nichols and Wray, pp. 412–14.

22. John Brownlow, *Memoranda; or Chronicles of the Foundling Hospital*, p. 196; Brownlow, *History and Objects of the Foundling Hospital*, pp. 60–61.

23. *32d Report of the Commissioners*, p. 784.

24. Coram to Colman, 13 September 1740, MHS, *Proceedings* 56:55.

BIBLIOGRAPHY

I. MANUSCRIPT SOURCES AND MAPS

1. *Relating to Captain Thomas Coram*

Athens, Ga. University of Georgia Library. Egmont Papers. Vol. 14203, pt 1. John Martin Bolzius to Captain Coram, 28 July 1737.

Boston, Mass. Boston Public Library. Department of Rare Books and Manuscripts. Complaint of Thomas Coram to the Superior Court of Judicature of Bristol County, 11 September 1701.

Boston, Mass. Houghton Library of Harvard University. HCL/MS Eng 549. 'To Her Royal Highness the Princess of Wales The Memorial and Petition of Thomas Coram Gent in behalf of great Numbers of Innocent Children daily exposed to Destruction'.

Boston, Mass. Massachusetts Historical Society.
Colman Papers. Vols 1 and 2.
Col. Edward Hutchinson Papers, 1679–1753.
Miscellaneous Bound Items. Vols 6 and 7.

Boston, Mass. Massachusetts State Archives Vols 3, 28, and 40.

Dorchester. Dorset County Record Office. Transcripts of Parish Registers of Lyme Regis, 1653–90.

London. Thomas Coram Foundation for Children. Foundling Hospital Library. Vols 6, 28, 42, and 98.

London. Public Record Office. PC 1/48. Petition of Thomas Coram for employment in the Royal Navy, 8 February 1727.

San Marino, California. Henry E. Huntington Library. Hastings Collection. HA1624. Thomas Coram to the Countess of Huntingdon, 15 September 1739.

Taunton, Mass. Bristol County Court House.
Records of the Inferior Court of Common Pleas for Bristol County, 1696–1702 and 1702–1720.

Records of the Court of General Sessions of the Peace for Bristol County, 1697–1701.

Taunton, Mass. Bristol County Register's Office.
Deed Books 3, 4, 31, and 41.

2. *Relating to the Foundling Hospital*

London. Thomas Coram Foundation for Children.
General Court Minutes. Vols 1–4, 1739–99.
General Committee Minutes. Vols 1–23, 1739–99.
Foundling Hospital Library. This library consists of a number of volumes of letters, reports, and other documents from the eighteenth and nineteenth centuries. Apparently John Brownlow, a nineteenth-century secretary of the Hospital, collected the items and had them bound in books but made no attempt to arrange them either chronologically or under any systems of classification. Moreover, in some volumes the pages are numbered consecutively; in others, each item is numbered but not each page; and in still others, neither pages nor items are numbered. Each volume, however, carries a number. Therefore, items in these volumes are cited by volume number, page or item number if any, and a description of the document. There is one exception: volume 24, a private notebook kept by Morris Lievesley, a secretary of the Hospital (1799–1849), which contains anecdotes, recollections, observations, and comments relating to the institution, has been referred to in footnotes as 'Lievesley' because it represents the work of a single author.

London. Greater London Record Office. Records of the Thomas Coram Foundation for Children (The Foundling Hospital). Ac. 54.38, 55.23, 57.72, 64.18, 64.27, 64.77, 65.58. These records have not as yet been catalogued, although interim lists of the main classes of materials have been prepared. Apart from the Subcommittee's Minutes, vols 1–23, therefore, the items cited in footnotes could only be listed descriptively. Although some of the records consist of bound volumes, not all have page numbers. Moreover, many items are loose documents tied up in bundles or placed in boxes. Difficulty in citing these materials arises from the fact that the bundles often contain documents from several nonconsecutive years, and no attempt has been made to prevent overlapping of dates among the bundles, for the archivists have, quite properly, preserved the bundles so far as possible in the form in which they were deposited. Until such time as cataloguing is complete, however, references to such items must necessarily be somewhat vague.

London. Greater London Record Office. Maps and Prints Room. John Rocque's Map of London, 1746, Section C1(a), and R. Horwood's Map of London, 1799, Section C.

All dates from manuscript sources are given in New Style unless otherwise indicated, and where quotations are made from such sources, the thorn (y) has been rendered as th.

II. Printed Sources

1. *Official*

Acts of the Privy Council of England, Colonial Series, 1713–1783. Edited by W. L. Grant and J. Munro. 6 vols. London, 1908–12.

Calendar of State Papers, Colonial Series, America and West Indies. Vols for 1701, 1712–14, 1714–15, 1716–17, 1717–18, 1728–29, 1731, 1734–35, 1735–36, and 1737.

The Colonial Records of the State of Georgia. Edited by Allen D. Candler. 26 vols. Atlanta, 1904–16.

The Journals of the House of Commons. Vols 18, 27, 28, 30, and 33.

The Parliamentary History of England from the Earliest Period to the Year 1803. Vol. 15 (1753–65). London, 1813.

Parliamentary Papers, Reports from Commissioners. Vol. 4, Part 1, *32d Report of the Commissioners for Inquiring Concerning Charities, Part IV.* London, 1840.

A Report of the Record Commissioners Containing Boston Births, Baptisms, Marriages, and Deaths, 1630–1699. Boston, 1883.

A Report of the Record Commissioners of the City of Boston Containing the Boston Marriages from 1700 to 1751. Boston, 1898.

2. *Historical Manuscripts Commission Reports*

Egmont MSS. Diary. Vol. 63, pts 1–3. 1920–23.
Morrison MSS. Ninth Report, app. II. 1883.
Portland MSS. Vol. 5. 1899.
Trinity House MSS. Eighth Report, app. I. 1881.

3. *Newspapers and Periodicals*

Annual Register
Daily Gazetteer
Daily Post
European Magazine and London Review
Gazetteer and London Daily Advertiser
Gentleman's Magazine
Guardian

Literary Magazine

London Advertiser

London Chronicle

London Daily Post and General Advertiser

London Evening Post

London Magazine

Morning Chronicle and London Advertiser

Penny London Post

Read's Weekly Journal

Remembrancer

Universal Museum

Whitehall Evening Post

All of these newspapers and periodicals were published in London. Most of the newspapers can be found in the Burney Collection at the British Library.

4. *Books, Pamphlets, Journals, Correspondence, and Documents*

Abregé Historique de l'Établissement de L'Hôpital des Enfans-Trouvés. Paris, 1753.

An Account of the Foundation and Government of the Hospital for Foundlings in Paris. Drawn up At the Command of her late Majesty Queen Caroline, and now published for the Information of those who may be concern'd in carrying on a like Design in this City. London, 1739.

An Account of the General Nursery or Colledg of Infants, Set up by the Justices of Peace for the County of Middlesex with the Constitution and Ends thereof. London, 1686.

An Account of the Hospital for the Maintenance and Education of Exposed and Deserted Young Children, Including the Charter, Act of Parliament, By-Laws and Regulations, and annual Accounts of all Receipts and Payments, from the Commencement of the Corporation, on the 17th Day of October, 1739, to the 31st Day of December, 1758. London, 1759.

An Account of the Institution and Proceedings of the Guardians of the Asylum or House of Refuge, situated on the Surry Side of Westminster-Bridge, for the Reception of Orphan Girls residing within the Bills of Mortality, whose Settlements cannot be found. London, 1763.

Account of the kitchen fitted up at the Foundling Hospital, under the direction of His Excellency Count Rumford. London, 1796.

Bernard, Thomas. *An Account of the Foundling Hospital in London, for the Maintenance and Education of Exposed and Deserted Young Children*. 2d ed. London, 1799.

———. *Of the Education of the Poor; Being the First Part of a Digest of the*

Reports of the Society for Bettering the Condition of the Poor: and Containing A Selection of Those Articles which have a Reference to Education. London, 1809. Reprint. New York, 1971.

[Bray, Thomas]. *A Memorial Concerning the Erecting in the City of London or the Suburbs thereof, an Orphanotrophy or Hospital for the Reception of Poor Cast-off Children or Foundlings.* N.p., n.d.

[Brocklesby, Richard]. *Private Virtue and publick Spirit display'd in a Succinct Essay on the Character of Capt. Thomas Coram.* London, 1751.

Cadogan, William. *An Essay upon Nursing, and the Management of Children, From their Birth to Three Years of Age.* 6th ed. London, 1753.

Candid Remarks on Mr. Hanway's Candid Historical Account of the Foundling Hospital, and A more useful Plan humbly Recommended, in a Letter to a Member of Parliament. 2d ed. London, 1760.

Cartwright, James J., ed. *The Wentworth Papers, 1705–1739, selected from the Private and Family Correspondence of Thomas Wentworth, Lord Raby, Created in 1711 Earl of Strafford.* London, 1883.

Cellier, Elizabeth. 'A Scheme for the Foundation of a Royal Hospital . . . for the Maintenance of a Corporation of skilful Midwives, and such Foundlings, or exposed Children, as shall be admitted therein: As it was proposed . . . by Mrs. Elizabeth Cellier, in the Month of June, 1687'. *The Harleian Miscellany.* 10 vols. London, 1808–13. Vol. 4:142–47.

Chapman, George. *A Treatise on Education. With a Sketch of the Author's Method.* Edinburgh, 1773.

Collyer, Joseph. *The Parent's and Guardian's Directory, and the Youth's Guide, in the Choice of a Profession or Trade.* London, 1761.

Considerations on the Fatal Effects to a Trading Nation of the present Excess of Public Charities. In which the Magdalene, Asylum, Foundling, Hospitals for Sick and Lame, Lying in Hospitals, Charity Schools, and the Dissenting Fund, are particularly considered. London, 1763.

Defoe, Daniel. *A Tour Thro' the whole Island of Great Britain.* 3 vols. London, 1724–26. Reprint (3 vols in 2). London, 1927.

de Paul, Saint Vincent. *Correspondance, Etretiens, Documents.* Edited by Pierre Coste. 15 vols. Paris, 1920–60.

'Documentary History of the State of Maine'. *Collections of the Maine Historical Society.* Second Series. Vols 9 and 11.

Dodington, George Bubb. *The Political Journal of George Bubb Dodington.* Edited by John Carswell and Lewis Arnold Dralle. Oxford, 1965.

Eden, Sir Frederic Morton. *The State of the Poor.* 3 vols. London, 1797.

Egmont, Earl of. *The Journal of the Earl of Egmont: Abstract of the Trustees Proceedings for Establishing the Colony of Georgia, 1732–1738.* Edited by Robert G. McPherson. Athens, Ga., 1962.

Fielding, Henry. *The History of Tom Jones, a Foundling*. The Modern Library. New York, 1950.

'From Liverpool to Worcester a Century and a Half Ago'. *Notes and Queries*. Twelfth Series, vol. 3 (1917): 64, 89.

Hanway, Jonas. *A Candid Historical Account of the Hospital For the Reception of Exposed and Deserted Young Children; representing The present Plan of it as productive of many Evils, and not adapted to the Genius and Happiness of this Nation*. London, 1759.

——. *The Genuine Sentiments of an English Country Gentleman, upon the Present Plan of the Foundling Hospital*. London, 1759.

——. *Letters on the Importance of the Rising Generation of the labouring part of our fellow-subjects; being an account of the miserable state of the infant parish poor; the great usefulness of the hospital for exposed and deserted young children properly restricted; the obligations of parochial officers; and an historical detail of the whole mortality of London and Westminster, from 1592 to this time*. 2 vols. London, 1767.

——. *A Proposal for saving £70,000 to £150,000 to the Public; at the same time rendering 5,000 young persons of both sexes more happy in themselves and more useful to their country, than if so much money were expended on their account*. London, 1764.

——. *A Reply to C-----A-------- Author of the Candid Remarks on Mr. Hanway's Candid Historical Account of the Foundling Hospital, With relation to the probable Advantages of this Institution, if confined to such Foundlings, Orphans, and Deserted Children, within the Bills of Mortality, as were usually sent to Parish Workhouses and Parish Nurses*. London, 1760.

——. *Solitude in Imprisonment, with proper profitable Labour and a spare Diet, the most humane and effectual Means of bringing Malefactors, who have forfeited their Lives, or are subject to Transportation, to a right Sense of their Condition; with Proposals for Salutary Prevention*. London, 1776.

Highmore, Anthony. *Pietas Londinensis: The History, Design, and Present State of the various Public Charities in and near London*. London, 1810.

An Historical Sketch of the Foundling Hospital; Including an Impartial Review of the conduct of the Children's Parents, and serious reflections on the evil tendency of Seduction. By a Foundling. London, [? 1800].

[Holliday, John]. *An Appeal to the Governors of the Foundling Hospital, on the Probable Consequences of Covering the Hospital Lands with Buildings*. London, 1787.

Holliday, John. *A Further Appeal to the Governors of the Foundling Hospital; and a Justification of their Conduct, in not having Covered the Hospital Lands with Buildings, since the Institution of the Charity*. London, 1788.

An Humble and Free Address To the Most Noble President, The Right

Honourable and Worthy Vice-Presidents, Governors, Trustees, and Guardians of the Foundling-Hospital. London, 1749.

Hutchinson, Thomas. *The History of the Colony and Province of Massachusetts-Bay.* Edited by Lawrence Shaw Mayo from 2d ed. of 1768. 3 vols. Cambridge, Mass., 1936.

The Information and Complaint made to the Last General Court, at the Hospital for the Maintenance and Education of Exposed and Deserted Young Children, By Dr. Mayo, One of their Physicians; with the Proceedings of the Committee of Enquiry Thereon. London, 1790.

Jones, George Fenwick, ed. *Henry Newman's Salzburger Letterbooks.* Athens, Ga., 1966.

Joyful News to Batchelors and Maids. Being a Song, In Praise of the Fondling Hospital, and the London Hospital Aldersgate Street. [London, ? 1760].

A Justification Of the Baptism of Foundling Infants. In Answer to the Argument and Objections In a late Pamphlet, intitled, An Humble and Free Address To the Most Noble President, The Right Honourable and Worthy Vice-Presidents, Governors, Trustees, and Guardians of the Foundling Hospital. London, 1750.

Kearsley, George. *Kearsley's Table of Trades, For the Assistance of Parents and Guardians, and for the Benefit of those Young Men, Who wish to prosper in the World, and become respectable Members of Society.* London, 1786.

'Letter of Jeremiah Dummer to the General Court of Massachusetts, April 8, 1720'. *Collections of the Massachusetts Historical Society.* Third Series, vol. 1:139–46.

'Letter of Thomas Coram to H. Newman, 20 November 1732'. *Notes and Queries.* Eighth Series, vol. 4 (1893): 266.

'Letters of Thomas Coram'. *Proceedings of the Massachusetts Historical Society* 56 (1922): 15–56.

Maitland, William. *The History of London, from its Foundation by the Romans, to the Present Time.* London, 1739.

Massie, J[oseph]. *Farther Observations concerning the Foundling-Hospital: Pointing out the ill Effects which such an Hospital is likely to have upon the Religion, Liberty, and domestic Happiness of the People of Great Britain . . . . To which are prefixed, Former Observations concerning the said Hospital.* London, 1759.

Nelson, James. *An Essay on the Government of Children Under Three General Heads: Viz. Health, Manners and Education.* 2d ed. London, 1756.

Nelson, Robert. *An Address to Persons of Quality and Estate.* London, 1715.

[Painter, John]. *A Scheme Designed to raise a Sum not exceeding Ten Thousand Pounds, for the Benefit of the Foundling-Hospital.* London, 1751.

Pelagius, Porcupinus [pseud.]. *The Scandalizade, a Panegyri-Satiri-Serio-Comi-Dramatic Poem.* London, 1750.

Perry, William Stevens, ed. *Historical Collections Relating to the American Colonial Church.* 5 vols. Hartford, 1870–73.

The Proceedings of the Select Committee for letting the Lands adjoining to the Foundling Hospital, on Building Leases. Reported to the General Quarterly Court, December 29, 1790. London, 1790.

Psalms, hymns & anthems used in the chapel of the Hospital for the Maintenance & Education of Exposed & Deserted Young Children. London, 1774.

Pugh, John. *Remarkable Occurrences in the Life of Jonas Hanway, Esq.* 3d ed. London, 1798.

Regulations For Managing the Hospital for the Maintenance and Education of exposed and deserted Young Children. London, 1759.

A Rejoinder to Mr. Hanway's Reply to C--A--'s Candid Remarks, ckmparing The New Plan of a Foundling Hospital, which is now offer'd by Mr. H; with the old one of our present Poor Laws : & pointing out a few of the many advantages, which would result to the community ; from the abolition of both, and establishing in lieu of 'em, National, or County Workhouses. London, 1760.

The Report of the Committee appointed by the Annual General Court of the Foundling Hospital, Of 12th May, 1790. London, 1790.

The Report of the General Committee for directing, managing, and transacting the Business, Affairs, Estate, and Effects of the Corporation of the Governors and Guardians of the Hospital for the Maintenance and Education of exposed and deserted Young Children Relating to the General Plan for executing the Purposes of the Royal Charter, establishing this Hospital. London, 1740.

The Report of the Special Committee appointed by the General Court of the Governors and Guardians of the Hospital for the Maintenance and Education of Exposed and Deserted Young Children. London, 1771.

The Rise and Progress of the Foundling Hospital Considered : And The Reasons for putting a Stop to the General Reception of All Children. London, 1761.

Sacred Musick, Composed by the late George Frederick Handel, Esq.; And Performed at the Chappel of the Hospital, for the Maintenance and Education of Exposed and Deserted Young Children ; on Thursday, the 24th May, 1759. In Grateful Memory Of his many Noble Benefactions to that Charity. London, 1759.

A Sketch of the General Plan For executing the Purposes of the Royal Charter Establishing an Hospital for the Maintenance and Education of exposed and deserted Young Children. London, 1740.

[Smith, Samuel]. *Publick spirit illustrated in the life and designs of the Reverend Thomas Bray, D. D. late minister of St. Botolph without Aldgate.* London, 1746.

The Society for Bettering the Condition and Increasing the Comforts of the Poor. *Reports.* Vols 1 and 4.

Some Considerations on the Necessity and Usefulness of the Royal Charter Establishing an Hospital for the Maintenance and Education of Exposed and Deserted Young Children. London, 1740.

Some Objections to the Foundling-Hospital, Considered By a Person in the Country to whom they were sent. London, 1761.

Stow, John. *A Survey of the Cities of London and Westminster.* Edited by John Strype. 2 Vols. London, 1720.

The Tendencies of the Foundling Hospital in its Present Extent considered In several Views. London, 1760.

Thompson, Sir Benjamin, Count Rumford. *Essays, Political, Economical, and Philosophical.* 3 Vols. London, 1800–1802.

Welch, Saunders. *A Proposal To render effectual a Plan, To remove the Nuisance of Common Prostitutes from the Streets of this Metropolis.* London, 1758.

White, Rev. Dr Stephen. *A Vindication of the Governors of the Foundling Hospital, for having determined to let the Land adjoining to the Hospital on Building Leases.* London, ca 1787–88.

Young, Arthur. *A Six Weeks Tour through the Southern Counties of England and Wales.* Dublin, 1768.

III. SELECTED SECONDARY WORKS

1. *Books and Articles*

Abbott, Grace, ed. *The Child and the State.* 2 vols. Chicago, 1938.

Allport, Gordon W. *The Nature of Prejudice.* Cambridge, Mass., 1954.

Ariès, Philippe. *Centuries of Childhood: A Social History of Family Life.* Translated by Robert Baldick. New York, 1962.

Ashton, T. S. 'Changes in Standards of Comfort in Eighteenth-Century England'. *Proceedings of the British Academy* 41 (1955): 171–87.

——. *Economic Fluctuations in England, 1700–1800.* Oxford, 1959.

Bailyn, Bernard, and Bailyn, Lotte. *Massachusetts Shipping, 1697–1714: A Statistical Study.* Cambridge, Mass., 1959.

Baker, James. *The Life of Sir Thomas Bernard, Baronet.* London, 1819.

Balch, Emily Green. 'Public Assistance of the Poor in France'. *Publications of the American Economic Association* 8 (1893): 7–179.

Barker, T. C., McKenzie, J. C., and Yudkin, John, eds. *Our Changing Fare: Two Hundred Years of British Food Habits.* London, 1966.

Beattie, John M. *The English Court in the Reign of George I.* Cambridge, 1967.

Benoiston de Chateauneuf, [Louis François]. *Considérations sur les Enfans Trouvés dans les Principaux États de l'Europe.* Paris, 1824.

Blunden, Edmund. *Christ's Hospital: A Retrospect.* London, 1923.

Brooks, E. St John. *Sir Hans Sloane, The Great Collector and his Circle.* London, 1954.

Brown, Ford K. *Fathers of the Victorians*. Cambridge, 1961.

Brownlow, John. *Hans Sloane. A Tale Illustrating the History of the Foundling Hospital in London*. London, 1831.

——. *The History and Objects of the Foundling Hospital with a Memoir of the Founder*. 4th ed. Revised by W. S. Wintle. London, 1881.

——. *Memoranda; or Chronicles of The Foundling Hospital, including Memoirs of Captain Coram*. London, 1847.

Burnett, John. *A History of the Cost of Living*. Harmondsworth: Penguin Books Ltd., A Pelican Original, 1969.

Caulfield, Ernest. *The Infant Welfare Movement in the Eighteenth Century*. New York, 1931.

Coats, A. W. 'Economic Thought and Poor Law Policy in the Eighteenth Century'. *Economic History Review*. Second Series, vol. 13 (1943): 39–51.

Cokayne, George Edward. *The Complete Peerage of England, Scotland, Ireland, Great Britain and the United Kingdom*. Edited by Hon. Vicary Gibbs. 2d ed. 13 vols. London, 1910–59.

Compston, Herbert Fuller Bright. *Thomas Coram, Churchman, Empire Builder and Philanthropist*. London, 1918.

Cowie, Leonard W. *Henry Newman, An American in London, 1708–43*. London, 1956.

Crane, Verner W. 'Dr. Thomas Bray and the Charitable Colony Project, 1730'. *William and Mary Quarterly*. Third Series, vol. 19 (1962): 49–63.

——. 'The Philanthropists and the Genesis of Georgia'. *The American Historical Review* 27 (1921): 63–69.

Creighton, Charles. *A History of Epidemics in Britain*. 2d ed. 2 vols. London, 1965.

deMause, Lloyd, ed. *The History of Childhood*. New York, 1974.

Dictionary of National Biography.

Drummond, J. C., and Wilbraham, Anne. *The Englishman's Food: A History of Five Centuries of English Diet*. London, 1939.

Dunlop, O. Jocelyn. *English Apprenticeship and Child Labour*. London, 1912.

Fant, H. B. 'Picturesque Thomas Coram, Projector of Two Georgias and Father of the London Foundling Hospital'. *The Georgia Historical Quarterly* 32 (1948): 77–104.

Fussell, G. E. *Village Life in the Eighteenth Century*. Worcester, 1948.

George, M. Dorothy. *London Life in the Eighteenth Century*. New York, 1925.

Gilboy, Elizabeth W. *Wages in Eighteenth Century England*. Harvard Economic Studies, vol. 45. Cambridge, Mass., 1934.

Gillis, John R. *Youth and History: Tradition and Change in European Age Relations, 1770-Present*. New York, 1974.

Greenwood, F. W. P. *A History of King's Chapel, in Boston; The First Episcopal Church in New England.* Boston, 1833.

Henriques, U. R. Q. 'Bastardy and the New Poor Law', pt I. *Past and Present*, no. 37 (1967), pp. 103–14.

Hill, Hamilton Andrews. *Thomas Coram in Boston and Taunton.* Worcester, Mass., 1892.

Howe, G. Melvyn. *Man, Environment and Disease in Britain.* New York, 1972.

Hufton, Olwen H. *The Poor of Eighteenth-Century France, 1750–1789.* Oxford, 1974.

Hunt, David. *Parents and Children In History: The Psychology of Family Life In Early Modern France.* New York, 1970.

Hutchins, John Herold. *Jonas Hanway, 1712–1786.* New York, 1940.

Jones, Charles C., Jr. *The History of Georgia.* 2 vols. Boston, 1883.

Jones, M. Gwladys. *The Charity School Movement: A Study of Eighteenth Century Puritanism in Action.* Cambridge, 1938.

Kassler, Jamie Croy. 'Burney's Sketch of a Plan for a Public Music-School'. *Musical Quarterly* 58 (1972): 210–34.

Kerridge, Eric. *The Farmers of Old England.* London, 1973.

King, Lester S. *The Medical World of the Eighteenth Century.* Chicago, 1958. Reprint. Huntington, N.Y., 1971.

Lallemand, Léon. *Histoire des Enfants Abandonnés et Délaissés.* Paris, 1885.

Lang, Paul Henry. *George Frideric Handel.* New York, 1966.

Laslett, Peter, and Oosterveen, Karla. 'Long-term Trends in Bastardy'. *Populations Studies* 27 (1973): 255–86.

Lawson, John, and Silver, Harold. *A Social History of Education in England.* London, 1973.

LeFanu, William R. 'The Lost Half-Century in English Medicine, 1700–1750'. *Bulletin of the History of Medicine* 46 (1972): 319–48.

London County Council. *Survey of London.* Vols 19 (1938) and 24 (1952).

Lonsdale, Roger. *Dr. Charles Burney: A Literary Biography.* Oxford, 1965.

Low, Sampson, Jr. *The Charities of London.* London, 1863.

Lydekker, John Wolfe. *Thomas Bray, 1658–1730, Founder of Missionary Enterprise.* Philadelphia, 1943.

McCleary, G. F. *The Early History of the Infant Welfare Movement.* London, 1933.

McCloy, Shelby T. *Government Assistance in Eighteenth-Century France.* Durham, N. C., 1946.

McClure, Ruth K. 'Johnson's Criticism of the Foundling Hospital and its Consequences'. *Review of English Studies.* New series, vol. 27 (1976): 17–26.

McCulloch, Samuel Clyde. 'Dr. Thomas Bray's Final Years at Aldgate, 1706–1730'. *Historical Magazine of the Protestant Episcopal Church of the U.S.A.* 14 (1945): 322–36.

Maechling, Charles, Jr. 'Count Rumford: Scientific Adventurer'. *History Today* 22 (1972): 245–54.

Marshall, Dorothy. *The English Poor in the Eighteenth Century*. London, 1926.

——. 'The Old Poor Law, 1662–1795'. In *Essays in Economic History*, edited by E. M. Carus-Wilson, vol. 1: 295–305. London, 1954.

Meroney, Geraldine. 'The London Entrepôt Merchants and the Georgia Colony'. *William and Mary Quarterly*. Third Series, vol. 25 (1968): 230–44.

Mingay, G. E. *English Landed Society in the Eighteenth Century*. London, 1963.

Moody, Robert E. 'The Proposed Colony of Georgia in New England, 1713–1733'. *Transactions of the Colonial Society of Massachusetts* 34 (1937–42): 255–73.

Neuburg, Victor E. *Popular Education in Eighteenth Century England*. London, 1971.

Nichols, R. H., and Wray, F. A. *The History of the Foundling Hospital*. London, 1935.

Nicolson, Benedict. *The Treasures of the Foundling Hospital*. Oxford, 1972.

Olsen, Donald J. *Town Planning in London: The Eighteenth & Nineteenth Centuries*. New Haven, 1964.

O'Malley, C. D. 'The English Physician in the Earlier Eighteenth Century'. In *England in the Restoration and Early Eighteenth Century*, edited by H. T. Swedenberg, Jr. Berkeley, 1972.

Owen, David. *English Philanthropy, 1660–1960*. Cambridge, Mass., 1964.

Paulson, Ronald. *Hogarth: His Life, Art, and Times*. 2 vols. New Haven, 1971.

Pearce, Ernest Harold. *Annals of Christ's Hospital*. 2d ed. London, 1908.

Pennington, Edgar Legare. *Anglican Beginnings in Massachusetts*. Boston, 1941.

Phillips, Hugh. *Mid-Georgian London*. London, 1964.

Pinchbeck, Ivy, and Hewitt, Margaret. *Children in English Society*. 2 vols. London, 1969– .

Rendle-Short, John. 'Infant Management in the 18th Century with Special Reference to the Work of William Cadogan'. *Bulletin of the History of Medicine* 34 (1960): 97–122.

Rendle-Short, Morwenna and John. *The Father of Child Care: Life of William Cadogan (1711–1797)*. Bristol, 1966.

Saye, Albert B. *A Constitutional History of Georgia, 1732–1945*. Athens, Ga., 1948.

Schofield, R. S. 'Dimensions of Illiteracy, 1750–1850'. *Explorations in Economic History* 10 (1973): 437–54.

Sedgwick, Romney. *The History of Parliament: The House of Commons, 1715–1754*. 2 vols. New York, 1970.

Sperling, John G. *The South Sea Company*. Cambridge, Mass., 1962.

Summerson, Sir John. *Georgian London*. Rev. ed. New York, 1970.

Taylor, James Stephen. 'Philanthropy and Empire: Jonas Hanway and the Infant Poor of London'. *Eighteenth-Century Studies* 12 (Spring, 1979): 285–305.

Thompson, H. P. *Thomas Bray*. London, 1954.

Turberville, A. S., ed. *Johnson's England*. 2 vols. Oxford, 1933.

Unwin, George. *Samuel Oldknow and the Arkwrights*. Manchester, 1924.

Warden, G. B. *Boston, 1689–1776*. Boston, 1970.

Webb, Sidney, and Webb, Beatrice. *English Poor Law History, Part I: The Old Poor Law*, Vol. 7 of *English Local Government*. London, 1927.

Webb, Sidney, and Webb, Beatrice. *English Poor Law History, Part II: The Last Hundred Years*, Vol. 8 of *English Local Government*. London, 1929.

Wilson, C. Anne. *Food and Drink in Britain*. New York, 1974.

2. *Unpublished Works*

Jennison, Samuel. 'Notes for a Biography of Thomas Coram'. Manuscript in the archives of the American Antiquarian Society, Worcester, Mass.

McClure, Ruth K. 'New Channels of Beneficence: A Portrait of Pre-Evangelical Associational Charity, 1739–1758'. Master's essay, Columbia University, 1968.

INDEX

FH indicates the London Foundling Hospital